Neuropsychology

A Review of Science and Practice, II

Neuropsychology

A Review of Science and Practice, II

Edited by

Sandra Koffler
Independent Practice
Philadelphia, Pennsylvania

Joel Morgan
Independent Practice
Morristown, New Jersey

Bernice Marcopulos
James Madison University
Harrisonburg, Virginia

Manfred F. Greiffenstein
Psychological Systems, Inc.
Royal Oak, Michigan

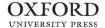
OXFORD
UNIVERSITY PRESS

OXFORD

UNIVERSITY PRESS

Oxford University Press is a department of the University of
Oxford. It furthers the University's objective of excellence in research,
scholarship, and education by publishing worldwide.

Oxford   New York

Auckland   Cape Town   Dar es Salaam   Hong Kong   Karachi
Kuala Lumpur   Madrid   Melbourne   Mexico City   Nairobi
New Delhi   Shanghai   Taipei   Toronto

With offices in

Argentina   Austria   Brazil   Chile   Czech Republic   France   Greece
Guatemala   Hungary   Italy   Japan   Poland   Portugal   Singapore
South Korea   Switzerland   Thailand   Turkey   Ukraine   Vietnam

Oxford is a registered trademark of Oxford University Press
in the UK and certain other countries.

Published in the United States of America by
Oxford University Press
198 Madison Avenue, New York, NY 10016

Library of Congress Cataloging-in-Publication Data
Neuropsychology : a review of science and practice / edited by Sandra Koffler, Joel Morgan,
Bernice Marcopulos, Manfred F. Greiffenstein.
volume cm
Includes bibliographical references and index.
ISBN 978-0-19-021557-6
1. Clinical neuropsychology.   2. Neuropsychiatry.   I. Koffler, Sandra, editor.
II. Morgan, Joel E, editor.   III. Marcopulos, Bernice, editor.   IV. Greiffenstein, Manfred F., 1952– editor.
RC341.N43557 2015
616.8—dc23
2014022176

1 3 5 7 9 8 6 4 2
Printed in the United States of America
on acid-free paper

CONTENTS

CONTRIBUTORS

Linas A. Bieliauskas
Mental Health Service
Ann Arbor VA Health
  Care System
Ann Arbor, Michigan

Elizaveta Bourchtein
Department of Psychology
Queens College
City University of New York
Flushing, New York

Lauren L. Drag
Stanford University Medical Center
Palo Alto, California

Daniel L. Drane
Emory University School of Medicine
Atlanta, Georgia

Daniel J. Goldman
NorthShore University Health System
Department of Psychiatry and
  Behavioral Sciences
Evanston, Illinois

Jeffrey M. Halperin
Department of Psychology
Queens College
City University of New York
Flushing, New York

Diane B. Howieson
The C. Rex and Ruth H. Layton Aging
  and Alzheimer's Disease Center
Oregon Health and Science University
Portland, Oregon

Peter T. Keenan
VA Illiana Health Care
  System
Danville, Illinois

Peter D. Leo
Columbia St. Mary's
Milwaukee, Wisconsin

Michael McCrea
Departments of Neurosurgery and
  Neurology
Medical College of Wisconsin
Milwaukee, Wisconsin

Lindsay D. Nelson
Departments of Neurosurgery and
  Neurology
Medical College of Wisconsin
Milwaukee, Wisconsin

Nathaniel W. Nelson
University of St. Thomas
Graduate School of Professional
  Psychology
Minneapolis, Minnesota

Melissa L. Ogden
Independent Practice
Mobile, Alabama

Sarah O'Neill
Department of Psychology
City College of New York
City University of
  New York
New York, New York

Ashley N. Simone
Department of Psychology
The Graduate Center
City University of New York
New York, New York

Robert Spencer
Ann Arbor VA Health
   Care System
Ann Arbor, Michigan

Jerry J. Sweet
NorthShore University Health System
Department of Psychiatry and
   Behavioral Sciences
Evanston, Illinois

David J. Williamson
College of Medicine
University of South Alabama
Mobile, Alabama

PREFACE TO THE SERIES

In Volume II of the Series the reader will once again find chapters by authors with distinguished credentials for summarizing recent research that has dominated the literature in neuropsychology and been prominent in workshops offered at professional conferences. This volume keeps to the promise of providing the profession with a resource for staying on top of the influential clinical and scientific studies of the past 12–15 months, for focusing on specific areas of interest, and for expanding the breadth and depth of awareness of the overall activity in the profession. The authors provide a rich consolidation of the important work that is being done in our centers, universities, and practices that would not otherwise be possible by perusing the literature alone. The range of topics included in Volume II likewise keeps to the mission of the Series of having applicability to practice, to the investigation of the science of neuropsychology, and to offer theoretical considerations to move the profession forward.

There has been a minor change in the name appended to the Series, which is now officially titled, **Neuropsychology: A Review of Science and Practice**. The editors believe this more clearly describes what the Series is about and what it purports to accomplish in this and future volumes. With this timely review neuropsychology now joins the medical and physical sciences that have long provided their readers with the means to be at the forefront of all that is new and significant in their professions.

Sandra Koffler, PhD
Joel Morgan, PhD
Bernice Marcopulos, PhD
Manfred F. Greiffenstein, PhD

PREFACE TO VOLUME II

In this second volume of *Neuropsychology: A Review of Science and Practice*, the reader is presented with comprehensive and timely summaries of recent literature that has dominated the professional journals in neuropsychology and allied disciplines.

Bieliauskas, Drag, and Spencer's comprehensive review of traumatic brain injury covers the recent literature regarding long-term cognitive, psychological, and medical outcomes. The authors discuss how premorbid and postinjury factors complicate outcomes, and they evaluate the research on current controversies, such as postconcussive syndrome, blast injuries and posttraumatic stress disorder, and chronic traumatic encephalopathy.

Howieson covers the recent literature on attention, a fundamental component of cognition that is impaired in a wide variety of neuropsychological conditions. Her review discusses current theories; methods of measuring attention; as well as neuroimaging, genetics, and neurochemistry studies. She evaluates the literature on the rehabilitation of attention disorders.

McCrea, Leo, and Nelson in their chapter review the literature on the incidence, epidemiology, and physiology of sport-related concussion. The acute and late effects of injury are examined through the recent research on neuropsychological diagnosis and assessment; the effects of multiple injuries and chronic traumatic encephalopathy; findings of studies with functional magnetic resonance imaging, electroencephalography, and the most recent noninvasive techniques; and the management of athletes who have suffered concussive trauma. The chapter concludes with consideration of the future direction for neuropsychology and its critical role in providing the science for understanding the effects of impact injuries.

Sweet and Goldman review contemporary scientific literature and legal commentary that is relevant to forensic neuropsychology practitioners. Topics addressed include the significance and admissibility of modern neuroimaging techniques, such as diffusion tensor imaging; evidentiary case law; performance and symptom validity testing; differential diagnosis of genuine from feigned presentations; and ongoing challenges to neuropsychological testimony.

Nelson and Keenan summarize and integrate the most recent literature in blast exposure. The focus is on the military, the nearly exclusive context for blast exposure since the invasions of Iraq and Afghanistan. They define blast injury carefully, review the remarkably long and complicated history of the concept, and draw out the similarities and differences between blast and related diagnoses. The recent literature that is reviewed includes such topics as comorbid psychopathology, screening and applicable neuropsychological methods, symptom constellations, differential diagnosis, and complicating factors that influence symptom course (e.g., secondary gain).

Williamson, Ogden, and Drane review the recent literature on psychogenic nonepileptic seizures, providing updates in relation to numerous psychogenic and neurogenic factors. Readers will find concise summaries of research with regard to psychogenic nonepileptic seizures and the history of trauma, depressive disorders, psychological testing, and neurologic comorbidities, among many others. Professionals working with patients with epilepsy will find this review an invaluable resource.

Halperin, O'Neill, Simone, and Bourchtein provide a review of one of the most studied areas in neuropsychology, reviewing the literature on executive dysfunction and attention-deficit/hyperactivity disorder. This extensive literature concerns multiple components of executive functioning as manifested in children with attention-deficit/hyperactivity disorder. Providing elucidation of what may perhaps be new or only vaguely familiar to readers, the authors' review is also a primer on the neurobiologic and psychological aspects of attention-deficit/hyperactivity disorder.

1

PSYCHOGENIC NONEPILEPTIC SEIZURES

An Update

David J. Williamson, Melissa L. Ogden, and Daniel L. Drane

Psychogenic nonepileptic seizures (PNES) have been with us for centuries. These episodes, also referred to as psychogenic nonepileptic spells, pseudoseizures, or nonepileptic events, have confounded patients, caregivers, and physicians due to the suffering that often accompanies them. They are marked by behavior that often superficially appears like that seen in epileptic seizures (e.g., paroxysmal movements or other transient behavioral changes) that are not accompanied by electrographic changes consistent with epilepsy. Their study has a long history in neuropsychology, as patients with PNES make up a substantial proportion of those evaluated in tertiary epilepsy centers, and neuropsychologists are often called upon to help with differential diagnosis or psychotherapeutic management. They are also the only major category of medically unexplained illness with a gold standard diagnostic technique, a video electroencephalogram (vEEG) of a spell recognized as "typical" by family members or caretakers.

It has been said that the understanding of a topic is inversely proportional to the amount written about it. A great deal has been written about individuals with PNES. Consistent with the maxim, this is an area in which experts have not even reached a consensus on terminology (LaFrance, 2010; Sethi, 2013), and there remain a variety of views on the true nature and etiology of PNES. Fortunately, the past few years have witnessed resurgence in interest in potential psychotherapeutic and medical treatment approaches for these individuals, many of whom have often generated a sense of either diagnostic skepticism or therapeutic nihilism in the past. The goal of this chapter is to provide the reader with an overview of the most relevant advances in the understanding of PNES and its treatment since 2012, focusing most specifically on advances in the understanding of etiology, semiology, diagnosis, and treatment.

METHODS

Methodologic issues are always important to keep in mind when reviewing a literature, and the techniques used to investigate PNES have evolved over the years. Progress has been made in terms of diagnosis. Nearly all studies of PNES now mention that the diagnosis of each subject included capture of at least one "typical" spell with video EEG (vEEG), and patients with spells of undetermined origin or mixed epileptic and nonepileptic origin are typically excluded or explicitly analyzed separately.

Other challenges remain, however. Small sample sizes remain common, with their attendant limitations on the ability of the results to generalize and the accurate estimation of effect sizes (Button et al., 2013). A challenge of more recent origin is deciding if and how to handle results of performance validity testing (PVT). There are those (present authors included) who believe that the literature now supports the idea that a substantial subgroup of patients with PNES do not or are for some reason less able to put forth their best performance on neurocognitive tests (Cragar, Berry, Fakhoury, Cibula, & Schmitt, 2006; Drane et al., 2006; Williamson, Drane, & Stroup, 2007); consequently, the data produced by these patients cannot be assumed to accurately reflect brain-behavior relationships. Other researchers have offered differing opinions (Dodrill, 2008). This is not to say that these patients are malingering or that their suffering is any less genuine; on the contrary, we have noted that there is likely more than one route to PVT failure (Drane, Coady, Williamson, Miller, & Benbadis, 2011; Drane et al., 2006). However, inferring deficits or building models based upon samples in which no attempt has been made to identify poor effort or exaggeration in a population in which it is known to occur on a regular basis at this point is, at best, perilous.

Inexplicably poor performance on PVT is beginning to emerge as an exclusionary criterion (Myers, Fleming, Lancman, Perrine, & Lancman, 2013; Myers, Matzner, Lancman, Perrine, & Lancman, 2013; Myers, Perrine, Lancman, Fleming, & Lancman, 2013; Strutt, Hill, Scott, Uber-Zak, & Fogel, 2011a), but this criterion is still present in only a minority of studies. The Myers and Strutt groups have used the Test of Memory Malingering (Tombaugh, 1996), but with varying results: the failure rates reported by the Myers group (8–18%) are consistent with that seen in other studies using the Test of Memory Malingering (Cragar et al., 2006; Hill, Ryan, Kennedy, & Malamut, 2003), whereas Strutt and colleagues reported a truly exceptional finding in which *none* of their 58 consecutive subjects (33 PNES, 25 left temporal lobe epilepsy) scored below cut-offs for valid performance. Of note, the sample studied by Strutt and colleagues differed substantially from that of Myers and colleagues according to comorbidities: in an effort to explore only the impact of the PNES diagnosis on cognition, Strutt and colleagues excluded patients with reported histories of substance abuse, chronic mental illness, head trauma, and a variety of comorbid medical conditions.

Should the use of PVTs as exclusionary (or even explanatory) criteria continue, an important topic meriting further study will be the differences between PVTs and how these differences are relevant to interpretation of study findings. As demonstrated in both this and other literatures, these techniques do not have identical diagnostic characteristics (Cragar et al., 2006; Gervais, Rohling, Green, & Ford, 2004), particularly when used with their originally published cutoffs. The Test of Memory Malingering, for instance, when used at its original cutoffs, appears less sensitive and more specific than does the Word Memory Test (WMT) at its original cutoffs (Gervais et al., 2004); however, cut-offs can be adjusted to make tests more comparable (Greve, Ord, Curtis, Bianchini, & Brennan, 2008). Thus, the situation threatens to become one of "being certain of the time with one watch but not so much with two." An alternative approach that remains untested in this literature is using multiple indicators and excluding those patients who fail more than one due to the increased likelihood of their results being a poor indication of true brain-behavior relationships (Larrabee, 2008). Failure of a validated PVT is clearly associated with poorer performance on cognitive tests, typically inexplicably poor in the absence of histories consistent with neurologic disease or insult. The optimal tests, cutoffs, or combination of tests for a given situation (e.g., empirical evaluation for the purpose of building cognitive models vs. a forensic evaluation) may reasonably vary a bit due to the associated costs of false-positive or false-negative errors. It is clear, however, that the moment in time has passed when the notion of less-than-full performance and the potential role of PVT in disentangling this issue could simply be ignored.

EMOTIONAL ADJUSTMENT

Patients with PNES consistently demonstrate poorer psychological adjustment than matched healthy control subjects (Mokleby et al., 2002). However, the extent to which they differ from patients with epilepsy in this regard is more variable. In some reports, patients with PNES report more depressive symptoms (LaFrance et al., 2011), whereas in others, significant differences are not found in Axis I pathology (Direk, Kulaksizoglu, Alpay, & Gurses, 2012), reported levels of depressed mood or anxiety (Salinsky, Evrard, Storzbach, & Pugh, 2012; Strutt, et al., 2011a; Strutt, Hill, Scott, Uber-Zak, & Fogel, 2011b; Testa, Krauss, Lesser, & Brandt, 2012), or reported frequency of stressful events (Testa et al., 2012). This question does not appear satisfactorily resolved yet, as methodologic findings could be contributing to differences across studies (e.g., Strutt and colleagues excluded many subgroups that would likely have reported higher emotional distress).

Despite this apparent lack of consistent differences in current levels of depression and anxiety, patients with PNES generally report worse health-related quality of life (HRQOL) than do patients with epilepsy (LaFrance et al., 2011). The reasons driving these differences have received attention of late. Direk et al. (2012) and Salinsky et al. (2012) noted in civilian and military samples, respectively, that although rates of Axis I pathology are relatively similar in patients with PNES and those with epilepsy, personality disorders are significantly more common in patients with PNES. Strutt and colleagues reported a similar finding, noting that although women with PNES and those with temporal lobe epilepsy did not differ in their reports of current anxiety or depression, signs of more chronic personality pathology were evident in those with PNES (Strutt et al., 2011b). Although no comparison was made to patients with epilepsy, Mitchell and colleagues demonstrated that self-reported difficulties related to dissociation contribute independently to the well-established contribution of depressive symptoms to HRQOL (Mitchell, Ali, & Cavanna, 2012). LaFrance and colleagues (2011) explored the notion that poor family function may contribute to these differences in HRQOL; however, both groups reported relatively poor family function, with this being more evident among men.

Other topics related to the emotional adjustment of patients with PNES have been explored. Two distinct but intertwined topics are how this group experiences emotion and how they deal with stress. A common perception is that patients with PNES (and somatoform disorders more generally) are less able to correctly identify the somatic signals of various emotions and consequently misattribute them to somatic causes. The dampened ability to recognize emotion, or alexithymia, in turn deprives the individual of salient emotional signals that those without this problem are able to harness more effectively to understand and deal with stressful situations. This notion rests on two fundamental assumptions: (1) patients with PNES are more likely to be alexithymic than those without somatoform-type issues, and (2) they are less able to deal effectively with stressful situations, potentially due to choosing more conflict-avoidant strategies rather than more assertive ones based on accurate understanding of the emotional issues at play.

As Myers, Matzner, et al. (2013) document, it turns out that the first of these assumptions may not be true. In fact, alexithymia is commonly observed across a range of different types of emotional difficulty (Celikel et al., 2010; Leweke, Leichsenring, Kruse, & Hermes, 2012). Myers and colleagues (2013) replicated the finding of Tojek, Lumley, Barkley, Mahr, and Thomas (2000) that alexithymia is *not* significantly more prevalent in patients with PNES than it is in patients with epilepsy, occurring in approximately 30% of both groups (but see Bewley, Murphy, Mallows, & Baker, 2005 for strikingly higher rates, although still without significant PNES/ES differentiation).

The notion that patients with PNES are more likely to default to an avoidant style of coping with stress has received mixed results as well (Myers, Fleming, et al., 2013; Testa, et al., 2012). Testa and colleagues examined self-reported modes of coping and emotional adjustment in a group of 40 patients with PNES, 20 patients with epilepsy, and 40 healthy control subjects. They found few differences between patients with PNES and those with epilepsy: those with PNES reported more distress concerning legal difficulties and health concerns, but distress associated with other domains of life did not differ significantly. Likewise, the groups did not differ in terms of the types of coping strategies they used. The PNES group reported using less active coping and planning than healthy control subjects; however, it was the group with epilepsy not the group with PNES that reported using avoidant strategies significantly more frequently than healthy control subjects.

Myers, Fleming, et al. (2013) also examined the relationships between coping style, reported history of trauma, and emotional adjustment in a sample of

82 patients with PNES. In this sample, relative to the normative population, 25% of the group underused task-oriented approaches relative to expectations, and only 16% overused avoidance-oriented strategies; in contrast, over 30% overused emotion-based strategies (i.e., reducing stress by self-oriented emotional reactions, such as fantasizing or self-preoccupation). Of the three approaches, emotion-based strategies were clearly related to the worst outcomes in terms of emotional adjustment. Task-oriented approaches, consistent with previous findings, appeared to be protective. Curiously, use of avoidant strategies correlated quite highly with use of task-oriented approaches ($r = .45$). Consistent with this high correlation, negative impact of avoidant strategies was generally absent: in fact, the impact of using avoidant strategies appeared minimal on emotional adjustment and similar to that of task-oriented approaches in terms of relationships with trauma symptoms, alexithymia, anger, and mood.

Taken together, the recent work exploring alexithymia and avoidant coping styles in patients with PNES is important but not completely helpful regarding the fundamental nature of PNES. The consistently lower ratings of quality of life combined with the greater prevalence of character pathology clearly suggest this is a population that interprets the world in a negative fashion, even more negatively than the average person with epilepsy. However, we clearly have not yet hit on a true "core" pathology that can be generalized across most patients suffering from PNES (if such a construct actually exists). Rather, the relative infrequency of avoidant coping, mixed results in terms of the impact of avoidant coping when it is present, and a lack of significant separation between patients with PNES and epilepsy in terms of alexithymia call into question the prime place these constructs are given in our theories of the etiology of PNES. They clearly appear to be relevant in a substantial minority of patients; however, there appears to be nothing special about PNES in this regard, as patients with clear-cut epilepsy demonstrate many of the same features.

REPORTED TRAUMA

The understanding of the complex relationship between reported trauma and PNES has continued to develop over the past few years. In contrast to the mixed results seen in investigations of alexithymia and coping styles, investigations of the relationships between reported trauma and patient presentation have been much more consistent. The particular salience of reported trauma to the clinical presentation of the patient with PNES is highlighted in a few recent publications. Williamson, Holsman, Chaytor, Miller, and Drane (2012) reported the surprising result that a reported history of trauma was associated with failure of a well-established PVT, the WMT (Green & Astner, 1995), whereas compensation-seeking was not. The authors noted that "any report of abuse, regardless of how many subtypes are reported, more than doubles the likelihood of WMT failure" (p. 6). No differences were seen between the different types of abuse, although it should be noted that the psychometric assessment of trauma in this study was quite rudimentary, limited as it was to single questions regarding physical, emotional, and sexual abuse, respectively, on a background questionnaire that was then referenced in a clinical interview. As expected, Minnesota Multiphasic Personality Inventory (MMPI)-2 scores indicated greater psychopathology in the group reporting trauma; however, in contrast to findings in other populations, WMT failure was *not* associated with exaggerated reports of emotional distress on the same measure.

Myers, Perrine, et al. (2013), who examined reported trauma in a much more comprehensive fashion, found that those patients with PNES who report trauma were more likely to have been diagnosed with posttraumatic stress disorder (PTSD) or a mood disorder and to have been involved in psychotherapy. Those diagnosed with PTSD, in particular, used antipsychotic medication more frequently, attempted suicide more frequently, and reported greater demoralization and depression on the MMPI-RF. Diagnoses of mood disorders were seen only in the context of PTSD in this sample.

Salinsky and colleagues (2012) expanded on this theme in a sample of veterans. These investigators compared consecutive samples of 50 patients with PNES and 37 patients with epilepsy, each from the Portland VA Medical Center, who were rigorously diagnosed with regard to their seizures. Psychiatric diagnoses were drawn from all available medical records. The investigators found that major depression and substance abuse were common to both groups. In contrast, in a logistic regression, only PTSD differentiated the two groups, being much more common in the PNES group. PTSD preceded PNES in 58% of the patients in this sample but epilepsy in only 13.5%. This rate is higher than that reported by Myers et al. (2013), suggesting that there may be important differences between veteran and civilian samples. This could include greater vulnerability and/or exposure to trauma in the military sample, or alternatively, greater environmental contingencies favoring the report of PTSD symptoms by veterans (McNally & Frueh, 2012).

Finally, in an examination of their proposed model of PNES etiology and maintenance, Bodde and colleagues (2013) also highlighted the role of reported trauma. Approximately one-third of this sample of 40 patients with PNES had comorbid epilepsy, and no effort was made to quantify data validity, so the ability of their results to generalize to other patients with PNES is indeterminate. Based upon a cluster analysis of results from 11 self-report and cognitive measures, the two core constructs determining PNES subtype were (1) reported history of trauma and (2) tendency toward somatization/overly sensitive personality. These two dynamics operated essentially independently, with the reported history of trauma being more tightly linked to more pervasive psychopathology.

In summary, recent research examining the relationship between reported trauma and PNES further supports the connection long noted in the literature. In contrast to general levels of depressive or anxiety symptoms, this connection is more specific to PNES than to epilepsy, and it appears to have a compelling impact on reported psychopathology. Most surprising is the suggestion that reported trauma appears to have an even greater impact on the likelihood of failing PVT and on the severity of reported psychopathology than does the act of seeking to obtain or renew financial compensation.

SEMIOLOGY

In addition to seeking to understand psychological commonalities between patients with PNES, efforts have been made to identify semiologic consistencies between non-epileptic seizures. Individual behaviors characteristic of PNES have been detailed in a recent review (Mostacci et al., 2011), and investigators have tried to systemize these behaviors into various PNES "subtypes." Several such efforts have been published in the past (Griffith et al., 2007; Groppel, Kapitany, & Baumgartner, 2000; Meierkord, Will, Fish, & Shorvon, 1991; Seneviratne, Reutens, & D'Souza, 2010). The relevance of understanding (and teaching) consistencies in PNES presentation was emphasized by Seneviratne and colleagues' exploration of how well healthcare professionals differentiate PNES events from epileptic seizures based purely on semiology (Seneviratne, Rajendran, Brusco, & Phan, 2012). Neurologists at a tertiary epilepsy center did rather well, discriminating at 89% accuracy. In contrast, emergency medicine residents were 66% accurate, barely above neuroscience nurses (62%).

Dhiman and colleagues, stating that a substantial portion of the PNES behavior they observed in their tertiary care center could not be categorized into existing systems, published an elaborated version of the system initially proposed by Seneviratne and colleagues (Dhiman, Sinha, Rawat, Harish, et al., 2013). This work categorized nonepileptic spells into categories marked by abnormal motor response, affective/emotional behavior, dialeptic type (i.e., nonresponsive), nonepileptic aura, and varying combinations of the above ("mixed pattern"). The value of any of these systems will be determined by (1) the extent to which other raters can reliably use them to rate most of their patients, and (2) the extent to which the identified subtypes provide information meaningful to the patients' management. To this end, Dhiman and colleagues noted that the dialeptic and nonepileptic aura subtypes were never observed to co-occur with epileptic seizures and thus may be more specific markers of PNES than the other subtypes.

PNES semiology in children has also received attention. This is important, as the behavioral manifestation of PNES in adults is not identical to that seen in children (Alessi, Vincentiis, Rzezak, & Valente, 2013). Alessi and colleagues noted that ictal eye closure, motor phenomena lasting longer than 2 minutes, postictal speech changes, pelvic thrusting, and vocalization during the "tonic-clonic" phase all occur significantly more frequently in adults than in children and adolescents. No behaviors were significantly more characteristic of childhood spells than adult spells. Extending their work with adults, Dhiman and colleagues reported on the utility of their system in children (Dhiman, Sinha, Rawat, Vijaysagar, et al., 2014).

Investigators have also noted that categorizing PNES according to semiologic subgroups may be informative to the extent that such categorization is correlated with other deficits. For instance, evidence is mounting that as PNES semiology becomes more physically extreme (e.g., has more dramatic gross motor components), both neuropsychological performance and self-rated emotional adjustment decline (Griffith, Smith, Schefft, Szaflarski, & Privitera, 2008; Griffith, et al., 2007; Hill & Gale, 2011). As noted by Hill and Gale (2011), a potentially interesting dynamic that has yet to be explored in studies taking this perspective is the extent to which inconsistent effort or poor motivation may vary systematically across this spectrum. In other therapeutic indications (e.g., multi traumatic brain injury [mTBI]), such signs are generally associated with more implausible behavior, worse performance on neurocognitive testing, and endorsement of higher levels of psychopathology. Although Williamson et al. (2012) have documented that these same expectations should not necessarily hold in patients with PNES (at least with regard to endorsement of higher levels of psychopathology), a possible relationship between more extreme behavior and worse PVT performance is easy to explore empirically, and the results of such a study would be quite informative.

DIAGNOSIS

Psychological Testing

Psychological testing is often used to evaluate patients with known or suspected PNES. Although vEEG monitoring capturing the typical spell is the diagnostic gold standard, personality testing informs psychotherapeutic efforts by increasing understanding of an individual's psychological adjustment and identifying target areas for treatment. In addition, for patients whose spells remain indeterminate following monitoring, personality variables can provide greater insight into their spells. There is an extensive body of literature investigating the usefulness of the MMPI and MMPI-2 in this population, with general consensus that patients with PNES often produce a profile consistent with features of somatization (e.g., elevations on scales 1 and 3; Wilkus & Dodrill, 1989). There is also empirical support for use of the MMPI to help differentiate individuals with PNES from those with ES (Cragar, Berry, Fakhoury, Cibula, & Schmitt, 2002; Wilkus & Dodrill, 1989; Williamson, et al., 2007).

More recently, the MMPI-2 RF, a restructured, shorter version of the original test with increased reliability and scale homogeneity, has been used to help differentiate individuals with ES from those with PNES. Locke et al. (2010) correctly classified about two-thirds of patients with the Somatic Complaints (RC1), Neurological Complaints (NUC), and Symptom Validity (FBS-r) scales from the MMPI-2 RF. Classification accuracy was slightly improved with supplementary MMPI-2 RF scales designed by Locke and Thompson (2011) to specifically differentiate individuals with ES from those with PNES. A combination of statistical analyses and clinical judgment was used to identify MMPI-2-RF items that were combined to create scales measuring Physical Complaints (PNES-pc) and Attitudes (PNES-a). In combination, the scales correctly classified 73% of patients with ES and PNES, representing an improvement of 5% over the highest published classification rate using any single, traditional MMPI-2-RF scale (RC1 = 68%; Locke et al., 2010).

The Personality Assessment Inventory (PAI; Morey, 2007) has gained recent interest as a means of assessing personality characteristics of individuals with PNES. An "NES (nonepileptic seizure) Indicator" scale was developed by using scores from two PAI subscales (Conversion minus Health Concerns) and initially showed promise as a means of accurately classifying patients with nonepileptic and epileptic seizures (Wagner, Wymer, Topping, & Pritchard, 2005). However, recent replications using the NES Indicator have shown it to have low specificity and to be only slightly better than chance at differentiating ES and PNES patient groups (Gale & Hill, 2012; Testa, Lesser, Krauss, & Brandt, 2011; Thompson, Hantke, Phatak, & Chaytor, 2010).

Testa and colleagues (2011) were the first to describe an entire modal PAI profile for groups of patients with ES and PNES. Relative to a group of normal control subjects, both patient groups produced significant elevations on the following PAI scales: Somatic Complaints, Anxiety, Depression, Schizophrenia, and Borderline Features. The profiles of both groups were similar in terms of overall endorsement of mood-related symptoms, disorganized thought processes, and level of somatic concern. However, the patient groups produced elevations on different subscales, suggesting that their experience of these symptoms differed. In particular, the PNES group produced higher scores on the Stress and Suicidal Ideation subscales and endorsed higher levels of physical symptoms of anxiety and depression.

Reported accuracy rates using the PAI in the differential diagnosis of PNES and ES have been promising. Using the Conversion subscale, classification rates for PNES patients have ranged from 74% to 79% (Locke et al., 2011; Thompson et al., 2010). In a prospective study, Locke et al. (2011) randomized consecutive epilepsy monitoring unit patients to receive either the MMPI-2 or the PAI. MMPI-2 results were rescored to obtain MMPI-RF variables for additional comparison. Among various scales from the individual measures, the MMPI-2 indicators produced the lowest classification rates (63% and 68%) and PAI indicators produced the highest classification rates (71% and 79%). Likelihood ratios were presented to allow creation of individualized calculations depending on the base rate of PNES in the population assessed.

In a head-to-head comparison of diagnostic predictive ability, the MMPI-2 and PAI were concurrently administered to a sample of 17 patients with epilepsy and 23 patients with PNES undergoing vEEG monitoring (Gale & Hill, 2012). The authors found similar levels of predictive value for each measure. The most accurate predictive model included a combination of Somatic Complaints and Health Concerns subscales from the PAI and MMPI-2 Scale 3 (Hysteria), with an overall classification rate of 85%. Administration of both measures would be cumbersome in the context of most evaluations and most clinicians will likely choose a single self-report measure. The higher classification rates reported for the PAI, in conjunction with several additional advantages over the MMPI-2 (e.g., lower reading level, shorter administration time), make the PAI an attractive option when assessing patients with PNES. To date, the PAI appears to have a slight edge over the MMPI-2-RF in terms of overall classification accuracy as well, although the possibility that the measures may be "picking up on different patients" remains a question that is as yet unexamined.

Neurodiagnostics

Continuous, long-term vEEG of a patient's typical events remains the gold standard for PNES diagnosis (LaFrance & Benbadis, 2011). vEEG produces a definitive diagnosis in up to 90% of patients and corrects inaccurate diagnosis in up to 79% of patients (Noe, Grade, Stonnington, Driver-Dunckley, & Locke, 2012; Smolowitz et al., 2007). Diagnosis of PNES on the basis of clinical history and outpatient studies alone can be difficult, with varying rates of accuracy that may be affected by the gender of the patient. In a retrospective study of epilepsy monitoring unit (EMU) admissions, an epileptologist classified a series of patients as having PNES or ES based on review of history and medical records (e.g., physical examination, outpatient testing results). Thirty-five percent of men with PNES were mistakenly predicted to have neurologically based seizures, whereas only 14% of women with confirmed PNES were misclassified (Noe et al., 2012). This may reflect a selection bias based on the fact that PNES occurs at a higher rate in women. Interestingly, Noe and colleagues (2012) also found that during 39% of male EMU admissions, a typical seizure event was not captured during vEEG monitoring. In contrast, there was failure to capture an event during vEEG in only 12% of female admissions. One possible explanation for lack of events during monitoring is that removal of the patient from his or her typical environment removes circumstances that may typically trigger an event. Why this would occur at a higher rate for men versus women is unclear. Regardless, it appears that PNES is not only less common in men, but also more difficult to identify clinically.

For some patients with suspected PNES, inpatient vEEG is not an option. This occurs for numerous reasons, including lack of conveniently located EMU, inadequate health insurance, or inability to leave a home or work environment for prolonged admission. As such, recent studies have investigated alternate means of accurately identifying PNES. Outpatient short-term vEEG monitoring represents a shorter, less expensive, and more convenient method of examining seizure events. This procedure typically lasts between 3 and 6 hours, which increases patient convenience but limits the likelihood of capturing typical events. Prior studies have shown diagnostic accuracy rates as high as 67% using outpatient short-term vEEG monitoring (Varela, Taylor, & Benbadis, 2007). In a more recent series of 175 patients seen in an Australian tertiary care hospital, outpatient short-term vEEG monitoring resulted in diagnosis change from ES to PNES in 29% of patients (Seneviratne et al., 2012). The rate of correct classification was lower than that found by the Varela group (37%), which may have stemmed from methodologic differences. In particular, verbal suggestion to induce seizure activity was not consistently used in the Seneviratne sample.

Based on previous research showing a differential pattern of rhythmic movement artifact on EEG between individuals with ES and PNES, Bayly and colleagues (2013) hypothesized that a movement-recording device worn on the wrist could effectively differentiate epileptic and nonepileptic events. Using this method, 93% of nonepileptic and 91% of epileptic events were correctly identified. However, only one-third of patients undergoing vEEG produced movements that could be meaningfully analyzed. Thus, although highly accurate, this technique appears to be most useful for only a minority of patients. However, depending upon the cost of the procedure, such a high-specificity/low sensitivity may still be useful if understood and used appropriately. The extent to which this technology improves diagnostic decision-making and the contexts in which this is true must be established. For instance, it is unlikely that such a method would add significantly to decisions made in an EMU, but it may be a helpful specific (yet not sensitive) tool for patients for whom there is diagnostic uncertainty and for whom an EMU is not an option.

The presence of certain medical comorbidities has also been examined as a means of differentiating PNES from ES. Gazzola and colleagues (2012) found a higher rate of chronic pain and prescription pain medication use (particularly opioids) in individuals with PNES, as compared to individuals with ES. Another recent study investigated the possibility that the presence of "functional somatic syndromes," including fibromyalgia, chronic pain syndrome, tension headaches, irritable bowel syndrome, asthma, migraine, and gastroesophageal reflux disease, could discriminate individuals with PNES from those with ES (Dixit, Popescu, Bagic, Ghearing, & Hendrickson, 2013). They found significantly more individuals with PNES (65.8%) than with ES (27%) had been diagnosed with at least one of these disorders. The presence of one of the listed syndromes resulted in a positive predictive value for PNES of 75%. A third of the PNES population reported prior diagnosis of two of these disorders (vs. only 6% of the ES group). Although diagnostic specificity increased in those patients with two of the disorders, sensitivity was lowered. These findings suggest that PNES should be suspected in individuals presenting with seizures and at least one functional somatic syndrome. These studies also suggest that there is overlap between PNES and other conditions that include medically unexplained symptoms. Along these lines, Hopp and LaFrance (2012) found numerous similarities between patients with PNES and those with psychogenic movement disorders. Although the physical manifestations of these conditions differed, the patient groups produced similar psychological profiles, including low levels of quality of life, self-efficacy, and overall psychological functioning. There is growing evidence that PNES and other medically unexplained symptoms are a manifestation of an underlying cause (or cluster of causes) that may be similar across disorders.

Use of a stuffed animal as a transitional object in adulthood is commonly referred to as "the teddy bear sign." This phenomenon has been associated with the presence of various types of psychopathology (Cardasis, Hochman, & Silk, 1997; Schmaling, DiClementi, & Hammerly, 1994) and shown to occur more often in PNES than ES (Burneo et al., 2003). In a recent series of 264 EMU patients aged 15 and older (including those with ES and PNES), 14% of the sample brought a stuffed animal to the EMU (Cervenka et al., 2013). A higher percentage of those who showed a positive teddy bear sign were diagnosed with ES than PNES (56% vs. 39%). Female patients and those with longer seizure duration were significantly more likely to bring a stuffed animal. In analyses that included only patients aged 18 and older, patients with stuffed animals were more likely to have PNES than ES, but only when other patient variables were controlled. Overall, the Cervenka et al. study suggests that the teddy bear sign is not as reliable of a predictor of PNES as was previously thought.

Physical signs exhibited ictally or peri-ictally can also inform diagnosis of PNES. In a meta-analysis and review of existing literature regarding diagnostic significance of tongue-biting in patients with ES and PNES, Brigo and colleagues (2012) found that general ictal tongue-biting did not add significant value to differential diagnosis of these populations. However, lateral tongue biting (as opposed to tip of the tongue biting) was strongly suggestive of ES. Post-ictal snoring is also highly suggestive of ES (Rosemergy, Frith, Herath, & Walker, 2013). In fact, in their sample of 72 seizure episodes in patients with ES and PNES, none of the nonepileptic episodes were accompanied by post-ictal snoring. Post-ictal breathing patterns in general differed between the groups, with return to normal respiratory rate twice as fast following nonepileptic versus epileptic events.

Presence of urinary incontinence and differences in heart rate have also been proposed as a potential means of differentiating patients with PNES and ES. Brigo and colleagues (2013) reviewed studies of urinary incontinence in seizure disorders and found that it did not help to differentiate PNES from ES. A recent study investing changes in heart rate as a potential biomarker of PNES found that although patients with PNES and ES showed differences in resting heart rate relative to control subjects, these were not of sufficient magnitude to aid in differential diagnosis (Ponnusamy, Marques, & Reuber, 2011).

Neuroimaging

Neuroimaging studies have investigated the possibility of defining neuroanatomic correlates of PNES. In a sample of 20 patients with PNES and 40 age- and gender-matched controls, Labate and colleagues (2012) performed whole-brain magnetic resonance imaging measurements, voxel-based morphometry, cortical thickness analysis, and neuropsychological testing. Per the subgroup descriptions described in the Semiology section, the descriptions provided by the authors suggest that these patients with PNES consisted primarily of the abnormal motor/major motor subtypes. As a group, the PNES patients showed abnormal cortical atrophy of the motor and premotor regions in the right hemisphere and the cerebellum, bilaterally. There was a significant association between level of depression and cortical thinning or atrophy in right premotor sites, although the precise sites identified by voxel-based morphometry and cortical thickness analyses varied a bit within this region. Neuropsychological assessment failed to reveal any significant differences between groups.

Other studies have focused on the connectivity of different regions during specific types of tasks. Van der Kruijs and colleagues reported no significant differences between a sample of 11 patients with PNES and 12 healthy control subjects in terms of absolute levels of functional magnetic resonance imaging activation on two cognitive tasks (picture encoding, Stroop paradigm). However, the groups differed from each other during the resting state, as patients with PNES demonstrated stronger connectivity between the insula and some parietal regions as well as some premotor regions. The authors noted that these findings were thematically consistent with other findings linking "limbic" regions with "motor" regions (e.g., Voon et al., 2010), thereby providing a putative rationale for a neurobiologic basis for at least some consistently observed features of PNES (van der Kruijs et al., 2012).

A persistent challenge in interpreting imaging findings is the frequency with which they rely on very small samples and on techniques in which relatively common events or decisions can have significant interpretive implications (Bedenbender et al., 2011; Satterthwaite et al., 2012; Satterthwaite et al., 2013). Thus, replication is critical to gaining confidence in the extent to which such differences are reliable between samples and may have clinical implications in terms of psychiatric or neurocognitive function.

DIAGNOSTIC TIMING

Numerous studies prior to 2011 have shown that an average of 7 years passes from the onset of spells to accurate diagnosis of PNES (Bodde et al., 2009; Reuber, Fernández, Bauer, Helmstaedter, & Elger, 2002). Bodde et al. (2012) described a subgroup of patients with PNES with a shorter duration from seizure onset to referral to an epilepsy center. The average referral time was approximately 4 years, with nearly 50% of the sample being referred within 2 years of seizure onset. This group of patients was characterized by a higher number of historical psychological/psychiatric complaints for which they actively sought diagnosis and treatment. The authors described these patients as having a "stronger drive for medical examinations and treatment," which may have contributed to a more expedient referral pattern. Even shorter diagnostic delays were noted in a sample of veterans and civilians who underwent vEEG monitoring at a Veterans Administration EMU (Salinsky, Spencer, Boudreau, & Ferguson, 2011). The authors found an average span of 60.5 months between symptom onset and EMU diagnosis in veterans and only 12.5 months in the civilian members of the sample. These averages are significantly shorter than averages reported in prior studies of diagnostic delay, and it is unclear why individuals in this sample were referred for EMU monitoring so much sooner than other, previously studied samples of patients. There was a significant difference between the diagnostic delay for civilians and veterans, which the authors hypothesized may have occurred due to assumptions that seizures in a veteran could stem from prior traumatic brain injury and associated assumptions that these patients were at risk for ES and/or decreased availability of epilepsy monitoring units in Veterans Administration systems (Salinsky et al., 2011).

Decreasing the time from spell onset to accurate diagnosis is critical in this patient population, because diagnosis alone can decrease health service utilization (especially emergency department visits), lower healthcare costs, and improve treatment outcome (Ahmedani et al., 2013; Jirsch, Ahmed, Maximova, & Gross, 2011; Razvi, Mulhern, & Duncan, 2012). In one series of patients (Ahmedani et al., 2013), overall healthcare costs were reduced by $1,800 per patient in the 12 months following PNES diagnosis delivery. Behavioral health service costs increased after PNES diagnosis in one hospital setting, but the costs were minimal and offset by a reduction of service use in other medical areas. Early diagnosis can also prevent unnecessary treatment with antiepileptic drugs (AEDs), which can produce deleterious side effects.

TREATMENT

Establishing a secure diagnosis is the first step toward effective treatment of individuals with PNES. Receiving a diagnosis of PNES represents the beginning of a paradigm shift for many patients who have operated under the assumption that they have epileptic seizures, sometimes for many years. As such, patients' perceptions of their condition tend to differ from that of the diagnosing treatment team. Patients tend to see their problem within a medical framework, often because they have been diagnosed with epilepsy and treated with AEDs. Once seizures are identified as non-epileptic in nature, the neurologist/epileptologist views the problem as one that is psychological in nature. In a survey of neurologists and psychiatrists, physicians from both specialties reported that patients with PNES have greater control over seizure events than patients with ES (Whitehead & Reuber, 2012). In another survey of healthcare professionals who treat PNES, 48% of nurses expressed a belief that PNES are voluntarily controlled (Sahaya, Dholakia, Lardizabal, & Sahota, 2012). This stands in contrast to the existing literature suggesting that, although an elevated proportion of patients with PNES perform poorly on SVT/PVT compared to patients with epilepsy, the majority perform within the valid range. Many of those who perform below expectation on PVTs appear to do so for reasons unrelated to compensation-seeking efforts that have been commonly associated with PVT failure in other patient populations (Williamson et al., 2012). The findings reported by Sahaya and colleagues shed light on the mixed opinions among professionals caring for patients with PNES. Differences in illness perception between patients and treating professionals likely contribute to the feelings of anger or confusion some patients report after receiving a diagnosis of PNES (Whitehead, Kandler, & Reuber, 2013).

The differences in illness perception between patient and physician may also serve to reduce physicians' level of comfort with delivering a diagnosis of PNES. Most neurologists surveyed report that communicating a diagnosis of PNES is a difficult process. Linguistic analyses of communications between neurologists and patients with PNES indicate that these conversations are often approached with delicacy and defensiveness (Monzoni, Duncan, Grunewald, & Reuber, 2011). Regardless, there is evidence that presentation of the diagnosis has the potential to serve as an effective therapeutic tool. Several standardized methods for delivering a PNES diagnosis were outlined in earlier studies. In a follow-up study of a diagnosis-delivery strategy designed by Hall-Patch and colleagues (2010), approximately 16% of patients were seizure free at 6-month follow-up (Mayor et al., 2012). An additional 23% of the patients showed greater than 50% reduction in seizure frequency. No change in reported ratings of healthcare utilization, physical health, or mental health occurred, underscoring the need for further psychological or psychiatric intervention in these patients even if they stop having PNES episodes (Mayor, et al., 2012). Other recent studies described spell remission rates following diagnosis alone ranging from 23% to 50% (Duncan, Razvi, & Mulhern, 2011; Nezadal et al., 2011). Additional early intervention strategies include provision of an informational brochure describing the nature of PNES and what patients and their families can expect (e.g., the brochure available from the University of South Florida: http://hsc. usf.edu/COM/epilepsy/PNESbrochure.pdf). In general, the impact of these efforts has not been formally studied.

A recent study conducted at Emory University randomized patients diagnosed with PNES events to one of three treatment groups (Ganesh et al., 2013), with each patient asked to maintain a daily log of any ongoing events: (A) standard care—the attending neurologist delivered the diagnosis and suggested that the patient follow-up in the community with mental health services; (B) scripted diagnosis and psychiatry consult—the diagnosis was made in a structured manner, the PNES patient was provided with the University of South Florida handout, and he or she was seen by the psychiatry service for a one-time consult; and (C) scripted diagnosis, psychiatry consult, and weekly scripted telephone calls—this intervention was the same as "b," except each patient was called on a weekly basis to reinforce the diagnosis and provide support in a structured manner. At the end of 8 weeks, all patients were evaluated by telephone interview, including some brief assessment scales (QOL, mood inventories) and a survey of outcome factors (e.g., numbers of events per week, utilization of health services related to the PNES events). Groups B and C both exhibited a significant decrease in event occurrence as compared to Group A. Group C also demonstrated gains in aspects of mood not evidenced by the other two groups. This rather simple study demonstrated that even some minimal interventions geared toward emphasizing diagnosis and providing an opportunity for feedback and minimal support can have an appreciable impact on outcome. This is useful knowledge, because formal treatment programs remain rare in most communities. A weakness in the study involved the inclusion of several strategies, making it difficult to know the relative value of each intervention.

At the request of the International League Against Epilepsy, a panel of internationally recognized PNES experts produced recommendations for management of PNES (LaFrance, Jr., Reuber, & Goldstein, 2013a). Formal psychiatric consultation was recommended to occur early in the diagnostic process, with goals of ruling out psychiatric conditions that may mimic PNES (e.g., panic disorder), identifying psychiatric comorbidities that may respond to psychopharmacologic efforts, characterizing background and psychiatric factors contributing to an individual's presentation that may not be emphasized during neurologic work-up, and addressing any acute risks. Only 42% of a sample of surveyed monitoring units certified by the National Association of Epilepsy Centers reported that they routinely obtain an inpatient psychiatric consultation for patients newly diagnosed with PNES. Approximately 30% of the referred patients refused psychiatric consultation. In lieu of this treatment option, 33% of the centers made referrals to an outpatient mental health provider. Change in treatment occurred in only one patient who received inpatient psychiatric consultation, leading the authors to conclude that inpatient psychiatric consultation should be performed on a case-by-case basis in patients with PNES and is best utilized in those with emergent psychiatric needs (Acton & Tatum, 2013). Psychiatric consultation may occur more frequently on an outpatient basis following discharge from the diagnostic admission.

Pharmacologic treatment of patients with PNES ideally begins with early discontinuation of any AEDs the patient may have been prescribed for previously assumed epileptic seizures. After communication of diagnosis, initiating the discontinuation of AEDs (if applicable) is the next step in treating patients with PNES. In addition to removing unnecessary medication with potential for side effects, withdrawing AEDs after PNES diagnosis reinforces communication that seizures do not have a medical etiology (LaFrance, Jr., et al., 2013a). AED withdrawal that occurs immediately following PNES diagnosis is more effective than later withdrawal and has been shown to double the likelihood that a patient will become seizure free after diagnosis delivery alone (Oto, Espie, & Duncan, 2010). Pharmacologic treatment may also target psychiatric comorbidities present in patients with PNES. A high percentage of patients with PNES meet diagnostic criteria for a mood disorder, suggesting that treatment appropriate to their comorbid psychiatric diagnoses may be helpful in this population.

To date, no medications have received Food and Drug Administration approval for the treatment of PNES or conversion disorder. Preliminary investigations have suggested some potential efficacy for selective serotonin reuptake inhibitors (SSRIs) in conversion disorders (Voon & Lang, 2005). To investigate the possibility that SSRIs may be an effective treatment for PNES, LaFrance (2010) conducted a small randomized, placebo-controlled trial. Of the 26 subjects who completed the trial, those who received sertraline (up to 200-mg doses) experienced a 45% reduction in seizure frequency. Individuals in the placebo arm of the study experienced an 8% increase in seizure frequency. Although this is a promising finding in terms of seizure reduction, the obvious caveats associated with small sample size are relevant, as is the fact that analysis of secondary outcome measures (e.g., quality of life, family functioning, psychosocial functioning) failed to reveal any significant difference between treatment and control groups. Depressive symptoms also failed to improve significantly in either group. Thus, additional trials are needed to determine the potential utility of SSRIs in PNES and whether they may be more relevant for some subgroups than others (Bravo et al., 2013).

There is more support for use of psychotherapy for treating PNES, as it is generally considered the best-validated approach for its treatment (LaFrance Jr., et al., 2013a). Nevertheless, evidence-based treatment in this area remains limited. Cognitive-behavioral therapy (CBT) has the most substantial body of literature supporting its use. Two approaches to CBT in this population (Goldstein et al., 2010; LaFrance et al., 2009; LaFrance, Jr., et al., 2013) have been organized in manuals for multicenter use, although the manuals are not currently available for outside clinicians. Nevertheless, elements are described in the original articles and could be adapted for use in clinical practice. Reductions in seizure frequency and improvements on measures of anxiety, depression, somatic symptoms, quality of life, and family functioning have been shown in open-label studies and a pilot randomized controlled trial using these approaches. Most recently, LaFrance and colleagues conducted a multicenter pilot randomized controlled trial using a 12-week CBT treatment model (LaFrance, Jr., et al., 2013b). Across three treatment sites, 35 patients were randomized into four treatment arms: (1) sertraline only, (2) CBT only, (3) CBT and medication, and (4) standard medical care that the authors likened to supportive therapy. The patients treated with CBT only showed a significant reduction in seizure frequency and improvements on secondary measures. Those treated with CBT and medication also showed improvements, but to a lesser degree than the CBT-only group, and those treated with medication only showed "trends toward improvement." The patients who received standard medical care did not show any seizure reduction or improvement in secondary outcomes. Several articles reviewing findings from prior CBT studies and other treatment approaches have been published in recent years (Baslet, 2012; Hopp & LaFrance, 2012; LaFrance, Jr., et al., 2013a), showing that psychotherapeutic efforts (particularly CBT) are a promising form of treatment for individuals with PNES.

Prior research using uncontrolled trials has produced support for use of psychodynamic therapy, group therapy, and family therapy for treatment of PNES, although no recent studies of these approaches have been published. Mayor and colleagues (2013) recently investigated the efficacy of a 4-week, standardized, psychoeducational program delivered by treating professionals with little to no psychotherapy experience. Approximately one-third of patients were seizure free at a 7-month follow-up survey and an additional 23% reported a 50% reduction in seizure frequency. Consistent with findings from LaFrance and colleagues (2013), these results indicate that a simple, psychoeducational program is not sufficient treatment for most patients with PNES. Most individuals require more intensive treatment that addresses predisposing, precipitating, and perpetuating factors (LaFrance, Jr., et al., 2013a).

Engaging patients in mental health treatment and maintaining treatment adherence are challenges common to the PNES population. Some patients may not initially accept a psychological explanation for their seizures and therefore decline referral to a mental health professional. Those who do initiate treatment are often unlikely to continue through to treatment completion, with reported treatment adherence rates ranging from 31% to 54% for patients with PNES (Baslet & Prensky, 2013; Mayor, et al., 2013), compared to an average treatment adherence rate of 80% for psychotherapy in general (Swift & Greenberg, 2012). In a small sample of surveyed therapists, preparation level for treating the complexities seen in many patients with PNES was low (Quinn, Schofield, & Middleton, 2010), which may contribute to unsuccessful treatment or increased drop-out rates. However, other contributory factors likely involve the comorbidities assoicated with many of these patients (e.g., chronic pain issues, psychiatric conditions), problems with transportation, and lack of health insurance.

To counteract the problem of inconsistent mental health follow-up, the International League Against Epilepsy recommendations encourage long-term follow-up with a physician who has knowledge of PNES. This may be especially helpful in patients who are reluctant to seek psychotherapy or other mental health care, as the physician may be able to introduce treatment options that promote social and functional improvements, but involve specialists other than a psychotherapist (e.g., occupational therapists, physiotherapists, rehabilitation experts). Likewise, psycho-educational and CBT-based programs managed by tertiary epilepsy centers may not be seen as strictly mental health interventions, and keep the patient in contact with familiar treatment providers. Coordination between treatment providers is encouraged to prevent unnecessary treatment and limit investigation of symptoms for which a medical cause is unlikely.

CONCLUSIONS

The quest to understand PNES and the patients who experience them remains vibrant. It is understood that these individuals tend to experience and report physical symptoms more frequently than others, that they are more likely to report having experienced abuse of various types, and that they characterize their quality of life as even worse than the patients with epilepsy, which their condition so closely mimics. It appears that those whose spells are more flamboyant also tend to report more psychopathology and perform less well on neurocognitive testing. Typical statements about motivation to perform optimally on neurocognitive testing learned from other groups do not appear to generalize as cleanly as we might have assumed, as compensation-seeking appears to be a less consistent driver of PVT failure among PNES patients (at least in tertiary epilepsy centers).

However, there is still much more to learn. There is now a variety of evidence-based "what" subgroup classification systems that quantify behaviorally different subtypes of spells. Unfortunately, there is little in the way of "why" subgroups that cut to the core reasons as to why a specific person is manifesting PNES. Trauma certainly seems to exacerbate the suffering associated with PNES, but not everyone with PNES reports having suffered trauma. Likewise, although alexithymia and avoidant coping styles are conceptually appealing as explanatory mechanisms, the available evidence does not make a terribly compelling case that these play a more central role in PNES than in a variety of other problems, some of which are not even marked by significant somatoform pathology.

Although limitations remain, the methods used to examine these questions continue to evolve. Rigorous definition of PNES samples is now *de riguer* in the literature, and early signs of taking validity of performance in mind when assembling samples are emerging. Limitations persist, such as small sample sizes, lack of control groups, limited generalizability, and variable definitions of diagnosis and outcome. However, the hope is that clinicians can continue to refine the models and the methods to chip away at the obstacles obscuring understanding of the critical features that are needed to comprehend in order to be of the most service to these patients seeking assistance.

REFERENCES

Acton, E. K., & Tatum, W. O. (2013). Inpatient psychiatric consultation for newly-diagnosed patients with psychogenic non-epileptic seizures. *Epilepsy Behav, 27*(1), 36–39. doi:10.1016/j.yebeh.2012.11.050

Ahmedani, B. K., Osborne, J., Nerenz, D. R., Haque, S., Pietrantoni, L., Mahone, D., et al. (2013). Diagnosis, costs, and utilization for psychogenic non-epileptic seizures in a US health care setting. *Psychosomatics, 54*(1), 28–34. doi:10.1016/j.psym.2012.08.005

Alessi, R., Vincentiis, S., Rzezak, P., & Valente, K. D. (2013). Semiology of psychogenic non-epileptic seizures: Age-related differences. *Epilepsy Behav, 27*(2), 292–295. doi:10.1016/j.yebeh.2013.02.003

Baslet, G. (2012). Psychogenic nonepileptic seizures: A treatment review. What have we learned since the beginning of the millennium? *Neuropsychiatr Dis Treat, 8*, 585–598. doi:10.2147/NDT.S32301

Baslet, G., & Prensky, E. (2013). Initial treatment retention in psychogenic non-epileptic seizures. *J Neuropsychiatry Clin Neurosci, 25*(1), 63–67. doi:10.1176/appi.neuropsych.11090223

Bayly, J., Carino, J., Petrovski, S., Smit, M., Fernando, D. A., Vinton, A., et al. (2013). Time-frequency mapping of the rhythmic limb movements distinguishes convulsive epileptic from psychogenic nonepileptic seizures. *Epilepsia, 54*(8), 1402–1408.

Bedenbender, J., Paulus, F. M., Krach, S., Pyka, M., Sommer, J., Krug, A., et al. (2011). Functional connectivity analyses in imaging genetics: Considerations on methods and data interpretation. *PLoS One, 6*(12), e26354. doi:10.1371/journal.pone.0026354

Bewley, J., Murphy, P. N., Mallows, J., & Baker, G. A. (2005). Does alexithymia differentiate between patients with nonepileptic seizures, patients with epilepsy, and nonpatient controls? *Epilepsy Behav, 7*(3), 430–437.

Bodde, N. M., Brooks, J. L., Baker, G. A., Boon, P. A., Hendriksen, J. G., Mulder, O. G., & Aldenkamp, A. P. (2009). Psychogenic non-epileptic seizures--definition, etiology, treatment and prognostic issues: a critical review. *Seizure, 18*(8), 543–553.

Bodde, N. M., van der Kruijs, S. J., Ijff, D. M., Lazeron, R. H., Vonck, K. E., Boon, P. A., et al. (2013). Subgroup classification in patients with psychogenic non-epileptic seizures. *Epilepsy Behav, 26*(3), 279–289. doi:10.1016/j.yebeh.2012.10.012

Bravo, T. P., Hoffman-Snyder, C. R., Wellik, K. E., Martin, K. A., Hoerth, M. T., Demaerschalk, B. M., et al. (2013). The effect of selective serotonin reuptake inhibitors on the frequency of psychogenic nonepileptic seizures: A critically appraised topic. *Neurologist, 19*(1), 30–33. doi:10.1097/NRL.0b013e31827c6bfd

Brigo, F., Nardone, R., Ausserer, H., Storti, M., Tezzon, F., Manganotti, P., et al. (2013). The diagnostic value of urinary incontinence in the differential diagnosis of seizures. *Seizure, 22*(2), 85–90. doi:10.1016/j.seizure.2012.10.011

Brigo, F., Nardone, R., & Bongiovanni, L. G. (2012). Value of tongue biting in the differential diagnosis between epileptic seizures and syncope. *Seizure, 21*(8), 568–572.

Burneo, J. G., Martin, R., Powell, T., Greenlee, S., Knowlton, R. C., Faught, R. E., et al. (2003). Teddy bears: an observational finding in patients with non-epileptic events. *Neurology, 61*(5), 714–715.

Button, K. S., Ioannidis, J. P., Mokrysz, C., Nosek, B. A., Flint, J., Robinson, E. S., et al. (2013). Power failure: Why small sample size undermines the reliability of neuroscience. *Nat Rev Neurosci, 14*(5), 365–376. doi:10.1038/nrn3475

Cardasis, W., Hochman, J. A., & Silk, K. R. (1997). Transitional objects and borderline personality disorder. *Am J Psychiatry, 154*(2), 250–255.

Celikel, F. C., Kose, S., Erkorkmaz, U., Sayar, K., Cumurcu, B. E., & Cloninger, C. R. (2010). Alexithymia and temperament and character model of personality in patients with major depressive disorder. *Compr Psychiatry, 51*(1), 64–70. doi:10.1016/j.comppsych.2009.02.004

Cervenka, M. C., Lesser, R., Tran, T. T., Fortuné, T., Muthugovindan, D., & Miglioretti, D. L. (2013). Does the teddy bear sign predict psychogenic nonepileptic seizures? *Epilepsy Behav, 28*(2), 217–220.

Cragar, D. E., Berry, D. T. R., Fakhoury, T. A., Cibula, J. E., & Schmitt, F. A. (2002). A review of diagnostic techniques in the differential diagnosis of epileptic and nonepileptic seizures. *Neuropsychology Review, 12*(1), 31.

Cragar, D. E., Berry, D. T., Fakhoury, T. A., Cibula, J. E., & Schmitt, F. A. (2006). Performance of patients with epilepsy or psychogenic non-epileptic seizures on four measures of effort. *Clin Neuropsychol, 20*(3), 552–566. doi:M5650304051282H2 [pii]10.1080/13854040590947380

Dhiman, V., Sinha, S., Rawat, V. S., Harish, T., Chaturvedi, S. K., & Satishchandra, P. (2013). Semiological characteristics of adults with psychogenic nonepileptic seizures (PNESs): An attempt towards a new classification. *Epilepsy Behav, 27*(3), 427–432. doi:10.1016/j.yebeh.2013.03.005

Dhiman, V., Sinha, S., Rawat, V. S., Vijaysagar, K. J., Thippeswamy, H., Srinath, S., et al. (2014). Children with psychogenic non-epileptic seizures (PNES): A detailed semiologic analysis and modified new classification. *Brain Dev, 36*(4), 287–293. doi:10.1016/j.braindev.2013.05.002

Direk, N., Kulaksizoglu, I. B., Alpay, K., & Gurses, C. (2012). Using personality disorders to distinguish between patients with psychogenic nonepileptic seizures and those with epileptic seizures. *Epilepsy Behav, 23*(2), 138–141. doi:10.1016/j.yebeh.2011.11.013

Dixit, R., Popescu, A., Bagic, A., Ghearing, G., & Hendrickson, R. (2013). Medical comorbidities in patients with psychogenic nonepileptic spells (PNES) referred for video-EEG monitoring. *Epilepsy Behav, 28*(2), 137–140. doi:10.1016/j.yebeh.2013.05.004

Dodrill, C. B. (2008). Do patients with psychogenic nonepileptic seizures produce trustworthy findings on neuropsychological tests? *Epilepsia, 49*(4), 691–695. doi:EPI1457 [pii]10.1111/j.1528-1167.2007.01457.x

Drane, D. L., Coady, E., Williamson, D. J., Miller, J. W., & Benbadis, S. R. (2011). Neuropsychological assessment of patients with psychogenic nonepileptic seizures. In M. R. Schoenberg & J. Scott (Eds.), *Black book of neuropsychology* (pp. 521–550). New York: Springer.

Drane, D. L., Williamson, D. J., Stroup, E. S., Holmes, M. D., Jung, M., Koerner, E., et al. (2006). Cognitive impairment is not equal in patients with epileptic and psychogenic nonepileptic seizures. *Epilepsia, 47*(11), 1879–1886.

Duncan, R., Razvi, S., & Mulhern, S. (2011). Newly presenting psychogenic nonepileptic seizures: Incidence, population characteristics, and early outcome from a prospective audit of a first seizure clinic. *Epilepsy Behav, 20*(2), 308–311. doi:10.1016/j.yebeh.2010.10.022

Gale, S. D., & Hill, S. W. (2012). Concurrent administration of the MMPI-2 and PAI in a sample of patients with epileptic or non-epileptic seizures: Implications for an inpatient epilepsy monitoring unit. *Epilepsy Behav, 25*(2), 181–184. doi:10.1016/j.yebeh.2012.07.012

Ganesh, G., Drane, D., Loring, D., Teagarden, D., Kress, K., & Laroche, S. (2013). Treatment strategies for psychogenic nonepileptic seizures: A pilot study. *Epilepsy Currents, 13*(Suppl. 1), 135–136.

Gazzola, D. M., Carlson, C., Rugino, A., Hirsch, S., Starner, K., & Devinsky, O. (2012). Psychogenic nonepileptic seizures and chronic pain: a retrospective case-controlled study. *Epilepsy Behav, 25*(4), 662–665.

Gervais, R. O., Rohling, M. L., Green, P., & Ford, W. (2004). A comparison of WMT, CARB, and TOMM failure rates in non-head injury disability claimants. *Archives of Clinical Neuropsychology, 19*(4), 475.

Goldstein, L. H., Chalder, T., Chigwedere, C., Khondoker, M. R., Moriarty, J., Toone, B. K., et al. (2010). Cognitive-behavioral therapy for psychogenic nonepileptic seizures: A pilot RCT. *Neurology, 74*(24), 1986–1994. doi:10.1212/WNL.0b013e3181e39658

Green, P., & Astner, K. (1995). *Manual for the Oral Word Memory Test*. North Carolina: CogniSyst.

Greve, K. W., Ord, J., Curtis, K. L., Bianchini, K. J., & Brennan, A. (2008). Detecting malingering in traumatic brain injury and chronic pain: A comparison of three forced-choice symptom validity tests. *Clin Neuropsychol, 22*(5), 896–918. doi:10.1080/13854040701565208

Griffith, N. M., Smith, K. M., Schefft, B. K., Szaflarski, J. P., & Privitera, M. D. (2008). Optimism, pessimism, and neuropsychological performance across semiology-based subtypes of psychogenic nonepileptic seizures. *Epilepsy Behav, 13*(3), 478–484. doi:10.1016/j.yebeh.2008.06.005

Griffith, N. M., Szaflarski, J. P., Schefft, B. K., Isaradisaikul, D., Meckler, J. M., McNally, K. A., et al. (2007). Relationship between semiology of psychogenic nonepileptic seizures and Minnesota Multiphasic Personality Inventory profile. *Epilepsy Behav, 11*(1), 105–111. doi:10.1016/j.yebeh.2007.04.021

Groppel, G., Kapitany, T., & Baumgartner, C. (2000). Cluster analysis of clinical seizure semiology of psychogenic nonepileptic seizures. *Epilepsia, 41*(5), 610–614.

Hall-Patch, L., Brown, R., House, A., Howlett, S., Kemp, S., Lawton, G., Mayor, R., Smith, P., Reuber, M., & NEST collaborators. (2010). Acceptability and effectiveness of a strategy for the communication of the diagnosis of psychogenic nonepileptic seizures. *Epilepsia, 51*(1), 70–78.

Hill, S. K., Ryan, L. M., Kennedy, C. H., & Malamut, B. L. (2003). The relationship between measures of declarative memory and the Test of Memory Malingering. *Journal of Forensic Neuropsychology, 3*, 1–18.

Hill, S. W., & Gale, S. D. (2011). Neuropsychological characteristics of nonepileptic seizure semiological subgroups. *Epilepsy Behav, 22*(2), 255–260. doi:10.1016/j.yebeh.2011.06.011

Hopp, J. L., & LaFrance, W. C., Jr. (2012). Cognitive behavioral therapy for psychogenic neurological disorders. *Neurologist, 18*(6), 364–372. doi:10.1097/NRL.0b013e31826e8ff5

Jirsch, J. D., Ahmed, S. N., Maximova, K., & Gross, D. W. (2011). Recognition of psychogenic nonepileptic seizures diminishes acute care utilization. *Epilepsy Behav, 22*(2), 304–307. doi:10.1016/j.yebeh.2011.06.031

Labate, A., Cerasa, A., Mula, M., Mumoli, L., Gioia, M. C., Aguglia, U., et al. (2012). Neuroanatomic correlates of psychogenic nonepileptic seizures: A cortical thickness and VBM study. *Epilepsia, 53*(2), 377–385. doi:10.1111/j.1528-1167.2011.03347.x

LaFrance, W. C., Jr. (2010). Psychogenic nonepileptic "seizures" or "attacks"? It's not just semantics: Seizures. *Neurology, 75*(1), 87–88.

LaFrance, W. C., Jr., Alosco, M. L., Davis, J. D., Tremont, G., Ryan, C. E., Keitner, G. I., et al. (2011). Impact of family functioning on quality of life in patients with psychogenic nonepileptic seizures versus epilepsy. *Epilepsia, 52*(2), 292–300. doi:10.1111/j.1528-1167.2010.02765.x

LaFrance, W. C., Jr., & Benbadis, S. R. (2011). Differentiating frontal lobe epilepsy from psychogenic nonepileptic seizures. *Neurol Clin, 29*(1), 149–162, ix. doi:10.1016/j.ncl.2010.10.005

LaFrance, W. C., Jr., Miller, I. W., Ryan, C. E., Blum, A. S., Solomon, D. A., Kelley, J. E., et al. (2009). Cognitive behavioral therapy for psychogenic nonepileptic seizures. *Epilepsy Behav, 14*(4), 591–596. doi:10.1016/j.yebeh.2009.02.016

LaFrance, W. C. Jr., Papandonatos, G. D., Blum, A. S., Machan, J. T., Ryan, C. E., et al. (2010). Pilot pharmacologic randomized controlled trial for psychogenic nonepileptic seizures. *Neurology*, *75*(13), 1166–1173.

LaFrance, W. C., Jr., Reuber, M., & Goldstein, L. H. (2013a). Management of psychogenic nonepileptic seizures. *Epilepsia*, *54*(Suppl. 1), 53–67. doi:10.1111/epi.12106

LaFrance, W. C., Jr., Webb, A. F., Blum, A. S., Keitner, G. I., Barry, J., & Szaflarski, J. P. (2013b). Multi-center treatment trial pilot for psychogenic nonepileptic seizures. *Epilepsy Currents*, *13*(1), 99.

Larrabee, G. J. (2008). Aggregation across multiple indicators improves the detection of malingering: Relationship to likelihood ratios. *Clin Neuropsychol*, *22*(4), 666–679. doi:10.1080/13854040701494987

Leweke, F., Leichsenring, F., Kruse, J., & Hermes, S. (2012). Is alexithymia associated with specific mental disorders? *Psychopathology*, *45*(1), 22–28. doi:10.1159/000325170

Locke, D. E., Kirlin, K. A., Thomas, M. L., Osborne, D., Hurst, D. F., Drazkowski, J. F., Sirven, J. I., & Noe, K. H. (2010). The Minnesota Multiphasic Personality Inventory-2-Restructured Form in the epilepsy monitoring unit. *Epilepsy Behav*, *17*(2), 252–258.

Locke, D. E., Kirlin, K. A., Wershba, R., Osborne, D., Drazkowski, J. F., Sirven, J. I., et al. (2011). Randomized comparison of the Personality Assessment Inventory and the Minnesota Multiphasic Personality Inventory-2 in the epilepsy monitoring unit. *Epilepsy Behav*, *21*(4), 397–401. doi:10.1016/j.yebeh.2011.05.023

Locke, D. E., & Thomas, M. L. (2011). Initial development of Minnesota Multiphasic Personality Inventory-2-Restructured Form (MMPI-2-RF) scales to identify patients with psychogenic nonepileptic seizures. *J Clin Exp Neuropsychol*, *33*(3), 335–343.

Mayor, R., Brown, R. J., Cock, H., House, A., Howlett, S., Singhal, S., et al. (2012). Short-term outcome of psychogenic non-epileptic seizures after communication of the diagnosis. *Epilepsy Behav*, *25*(4), 676–681. doi:10.1016/j.yebeh.2012.09.033

Mayor, R., Brown, R. J., Cock, H., House, A., Howlett, S., Smith, P., et al. (2013). A feasibility study of a brief psycho-educational intervention for psychogenic nonepileptic seizures. *Seizure*, *22*(9), 760–765. doi:10.1016/j.seizure.2013.06.008

McNally, R. J., & Frueh, B. C. (2012). Why we should worry about malingering in the VA system: Comment on Jackson et al. (2011). *J Trauma Stress*, *25*(4), 454–456; author reply 457–460. doi:10.1002/jts.21713

Meierkord, H., Will, B., Fish, D., & Shorvon, S. (1991). The clinical features and prognosis of pseudoseizures diagnosed using video-EEG telemetry. *Neurology*, *41*(10), 1643–1646.

Mitchell, J. W., Ali, F., & Cavanna, A. E. (2012). Dissociative experiences and quality of life in patients with non-epileptic attack disorder. *Epilepsy Behav*, *25*(3), 307–312. doi:10.1016/j.yebeh.2012.08.022

Mokleby, K., Biomhoff, S., Malt, U. F., Dahlstrom, A., Tauboll, E., & Gjerstad, L. (2002). Psychiatric comorbidity and hostility in patients with psychogenic nonepileptic seizures compared with somatoform disorders and healthy controls. *Epilepsia*, *43*(2), 193–198.

Monzoni, C. M., Duncan, R., Grunewald, R., & Reuber, M. (2011). How do neurologists discuss functional symptoms with their patients: A conversation analytic study. *J Psychosom Res*, *71*(6), 377–383. doi:10.1016/j.jpsychores.2011.09.007

Morey, L. C. (2007). *Personality Assessment Inventory professional manual* (2nd ed.). Lutz, FL: Psychological Assessment Resources.

Mostacci, B., Bisulli, F., Alvisi, L., Licchetta, L., Baruzzi, A., & Tinuper, P. (2011). Ictal characteristics of psychogenic nonepileptic seizures: What we have learned from video/EEG recordings—a literature review. *Epilepsy Behav, 22*(2), 144–153. doi:10.1016/j.yebeh.2011.07.003

Myers, L., Fleming, M., Lancman, M., Perrine, K., & Lancman, M. (2013). Stress coping strategies in patients with psychogenic non-epileptic seizures and how they relate to trauma symptoms, alexithymia, anger and mood. *Seizure, 22*(8), 634–639. doi:10.1016/j.seizure.2013.04.018

Myers, L., Matzner, B., Lancman, M., Perrine, K., & Lancman, M. (2013). Prevalence of alexithymia in patients with psychogenic non-epileptic seizures and epileptic seizures and predictors in psychogenic non-epileptic seizures. *Epilepsy Behav, 26*(2), 153–157. doi:10.1016/j.yebeh.2012.11.054

Myers, L., Perrine, K., Lancman, M., Fleming, M., & Lancman, M. (2013). Psychological trauma in patients with psychogenic nonepileptic seizures: Trauma characteristics and those who develop PTSD. *Epilepsy Behav, 28*(1), 121–126. doi:10.1016/j.yebeh.2013.03.033

Nezadal, T., Hovorka, J., Herman, E., Nemcova, I., Bajacek, M., & Stichova, E. (2011). Psychogenic non-epileptic seizures: Our video-EEG experience. *Neurol Res, 33*(7), 694–700. doi:10.1179/1743132811Y.0000000003

Noe, K. H., Grade, M., Stonnington, C. M., Driver-Dunckley, E., & Locke, D. E. (2012). Confirming psychogenic nonepileptic seizures with video-EEG: sex matters. *Epilepsy Behav, 23*(3), 220–223.

Oto, M., Espie, C. A., & Duncan, R. (2010). An exploratory randomized controlled trial of immediate versus delayed withdrawal of antiepileptic drugs in patients with psychogenic nonepileptic attacks (PNEAs). *Epilepsia, 51*(10), 1994–1999. doi:10.1111/j.1528-1167.2010.02696.x

Ponnusamy, A., Marques, J. L., & Reuber, M. (2011). Heart rate variability measures as biomarkers in patients with psychogenic nonepileptic seizures: potential and limitations. *Epilepsy Behav, 22*(4), 685–691.

Quinn, M. C., Schofield, M. J., & Middleton, W. (2010). Permission to speak: Therapists' understandings of psychogenic nonepileptic seizures and their treatment. *J Trauma Dissociation, 11*(1), 108–123. doi:10.1080/15299730903491322

Razvi, S., Mulhern, S., & Duncan, R. (2012). Newly diagnosed psychogenic nonepileptic seizures: Health care demand prior to and following diagnosis at a first seizure clinic. *Epilepsy Behav, 23*(1), 7–9. doi:10.1016/j.yebeh.2011.10.009

Reuber, M., Fernández, G., Bauer, J., Helmstaedter, C., & Elger, C. E. (2002). Diagnostic delay in psychogenic nonepileptic seizures. *Neurology, 58*(3), 493–495.

Rosemergy, I., Frith, R., Herath, S., & Walker, E. (2013). Use of postictal respiratory pattern to discriminate between convulsive psychogenic nonepileptic seizures and generalized tonic-clonic seizures. *Epilepsy Behav, 27*(1), 81–84. doi:10.1016/j.yebeh.2012.12.024

Sahaya, K., Dholakia, S. A., Lardizabal, D., & Sahota, P. K. (2012). Opinion survey of health care providers towards psychogenic non epileptic seizures. *Clin Neurol Neurosurg, 114*(10), 1304–1307. doi:10.1016/j.clineuro.2012.03.047

Salinsky, M., Evrard, C., Storzbach, D., & Pugh, M. J. (2012). Psychiatric comorbidity in veterans with psychogenic seizures. *Epilepsy Behav, 25*(3), 345–349. doi:10.1016/j.yebeh.2012.07.013

Salinsky, M., Spencer, D., Boudreau, E., & Ferguson, F. (2011). Psychogenic nonepileptic seizures in US veterans. *Neurology, 77*(10), 945–950.

Satterthwaite, T. D., Wolf, D. H., Loughead, J., Ruparel, K., Elliott, M. A., Hakonarson, H., et al. (2012). Impact of in-scanner head motion on multiple measures of functional connectivity: Relevance for studies of neurodevelopment in youth. *Neuroimage, 60*(1), 623–632. doi:10.1016/j.neuroimage.2011.12.063

Satterthwaite, T. D., Wolf, D. H., Ruparel, K., Erus, G., Elliott, M. A., Eickhoff, S. B., et al. (2013). Heterogeneous impact of motion on fundamental patterns of developmental changes in functional connectivity during youth. *Neuroimage, 83C*, 45–57. doi:10.1016/j. neuroimage.2013.06.045

Schmaling, K. B., DiClementi, J. D., & Hammerly, J. (1994). The positive teddy bear sign: transitional objects in the medical setting. *J Nerv Ment Dis, 182*(12), 725.

Seneviratne, U., Rajendran, D., Brusco, M., & Phan, T. G. (2012). How good are we at diagnosing seizures based on semiology? *Epilepsia, 53*(4), e63–66. doi:10.1111/j.1528-1167.2011.03382.x

Seneviratne, U., Reutens, D., & D'Souza, W. (2010). Stereotypy of psychogenic non-epileptic seizures: Insights from video-EEG monitoring. *Epilepsia, 51*(7), 1159–1168. doi:10.1111/j.1528-1167.2010.02560.x

Sethi, N. K. (2013). Psychogenic nonepileptic seizure: The name matters. *Journal of the American Medical Association Neurology, 70*(4), 528–529.

Smolowitz, J. L., Hopkins, S. C., Perrine, T., Eck, K. E., Hirsch, L. J., & O'Neil Mundinger, M. (2007). Diagnostic utility of an epilepsy monitoring unit. *Am J Med Qual, 22*(2), 117–122.

Strutt, A. M., Hill, S. W., Scott, B. M., Uber-Zak, L., & Fogel, T. G. (2011a). A comprehensive neuropsychological profile of women with psychogenic nonepileptic seizures. *Epilepsy Behav, 20*(1), 24–28. doi:10.1016/j.yebeh.2010.10.004

Strutt, A. M., Hill, S. W., Scott, B. M., Uber-Zak, L., & Fogel, T. G. (2011b). Motivation, psychopathology, locus of control, and quality of life in women with epileptic and non-epileptic seizures. *Epilepsy Behav, 22*(2), 279–284. doi:10.1016/j.yebeh.2011.06.020

Swift, J. K., & Greenberg, R. P. (2012). Premature discontinuation in adult psychotherapy: a meta-analysis. *J Consult Clin Psychol, 80*(4), 547–559.

Testa, S. M., Krauss, G. L., Lesser, R. P., & Brandt, J. (2012). Stressful life event appraisal and coping in patients with psychogenic seizures and those with epilepsy. *Seizure, 21*(4), 282–287. doi:10.1016/j.seizure.2012.02.002

Testa, S. M., Lesser, R. P., Krauss, G. L., & Brandt, J. (2011). Personality Assessment Inventory among patients with psychogenic seizures and those with epilepsy. *Epilepsia, 52*(8), e84–88. doi:10.1111/j.1528-1167.2011.03141.x

Thompson, A. W., Hantke, N., Phatak, V., & Chaytor, N. (2010). The Personality Assessment Inventory as a tool for diagnosing psychogenic nonepileptic seizures. *Epilepsia, 51*(1), 161–164. doi:10.1111/j.1528-1167.2009.02151.x

Tojek, T. M., Lumley, M., Barkley, G., Mahr, G., & Thomas, A. (2000). Stress and other psychosocial characteristics of patients with psychogenic nonepileptic seizures. *Psychosomatics, 41*(3), 221–226. doi:10.1176/appi.psy.41.3.221

Tombaugh, T. N. (1996). *Test of Memory Malingering*. North Tonawanda: Multi-Health Systems, Inc.

van der Kruijs, S. J., Bodde, N. M., Vaessen, M. J., Lazeron, R. H., Vonck, K., Boon, P., et al. (2012). Functional connectivity of dissociation in patients with psychogenic non-epileptic seizures. *J Neurol Neurosurg Psychiatry, 83*(3), 239–247. doi:10.1136/jnnp-2011-300776

Varela, H. L., Taylor, D. S., & Benbadis, S. R. (2007). Short-term outpatient EEG-video monitoring with induction in a veterans administration population. *J Clin Neurophysiol, 24*(5), 390–391.

Voon, V., Gallea, C., Hattori, N., Bruno, M., Ekanayake, V., & Hallett, M. (2010). The involuntary nature of conversion disorder. *Neurology, 74*(3), 223–228. doi:10.1212/WNL.0b013e3181ca00e9

Voon, V., & Lang, A. E. (2005). Antidepressant treatment outcomes of psychogenic movement disorder. *J Clin Psychiatry, 66*(12), 1529–1534.

Wagner, M. T., Wymer, J. H., Topping, K. B., & Pritchard, P. B. (2005). Use of the Personality Assessment Inventory as an efficacious and cost-effective diagnostic tool for nonepileptic seizures. *Epilepsy Behav, 7*(2), 301–304. doi:S1525-5050(05)00209-X [pii]10.1016/j.yebeh.2005.05.017

Whitehead, K., Kandler, R., & Reuber, M. (2013). Patients' and neurologists' perception of epilepsy and psychogenic nonepileptic seizures. *Epilepsia, 54*(4), 708–717. doi:10.1111/epi.12087

Whitehead, K., & Reuber, M. (2012). Illness perceptions of neurologists and psychiatrists in relation to epilepsy and nonepileptic attack disorder. *Seizure, 21*(2), 104–109. doi:10.1016/j.seizure.2011.09.012

Wilkus, R. J., & Dodrill, C. B. (1989). Factors affecting the outcome of MMPI and neuropsychological assessments of psychogenic and epileptic seizure patients. *Epilepsia, 30*, 339–347.

Williamson, D. J., Drane, D. L., & Stroup, E. S. (2007). Symptom validity tests in the epilepsy clinic. In K. B. Boone (Ed.), *Assessment of feigned cognitive impairment: A neuropsychological perspective* (pp. 346–365). New York: Guilford.

Williamson, D. J., Holsman, M., Chaytor, N., Miller, J. W., & Drane, D. L. (2012). Abuse, not financial incentive, predicts non-credible cognitive performance in patients with psychogenic non-epileptic seizures. *Clin Neuropsychol, 26*(4), 588–598. doi:10.1080/13854046.2012.670266

2

LONG-TERM OUTCOMES FROM TRAUMATIC BRAIN INJURY

Linas A. Bieliauskas, Lauren L. Drag, and Robert Spencer

INTRODUCTION

Traumatic brain injury (TBI) is a significant public health concern. Approximately 1.7 million TBIs occur in the United States annually, resulting in 52,000 deaths, 275,000 hospitalizations, and 1,365,000 emergency room visits (Faul, Xu, Wald, & Coronado, 2010). These injuries are generally mild—the World Health Organization reported that 70–90% of all head injuries are mild in severity (Cassidy et al., 2004)— but unfortunately common. There is an estimated population-based base rate of TBI of 600 per 100,000 individuals and this rate increases in athletes (Cassidy et al., 2004). Historically, the majority of research has focused on understanding the acute or sub-acute effects of TBI on cognitive, functional, and health outcomes in the days, weeks, and sometimes months following the injury. However, a better understanding of the long-term prognosis of TBI survivors is essential, particularly as more individuals are surviving their injuries due to advances in emergency care and treatment. As of 2005, there are an estimated 3.17 million people living with a long-term disability secondary to TBI (Zaloshnja, Miller, Langlois, & Selassie, 2008). In addition, as the population ages there will be an increasing number of older adults with a history of head injury, making it critical to identify the long-term consequences of TBI.

Outcomes from head injury are highly variable but clinical axiom has suggested that symptoms typically improve before eventual stabilization (and full recovery in the case of mild injuries). However, there is some suggestion that the trajectory of outcomes may be more variable, ranging from continued improvement resulting in full recovery to progressive decline resulting in a significant disability (see Corrigan & Hammond, 2013 for review). For example, Himanen and colleagues (2006) examined 30-year follow-ups of 61 patients with TBI of variable severity who experienced postconcussive symptoms following the injury and found that approximately half of the patients showed cognitive decline over the 30-year period, whereas others showed improvement or stayed the same. However, there was no control group in this study, a significant shortcoming. In another large sample of individuals with severe TBI assessed at 18 years postinjury, twice as many patients showed a negative trajectory than a positive trajectory on the Glasgow Outcomes Scale (30% compared to 14% of the sample; Millar, Nicoll, Thornhill, Murray, & Teasdale, 2003). A more in-depth review of the trajectory of cognitive outcomes following TBI is provided below but these studies illustrate the need to reconcile inconsistencies in the literature in order to draw conclusions about prognosis and expectations following TBI.

Our initial goal in conceptualizing this chapter was to identify how TBI interacts with the normal aging process to influence a variety of cognitive, psychological, functional, and neurologic outcomes. Namely, we were interested in how patients fared years to decades postinjury and how the injury interacted with normal aging given that both TBI and normal aging increase risk for negative outcomes. The literature has been relatively sparse regarding true long-term outcomes in TBI, understandably, as this type of information is best gleaned from large prospective studies. A focus on the months, or more rarely years, following the injury is more typical. For example, one study examining "longitudinal changes" in TBI compared neuroimaging scans at 2 months postinjury and 13 months postinjury (Bendlin et al., 2008). Another study examining "long-term outcomes" examined patients 3 months postinjury (Ponsford, Cameron, Fitzgerald, Grant, & Mikocka-Walus, 2011). We found that studies examining outcomes over 5 or more years are fairly rare. Therefore, in some cases, we describe research examining outcomes over a several-year period as information on more chronic sequelae is unavailable. We also focused solely on TBI in adults given that pediatric head injury is qualitatively different than adult head injury and can fill an entire chapter on its own. In addition, this chapter does not intend to provide an in-depth review of TBI occurring in older adulthood. We first discuss general considerations in TBI research before turning to the status of current research examining outcomes including dementia, chronic traumatic encephalopathy (CTE), and neurologic disorders. A brief review is also provided of psychiatric, health, and psychosocial outcomes.

GENERAL RESEARCH CONSIDERATIONS

There has been large amount of research in TBI in recent years: a PubMed search for "traumatic brain injury" yielded 30,211 studies published in the past 10 years. However, there are also significant inconsistencies in the literature, due at least in part to the difficulties inherent in TBI research. For example, TBI may cause subtle changes not picked up by conventional clinical methods that are exacerbated by either the normal aging process or subsequent environmental stressors, resulting in negative outcomes years to decades postinjury. There is also a host of other factors that can affect the aging process, with TBI being just one. Some of these factors may have a positive influence on aging (e.g., cognitive reserve), whereas others, such as TBI, may speed up or qualitatively alter the process (e.g., hypertension, psychiatric disorders; see Drag & Bieliauskas, 2010 for review). From a clinical standpoint, it is important to identify factors other than head injury that may be impacting a patient's functioning at a later age. From a research standpoint, it is important to identify, measure, and control for these confounds in order to truly isolate the effects of TBI on outcomes. In many cases, a carefully selected control group, although essential to isolate the effects of TBI and draw meaningful conclusions, is not always used.

As a group, patients with TBI are heterogeneous, which can explain some of the inconsistency in the literature. There are multiple factors that vary across individuals and moderate outcomes, including substance use, smoking, cardiovascular health, cognitive stimulation, and genetics. In addition, there is substantial variability in injury mechanism, severity, and number. For example, although many individuals with a more severe head injury report full return to function, others with only a mild TBI (mTBI) report the persistence of symptoms over time (although persisting symptoms with mTBI are unlikely to be neurologically based; see Binder, 1997, among others). It is generally accepted that resolution of symptoms is most common following mTBI (described in more detail later) with chronic deficits more typical of moderate to severe TBI. While outcomes clearly vary across severity levels, it is also quite likely that the underlying etiology of these outcomes also varies, ranging from psychological comorbidities to diffuse axonal shearing and cerebral edema. Unfortunately, many studies treat "TBI" as a unidimensional clinical phenomenon, including TBIs of varying severities in analyses. This delimits elucidation of the role of injury severity as a moderating variable in outcome research.

Much inconsistency in the literature is also likely due to differences in study methodology (e.g., cross-sectional vs. longitudinal) as well as operationalization of variables of interest. In particular, the definition of mild versus moderate versus severe TBI can vary widely in the literature, making it difficult to compare samples across studies and draw any firm conclusions. For example, the American Congress of Rehabilitation Medicine has set forth a definition of mTBI that includes any period of loss of consciousness less than 30 minutes, any loss of memory for events immediately before or after the injury less than 24 hours, any alternation in mental state at the time of injury, or focal neurologic deficits that may or may not be transient (Kay et al., 1993). Many researchers as well as the Veterans Affairs (VA) system have adopted this definition. Nevertheless, others have used different definitions for a "mild" injury, including "brain concussion without structural damage" (Yeh, Chen, Hu, Chiu, & Liao, 2013) or a Glasgow Coma Scale (GCS) score higher than 13 (e.g., Ponsford et al., 2011). One study defined mTBI as a GCS of 14 or 15, resulting in a sample inclusive of patients with skull fracture and intracranial hemorrhage—seemingly more severe than a mild injury from a clinical standpoint (i.e., complicated mild; Zumstein et al., 2011). It has been demonstrated that simply varying the inclusion and exclusion criteria in studies of TBI results in significant differences in demographics and injury-related characteristics in the resulting samples (Luoto et al., 2013).

Even when keeping the inclusion criteria constant, it is difficult to identify what constitutes an mTBI. There is a lack of tangible and reliable biomarkers that are often more salient for moderate and severe injuries (Larrabee, Binder, Rohling, & Ploetz, 2013). This leads to significant variability in mTBI samples; following the American Congress of Rehabilitation Medicine criteria, one individual may have hit his head after tripping over a rock, feeling dazed for a few minutes but with no other symptoms. Another individual may have fallen down three flights of stairs and been knocked unconscious for 45 minutes with 22 hours of posttraumatic amnesia. Both would be diagnosed as sustaining an mTBI. Advanced neuroimaging may provide a method for investigating subtle neurologic alterations following mTBI (Bouix et al., 2013), but such methods are not yet fully developed or available for routine clinical examination. Thus, even "mTBI" can encompass a range of injury severities across studies.

In addition, there are often sample biases in research, primarily with mTBI. Whereas the severity of the moderate or severe head injury usually dictates seeking immediate medical attention and participating in subsequent rehabilitation, there is less of an impetus for those with mTBI; although many seek treatment, many others do not. Some may minimize or deny symptoms (i.e., the athlete reluctant to leave a game after a head injury, or the soldier unwilling to abandon his or her comrades). Many US military service members believe that disclosure of a head injury or mental health problem upon return from deployment will delay reuniting with their families in the short-term, or limit opportunities for career advancement later on. Within the VA, screening procedures for TBI are also broad and overly inclusive. In our experience with veterans undergoing follow-up assessments for TBI, many *screen* "positive" for TBI but, upon closer examination, never actually suffered any sort of head trauma. Thus, some samples may not be a representative cross-sample of all individuals who have sustained an mTBI but essentially composed of those seeking care for it, some of whom may not have actually sustained a TBI. Finally, research on long-term outcomes often uses a cross-sectional design and asks participants to retrospect on details of a head injury. This process is prone to faulty recollection and bias. This can be partially addressed by requiring corroboration from medical records or family members or use of a prospective study design.

Despite the difficulties inherent in TBI research, there have been multiple noteworthy attempts to gather large-scale data on TBI. In 1987, the National Institute of Disability and Rehabilitation Research Model Systems program created a TBI National Database in collaboration with the VA. This Model Systems program monitors outcomes in patients who sustained a moderate or severe TBI and received both acute hospital care and comprehensive rehabilitation following the injury. As of 2010, the Model Systems program includes more than 8,778 patients (Dijkers, Harrison-Felix, & Marwitz, 2010) and will likely be a valuable source of information for years to come. In addition, the Department of Defense announced in June of 2013 that it had established the Center for Neuroscience and Regenerative Medicine Brain Tissue Repository for Traumatic Brain Injury in Bethesda, marking the first brain tissue repository devoted to researching the neuropathologic effects of TBI in service members (US Department of Defense, 2013). These research databases, in addition to future studies, should in time yield clinically relevant findings based on sound methodology. We now turn to a variety of cognitive, medical, and mental health long-term outcomes that have been attributed to TBI and review the recent evidence for each.

COGNITIVE OUTCOMES

Neuropsychological Outcomes

Mild TBI

The impact of TBI on cognitive functioning can understandably depend on numerous factors, among which are personal demographics, severity of injury, age at injury, and comorbid factors. Although it is not surprising that cognitive deficits often follow a moderate or severe injury, research on cognitive functioning following mTBI is much more inconsistent (and controversial) but generally demonstrates that mTBI alone does not lead to persistent cognitive deficits. The effect of mTBI on neuropsychological outcomes has been comprehensively documented elsewhere (for review see Iverson, 2005; McCrea et al., 2009) but we briefly cover a few of the main issues here. Cognitive symptoms are most severe immediately following injury with gradual recovery in the days to weeks following injury. Effect sizes shrink as time since injury increases (Iverson, 2005). Most mTBI patients show full recovery after the subacute period and symptoms that persist are generally thought to be attributable to other factors (postconcussion syndrome [PCS]; Carroll et al., 2004). In addition, a late onset of symptoms following injury is infrequent and likely not attributable to injury-related mechanisms. For example, the updated Diagnostic and Statistical Manual of Mental Disorders, 5th Edition (DSM-V) definition for neurocognitive disorder due to TBI requires an immediate onset of symptoms (American Psychiatric Association, 2013).

In 2013, the VA Health Services Research and Development Service published the results of an exhaustive review of the literature on complications of mTBI in service members and veterans (O'Neil et al., 2013). This literature review encompassed 31 studies and found no consistent support for an association between mTBI and cognitive functioning. Other large reviews and meta-analyses have also yielded minimal, if any, significant effect sizes following the subacute injury period. For example, a meta-analysis that included 25 studies and 2,929 patients found no significant effect sizes in any cognitive domain after 3 months postinjury (Rohling et al., 2011). Similarly, in a comprehensive review of the mTBI literature, Iverson (2005) reported that effect sizes of mTBI on neuropsychological functioning are minimal and much lower than those found in a variety of other conditions including depression, chronic benzodiazepine use, and attention-deficit/hyperactivity disorder.

Vanderploeg, Curtiss, and Belanger (2005) examined a large military sample of individuals with mTBI (on average 8 years postinjury) compared to individuals with a non-TBI injury (injured control subjects) and a noninjured control group. They found no group differences on a comprehensive neuropsychological battery of 15 measures and the average effect size of mTBI on neuropsychological functioning was −0.3. Another study by Ettenhofer and Abeles (2009) examined individuals with mTBI approximately 3 years postinjury compared to a group of orthopedic control subjects. They found no differences in cognitive functioning across a comprehensive neuropsychological battery that included verbal fluency, verbal memory, executive functioning, and attention and inhibition. These authors concluded that a single mTBI is "of little clinical significance" to long-term cognitive outcomes.

Some investigators have examined whether blast-related injuries differ from more traditional methods of sustaining a TBI (i.e., a direct blow to the head). In contrast to the general conclusion that mTBI produces an initial cognitive decline, followed by symptom resolution within 3 months, some researchers have contended that blast injuries can cause lasting problems, and even delayed effects. Macera, Aralis, Rauh, and MacGregor (2013) found that individuals who sustained blast injuries reported diminished functioning over time, and that this decline was more apparent among those individuals who also had posttraumatic stress disorder (PTSD), which suggests psychiatric contributions may be of significance. Similarly, Nelson et al. (2012) examined individuals with blasted-related mTBI, Axis I diagnoses, both mTBI and Axis I diagnoses, and control participants approximately 3.5 years after blast exposure (for the mTBI group). Despite exposure to multiple blasts (mean, 10.5; range, 1–150 exposures), the mTBI group did not differ significantly from a control group on a comprehensive neuropsychological battery that covered working memory, visuospatial functioning, executive functioning, and visual and verbal memory. In contrast, individuals with Axis I diagnoses performed worse than control subjects, with no difference between the Axis I group and the Axis I/mTBI group. Both the Macera et al. and the Nelson et al. studies suggest a psychological contribution to the cognitive sequelae of blast injury and given the stressful nature of blast exposures themselves, it is very difficult to disentangle the potential cognitive effects of the injury itself from comorbid psychiatric symptoms. The bulk of the research on this topic has concluded that although blast-induced TBI is real, it confers no more resulting symptomatology or cognitive decline than blunt-force TBI (Eskridge et al., 2013; Luethcke, Bryan, Morrow, & Isler, 2011). Lange et al. (2012) found that those with blast-induced TBI reported greater levels of depression, but that after accounting for depression and distress, blast-induced TBI had no more effect than blunt trauma.

Overall, most evidence suggests that mTBI is not associated with any long-standing cognitive effects. There is inconsistent evidence for cognitive sequelae following blast injuries but research suggests they are generally attributable to psychiatric symptoms.

Moderate and Severe TBI

Not surprisingly, however, individuals with moderate to severe TBI can show persistent neuropsychological deficits years and decades following the injury (e.g., Colantonio et al., 2004). In addition to the acute effects of the injury, there is some evidence that cognitive functioning may continue to decline over time in some of these individuals. Corkin et al. were one of the first to look at long-term cognitive functioning in TBI using a sample of World War II veterans with penetrating head injuries (Corkin, Rosen, Sullivan, & Clegg, 1989). Compared to non–TBI-injured veterans, the TBI veterans showed a greater decline in intellectual functioning and visuospatial functioning between the period of 10 years and 30 years postinjury and this decline was more pronounced for older veterans. Vocabulary knowledge, in contrast, remained stable.

Senathi-Raja, Ponsford, and Schönberger (2010) examined 112 patients with a range of injury severity (but almost half of the patients had a GCS score of 8 or less). Over one decade postinjury, the TBI group performed worse than the control group on measures of processing speed, working memory, attention, and executive functioning. Again, poorer cognitive functioning was associated with older age at the time of injury. A longitudinal study of inpatient rehabilitation patients with TBI ranging from complicated mild to severe demonstrated significant variability in trajectories of cognitive functioning during this period (Millis et al., 2001). They found that although 22% of patients improved, 15% declined and 63% percent were unchanged.

These findings suggest that continued recovery (or even stabilization) is not always a given, and that some patients may show decline over time. It appears that increasing age places individuals at an increased risk for cognitive decline. Given that continued recovery or stabilization cannot be an assumed trajectory, neuropsychological assessment is an important part of the long-term care in TBI to monitor functioning over time. Assessment is also important because subjective reports are not always aligned with objective performance. Draper and Ponsford (2009) examined subjective reports of functioning in 54 patients with TBI and a close informant approximately 10 years postinjury. They found that although ratings of cognitive functioning between the patient and the informant were in strong agreement, there was no relationship between the subjective reporting and objective performance on a comprehensive neuropsychological battery. However, there was a strong relationship between subjective reports of cognitive functioning and emotional state. Our group previously demonstrated that self-reported cognitive problems were associated with psychiatric symptoms but not neuropsychological performance in mTBI (Spencer, Drag, Walker, & Bieliauskas, 2010).

Dementia

As noted, moderate to severe TBI, but not mTBI, has been associated with reduced cognitive performance over time. There has also been interest in whether a history of head injury places older adults at increased risk for a formal dementia disorder. Retrospective studies tend to show an increased dementia risk following TBI with findings from prospective studies less clear (Starkstein & Jorge, 2005). Meta-analyses have failed to yield consistent findings. For example, although an early meta-analysis of seven studies found a minor relative risk of 1.82 (less than double) for Alzheimer Disease (AD) in individuals with TBI associated with loss of consciousness, this finding was only significant in males (Mortimer et al., 1991). Furthermore, a later meta-analysis of seven new studies published since this original finding failed to find any increased risk (Fleminger, 2003).

Inconsistent findings may reflect differences in severity of injury. For example, although Fleminger used loss of consciousness as an inclusion criterion, it can still be assumed that there was a great deal of variability in injury severity even within this sample. Severity of TBI appears to affect risk for subsequent dementia with only more severe injuries increasing this risk (Shively, Scher, Perl, & Diaz-Arrastia, 2012). In general, there is little or no evidence for such an association with mTBI. Plassman and colleagues (2000), who examined World War II veterans, found that moderate to severe head injuries were associated with an increased risk of AD (hazard ratios, 2.32 and 4.51, respectively), but failed to find a conclusive association between mild injuries and AD. This was similar to findings in a recent case-control study by Sayed, Culver, Dams-O'Connor, Hammond, and Diaz-Arrastia (2013). They examined 877 individuals with dementia and TBI from the National Alzheimer's Coordinating Center Uniform Data Set and found that TBI associated with either a brief or extended loss of consciousness was not associated with an increased risk of dementia. A large survey of 2,552 retired National Football League (NFL) players found that although 61% of players self-reported a history of concussion, less than one-fifth of these players believe that the concussion led to any permanent effect on thinking or memory skills (Guskiewicz et al., 2005). Neither history of concussion (vs. no concussion) nor a history of multiple concussions (vs. a single concussion) was significantly associated with an increased prevalence of AD. Consistent with these individual studies, a review of recent studies by the Institute of Medicine failed to find convincing evidence that an isolated mTBI is associated with subsequent dementia (Institute of Medicine Committee on Gulf War and Health, 2009).

Overall, although research has not been entirely consistent, it has generally suggested that moderate and severe TBI (but not mTBI) are associated with some increased risk of dementia (for further review, see Shively et al. [2012]). Variability in research findings may be due to methodologic differences (e.g., prospective vs. retrospective, differences in TBI severity) as well as the inherent difficulty in case-control studies that require an individual with documented memory difficulties to recall information about a remote head injury. In addition, the relationship between TBI and dementia likely reflects complex, synergistic interactions. Individuals with a history of TBI do not invariably develop dementia and not all patients with dementia have a history of TBI. There are likely a multitude of factors that contribute to an individual's likelihood of experiencing neurodegenerative and cognitive decline meeting criteria for dementia. Apolipoprotein E (ApoE) status is an obvious candidate for a moderating factor (discussed in more detail later) but other variables of interest include comorbid medical disorders, cognitive reserve (e.g., intellectual functioning, level of education), genetic predispositions, psychosocial factors (e.g., social engagement, occupation), and substance use.

Why might a TBI place an individual at risk for subsequent dementia? TBI might cause neuropathologic changes that trigger a cascade of neurodegenerative processes similar to that found in AD and other neurodegenerative processes (e.g., Irwin & Trojanowski, 2013). It has been demonstrated that beta-amyloid plaques can develop in the brain following TBI. Beta-amyloid plaques are a hallmark feature of AD but they can also be found in other chronic neurologic diseases and may reflect response to neurodegenerative process (Blennow, Hardy, & Zetterberg, 2012). Diffuse beta-amyloid plaques or deposits (similar to those found in AD) have been identified acutely postinjury as well as several years to decades after injury (Ikonomovic et al., 2004; Johnson, Stewart, & Smith, 2010, 2012). Johnson et al. (2010) hypothesized that these plaques may result from cytoskeletal disruptions (secondary to axonal swelling) that result in an accumulation of proteins, such as amyloid precursor protein, a precursor of beta-amyloid. Neurofibrillary tangles (NFTs), another common finding in AD, have also been demonstrated in a subset of survivors of TBI with increased prevalence rates particularly in younger patients (Ikonomovic et al., 2004; Johnson et al., 2012). These possibilities and potential links to dementia require further investigation.

Multiple mTBIs

As discussed, the research on the long-term effects of a single TBI suggests that single head injuries of mild severity are not associated with long-term cognitive effects (dementia or otherwise). However, this may not necessarily be the case when describing repetitive head injuries. Research has shown variable neuropsychological outcomes in individuals with multiple concussions. In the study of NFL players described previously by Guskiewicz et al. (2005), a history of three or more concussions was associated with a fivefold prevalence of physician-diagnosed Mild Cognitive Impairment and a threefold prevalence of subjective memory problems. Wall et al. (2006) demonstrated that jockeys with multiple concussions that were sustained on average 7 years prior to testing showed decrements in response inhibition and divided attention when compared to jockeys with a single concussion. In contrast to these studies, Silverberg and colleagues (2013) examined 105 participants who experienced an mTBI with a history of zero, one, or more than one prior head injuries and found that a history of previous mTBI was not associated with worse postconcussive outcomes following a subsequent mTBI. Belanger, Spiegel, and Vanderploeg (2010) performed a meta-analysis of studies comparing single to multiple self-reported mTBI in the months after injury and found that although the effect of repetitive head injuries on overall neuropsychological functioning was minimal (effect size, 0.06), multiple injuries were associated with poorer performance on individual measures of delayed memory and executive functioning, yielding small to medium effect sizes. It should be noted that the studies included in this meta-analysis did not all report time since injury and in those that did, the time period was 9 months or less. Thus, these data do not necessarily speak to longer-term prognoses. Overall, these studies provide variable evidence that there may be mild (if any) long-term neuropsychological effects following multiple mild head injuries. Despite this general finding, there has been significant interest in a small subset of individuals who have experienced a striking change in functioning following repetitive head injuries.

CTE

The idea of a syndrome of cognitive, motor, and behavioral abnormalities caused by multiple blows to the head has been around for more than 75 years. Martland (1928) first described this constellation of symptoms in boxers, naming it "punch drunk syndrome." This was later termed "dementia pugilistica" and more recently CTE. Martland noted that this syndrome was most common in "poor boxers who take considerable head punishment" or "second rate fighters used for training purposes." According to Martland, the degree of facial disfigurement could serve as an index of susceptibility to punch drunk syndrome (with the idea that the greater the disfigurement, the greater the injuries sustained). One of the earliest descriptions of CTE was provided by Mawdsley and Ferguson (1963) who presented case studies of 10 boxers with symptoms including dysarthria, ataxia, tremors, dementia, impotence, and personality changes. Findings of brain atrophy and cavum septum pellucidum were also noted. These symptoms were progressive with a relatively young age of onset near the end of the boxers' careers. Nine of the ten cases were in a lighter weight division, causing the authors to surmise, in line with the hypothesis of Martland, that less skillful boxers were more likely to become punch drunk.

Recent Research

As awareness of the detrimental effects of repetitive head injuries grew, researchers expanded the findings of CTE from boxers to include hockey players, soccer players, football players, and even jockeys. Omalu and colleagues have presented a series of three cases of presumed CTE in retired NFL players (Omalu et al., 2005; Omalu, Hamilton, Kamboh, DeKosky, & Bailes, 2010; Omalu et al., 2006). The first case was a 50-year-old player with a history of memory and judgment problems, parkinsonism, and dysthymic disorder who died of coronary atherosclerotic disease. The second case involved a 45-year-old player with symptoms that included paranoia, social withdrawal, risky business decisions, and mood and personality changes that resulted in several suicide attempts as well as a suicide completion. The third player died at age 44, also by suicide. His symptoms included chronic pain and headaches, forgetfulness, social withdrawal, a tendency to anger easily and overreact to minor situations, insomnia, paranoia, and depression with suicidal ideation as well as attempts. Although all three players had a history of cognitive impairment, depression, and behavioral changes, neuropathology was variable upon autopsy. NFTs and neuropil threads (NTs) in the absence of any gross brain atrophy were found in all three players. Two of the cases had NFTs and NTs in the hippocampus and/or entorhinal cortex, which is a pattern found in AD. Diffuse amyloid plaques were present in only one of the cases.

The research in CTE has traditionally focused on athletes and we are aware of only one study examining CTE in a military population. This dearth of research is not surprising given the recency of the Operation Enduring Freedom/Operation Iraqi Freedom conflicts and relatively young age of most service members. Goldstein and colleagues (2012) published the first report of postmortem brains of military veterans with TBI. They examined the brains of four veterans, ranging in age from 22 to 45 years, with a history of multiple blast injuries and/or concussions and subsequent mood, cognitive, and personality changes. Of note, each of these cases developed symptoms within a few years of their most recent concussion, which is somewhat of a shorter latency than that typically found in other athlete samples (Omalu et al., 2011). Although this inconsistency could suggest differences between athletic versus combat-related head injuries, it may also reflect the variability inherent in very small sample sizes. The brains of these four veterans were compared to the brains of four athletes with a history of repetitive concussions (who either died from their injuries, suicide, or drug overdose) and also brains from four control subjects without a history of head injury. The brains of both the veterans and athletes contained perivascular foci of NFT, axon degeneration and damage, and glial tangles, considered to be representative of CTE. This led the authors to conclude that CTE induced by different mechanisms can still have common pathogenic mechanisms leading to similar neuropathology.

Goldstein et al. (2012) also developed a mouse model of CTE following blast trauma, demonstrating the presence of CTE neuropathology in mice brains within 2 weeks following a single blast exposure. This neuropathology included neuroinflammation, tauopathy, axonal damage, microvascular change, and neurodegeneration. These neuropathologic changes were accompanied by impairment in spatial learning and memory. Given the recent establishment of the Center for Neuroscience and Regenerative Medicine Brain Tissue Repository for Traumatic Brain Injury by the Department of Defense, it is to be expected that the understanding of neuropathologic changes associated with head injury in service members will grow exponentially in the future.

Traditionally, CTE has been examined at autopsy; however, a recent study used positron emission tomography (PET) to identify markers of CTE-like pathology in living brains. Small and colleagues (2013) used a PET method for measuring tau in vivo in humans. PET scans were conducted in five retired NFL players (ages 45–73) referred for cognitive and/or mood symptoms with diagnoses of MCI, MCI and depression, and normal aging. Compared to nonathlete control subjects (and covarying for body mass index, education, age, and a family history of dementia), the players had higher levels of depression and lower scores on the Mini Mental State Examination. The players demonstrated higher abnormal biomarker signals in the caudate, putamen, thalamus, subthalamus, midbrain, and cerebellar white matter. There was generally no difference in cortical regions. The authors noted that this pattern is consistent with CTE tauopathy patterns seen in autopsy studies and different from that found in AD. Also, the player with the most concussions (20) had the greater biomarker abnormality. This study shows some promise for in vivo imaging of CTE, although caution is warranted given the small sample size, lack of autopsy confirmation of CTE, and the caveat that the biomarkers used are not specific to tauopathy.

CTE as a Diagnostic Entity

There are currently no consensus criteria for the diagnosis of CTE. However, Omalu et al. (2011) and McKee et al. (2009) each attempted to provide a description of a typical CTE clinical and neuropathologic profile by reviewing 17 and 51 autopsy-confirmed cases, respectively, with generally consistent results. The general clinical profile of CTE is described as a symptom onset between 25 and 76 years with a long latency period between the initial athletic activity and manifestation of symptoms and a long progression of symptoms over years to decades. Symptoms include progressive deterioration in a variety of domains that include social and cognitive functioning (e.g., money management, memory impairments, confusion, speech abnormalities), mood and behavioral functioning (e.g., paranoid ideation, suicidal thoughts, insomnia, aggressive outbursts, dysfunction in interpersonal relationships), motor abnormalities (e.g., parkinsonism, gait abnormalities, slurred speech), and headaches. It should be noted that CTE is not simply persistent PCS. Unlike PCS, the clinical symptoms of CTE do not appear until years after the initial injury. Thus, CTE cannot merely reflect the acute or subacute side effects of the original injury mechanism or the accumulation of symptoms over time. Frontotemporal dementia and AD are common differential diagnoses. The behavioral symptoms and young age of onset of frontotemporal dementia are most similar to CTE. However, Baugh and colleagues (2012) noted that CTE can present earlier than frontotemporal dementia, have a slower progression, and is not associated with a positive family history.

Omalu et al. and McKee et al. also noted that neuropathology associated with CTE includes reduction in brain weight, enlargement of lateral and third ventricles, presence of NFTs and NTs, thinning of corpus callosum, cavum septum pellucidum with fenestrations, and scarring and neuronal loss of the cerebellar tonsils. Beta-amyloid plaques, the hallmark pathology of AD, are only variably seen in CTE and not a central component of the disorder. McKee and colleagues (2013) have noted that CTE pathology typically starts focally in perivascular regions at the depths of the sulci in the cerebral cortex and later spreads to involve more widespread regions. Omalu et al. reported that neuropathology was more variable in their sample with four histologic phenotype groupings based on the distribution of NFTs and NTs in the cortex, brainstem, subcortical nuclei/basal ganglia, and cerebellum and the presence of amyloid plaques in the cortex. Compared to the more uniform distribution of cortical NFTs in AD, NFTs in CTE are more unevenly distributed throughout the frontal, temporal, and insular cortex. More research is needed to distinguish the pathophysiologic changes seen in CTE from those found in normal aging and AD. Further reading on CTE can be found in recent comprehensive reviews (Baugh et al., 2012; Costanza, Weber, & Gandy, 2011; Gavett, Stern, & McKee, 2011; Gavett, Cantu, et al., 2011; Heilbronner et al., 2009; Stern et al., 2011).

The Need for Further Research

Repetitive head injury has also become a topic of increasing interest in the popular press. Several retired professional football players have filed lawsuits against the NFL, claiming long-term neurologic damage as the result of repeated concussions. There has also been a spotlight on returning Operation Enduring Freedom/Operation Iraqi Freedom combat veterans who have suffered multiple blast exposures and report a variety of persistent cognitive and mental health symptoms. Although investigation of long-term effects of repeated concussions is growing, definitive understanding of such effects has not yet been achieved. Boston University has started a Center for the Study of Traumatic Encephalopathy which, as of June 2013, has examined the brains of 19 deceased formal NFL players, 18 of whom were deemed positive for CTE (BU Center for the Study of Traumatic Encephalopathy: Case Studies, n.d.). Although this figure may seem alarming at first glance, it is important to keep in mind that there is a very strong selection bias for who chooses to donate their brains to a brain bank for postmortem analysis. More specifically, this is not likely a representative sample of retired football players but rather players with notable cognitive impairment and/or personality changes that are a cause of concern.

The current research on CTE is provocative, but inconclusive, and the sensationalism surrounding CTE has far outpaced the science. At present, clinical or pathologic diagnostic criteria for CTE are lacking (Gavett, Stern, et al., 2011). The biologic mechanisms of CTE are not yet confirmed and an understanding of the necessary precipitating factors (e.g., subconcussive impacts vs. more severe injuries, a single injury vs. repetitive injuries) is lacking. For example, CTE has traditionally been thought to follow repetitive injuries but the mouse model by Goldstein (2012) demonstrated CTE pathology following a single (but significant) blast exposure. Identification of biomarkers of CTE has thus far been unfruitful but remains an important topic for research (Turner et al., 2012).

Research has also been marked by several methodologic issues. Sound CTE research requires postmortem analysis (or sophisticated neuroimaging), carefully selected control groups, representative samples of the population being studied, large sample sizes, and longitudinal methods. Understandably but unfortunately, most of the current studies have relied on case studies or very small sample sizes. This is a methodology helpful in highlighting issues in need of further research but not amenable to drawing any firm conclusions. There is also a clear selection bias in this type of research. These studies are not examining a representative sample of all individuals with a history of repetitive concussions or all individuals with cognitive, behavioral, and psychological changes. Rather, they are examining only those individuals with both a history of concussions and current symptomatology who are seeking medical care. Thus, the frequency of CTE pathology in individuals without symptoms or even without a history of head injury is also unclear. For example, the presence of CTE pathology in retired football players with a history of multiple concussions but without clinical symptoms is unknown and would be extremely important to identify. Thus, without a clear understanding of whether this pathology is specific to the behavioral profile of CTE or even head injuries in general, firm conclusions cannot be drawn.

Research on CTE has also been difficult due to multiple inherent confounds; unfortunately, it is often difficult to truly isolate the effects of head injury on outcomes from other influences. For example, NFL players are a seemingly ideal population for exploring the chronic effects of multiple concussions. Nevertheless, it is fairly clear that a history of concussions is not the only thing differentiating professional football players from the rest of the population. This is problematic when comparing an NFL "CTE" sample to a nonathlete "control" sample. Factors unique to professional athletes need to be accounted for, which can include non-TBI injuries, substance use, steroid use, body mass index, level of physical fitness and cardiovascular strain, and chronic pain. Thus, a well-matched control group is critical to study design.

Also of importance is that head injuries appear to be necessary but not sufficient to cause CTE, as not all ex-boxers, ex-football players, or even ex-jockeys go on to develop this symptom constellation (or any symptom constellation for that matter; Porter & Fricker, 1996; Savica, Parisi, Wold, Josephs, & Ahlskog, 2012). It has been suggested that a certain number of neurons must be damaged to result in CTE. This damage can be due to a combination of etiologies other than head injury (e.g., aging, health conditions—particularly inflammatory processes, such as hypertension) and affected by many factors (e.g., cognitive reserve, genetics, age at exposure, duration of exposure period). Thus, there are several factors that are likely involved in determining whether the brain damage sustained by head injuries crosses the critical "threshold" (Heilbronner et al., 2009).

Other criticisms that have been raised concerning CTE as an entity and etiology for cognitive decline include a lack of cross-sectional or prospective studies, minimal consideration of age-related changes, and the lack of a definitive animal model (Dashnaw, Petraglia, & Bailes, 2012; McCrory, Meeuwisse, Kutcher, Jordan, & Gardner, 2013). Common sense dictates that if CTE were a consistent cause of cognitive decline in individuals subjected to repetitive head injuries, we would be literally surrounded by demented former football players as the NFL has been in existence since 1920. This is clearly not the case as we see former quarterbacks and other players constantly on television as lucid spokespersons for commercial products, news and sports commentators, and businesspersons. It has been estimated that college football players sustain approximately 500–1,400 head impacts per season (Crisco et al., 2010; Faul et al., 2010; Guskiewicz et al., 2007; Schnebel, Gwin, Anderson, & Gatlin, 2007). Despite these repetitive injuries, certainly not all college players go on to develop CTE. Nevertheless, there is some suggestion that a subset of such players may be experiencing some untoward effects of multiple mTBIs, even though most are cognitively normal (Hart et al., 2013). Further controlled research is necessary before the etiology, entity, or outcome of CTE can be accepted as definitive. Ideally, individuals would be identified immediately following their injuries and followed over time to assess the trajectory of recovery. Control groups could comprise both a head-injured group without symptoms as well as a non–head-injured group, both as closely matched to the clinical sample as possible. An ideal study would also need to take into account the variety of factors that affect both performance and prognosis, including premorbid functioning, substance use, and psychiatric symptoms as well as effort and motivation.

NEUROLOGIC OUTCOMES

Epilepsy

The link between TBI and epilepsy has been well-established with posttraumatic epilepsy being one of the most common forms of acquired epilepsy (Lowenstein, 2009).

Although risk of TBI-related epilepsy is highest within the 1 year following injury, around one-quarter of seizures can first appear several years later (Asikainen, Kaste, & Sarna, 1999; Raymont et al., 2010; Yeh et al., 2013). As the severity of head injury increases, so does the likelihood of developing posttraumatic epilepsy (Yeh et al., 2013). For example, Herman (2002) found that the relative risk of posttraumatic epilepsy jumps from 1.5 in mild injuries to 4 for moderate injuries to 29 for severe injuries. In general, mTBI is associated with barely increased risk of developing epilepsy compared to the general population, whereas severe head trauma leads to epilepsy in about 15% of adults (Stanford Epilepsy Center, 2013). The rates of epilepsy associated with severe TBI were second only to brain tumor and subarachnoid hemorrhage. A recent retrospective study of 5- to 8-year follow-up of 19,336 patients with TBI found an epilepsy hazard risk of 10.6 for skull fractures, 5.05 for severe head injury (operationalized as TBI with structural brain injury), and 3.02 for mild head injuries (operationalized as TBI without structural brain injury; Yeh et al., 2013). The risk of posttraumatic epilepsy is particularly high for penetrating TBI compared to closed head injuries. A study examining posttraumatic epilepsy found an incidence around 50% in soldiers with missile wounds (Lowenstein, 2009). The Vietnam Head Injury Study, a longitudinal research program in a large sample of Vietnam veterans with penetrating head injuries, has demonstrated a high rate of posttraumatic epilepsy up to 35 years after injury (Raymont et al., 2010; Salazar et al., 1985). Around half of the sample had posttraumatic epilepsy, which was associated with brain volume loss and greater decline on intelligence testing over time. Although most participants had a seizure onset within 1 year, approximately one-quarter had an onset of 5 years or more with 13% of one sample having an onset more than 14 years after injury. mTBI may also result in an increased risk of seizure, although the absolute risk is still low (i.e., <1%; Annegers, Hauser, Coan, & Rocca, 1998; Herman, 2002). Much less is known about risk secondary to TBI due to blast exposures, an area in need of further research (Bazarian, Cernak, Noble-Haeusslein, Potolicchio, & Temkin, 2009).

Amyotrophic Lateral Sclerosis

Some studies have demonstrated that soccer players have increased incidence of amyotrophic lateral sclerosis (ALS; e.g., Chio, Benzi, Dossena, Mutani, & Mora, 2005), raising concern about an association between head injury and ALS. However, research has been inconsistent and has not strongly supported this hypothesis. A case-control study of 109 patients with ALS found that a history of multiple head injuries *or* a head injury within the past 10 years was associated with a threefold higher risk of ALS. The risk elevation was nearly 11-fold for individuals with multiple head injuries within the past 10 years. However, having an overall history of a TBI was not significantly associated with increased risk (Chen, Richard, Sandler, Umbach, & Kamel, 2007). These findings are similar to those of Schmidt, Kwee, Allen, and Oddone (2010) who found that head injury was associated with a more than twofold increased risk of ALS; however, this was only for head injuries occurring within the 15 years prior to ALS diagnosis. The relationship between head injury and ALS was not significant for injuries over 15 years. Thus it may be that head injuries are actually secondary consequences of prodromal symptoms of ALS, affecting balance and gait, rather than a cause of the disorder. Chen and colleagues also completed a meta-analysis of eight studies and found that head injury was associated with a 1.7 times increased risk of ALS. However, the results varied significantly across studies with seven of the eight studies having an odds ratio with a confidence interval including 1.0 or below (Chen et al., 2007). Additional research has not supported a link between ALS and TBI. A case-control study of 4,004 patients with ALS found no support for an etiologic relationship between severe head injury and subsequent ALS risk (Peters et al., 2013). Similarly, a comprehensive literature review of neurologic outcomes and TBI found limited or insufficient evidence of a link between TBI and ALS (Bazarian et al., 2009).

Multiple Sclerosis

There has been relatively minimal focus on a potential causal role of TBI in multiple sclerosis (MS), although the research that exists has generally found little evidence supporting this relationship. The American Academy of Neurology has specifically addressed the relationship between physical trauma and psychological stress and MS and concludes the "preponderance of Class II evidence (provided by one or more well-designed clinical studies) supports no association between physical trauma and either MS onset or MS exacerbation" (Goodin et al., 1999). There have also been multiple cohort studies that find no evidence linking head trauma to MS (e.g., Goldacre, Abisgold, Yeates, & Seagroatt, 2006; Pfleger, Koch-Henriksen, Stenager, Flachs, & Johansen, 2009; Siva et al., 1993), although this has not always been consistent (e.g., Kang & Lin, 2012).

Parkinson Disease

Research has tenuously supported an association between Parkinson disease (PD) and TBI, although this relationship is moderated by injury severity. Several studies, including a meta-analysis of 22 studies and 18,344 cases, have demonstrated that a head injury resulting in loss of consciousness leads to an increased risk of PD with odds ratios varying from 1.57 to 11.0 (Bower et al., 2003; Harris, Shen, Marion, Tsui, & Teschke, 2013; Jafari, Etminan, Aminzadeh, & Samii, 2013). Findings from studies of mTBI without loss of consciousness have been more mixed with some studies finding increased risk (Harris et al., 2013) and others not (Bower et al., 2003). Risk is also increased with more than one TBI leading to loss of consciousness (odds ratio, 1.39 for one head injury; odds ratio, 2.53 for more than one head injury; Dick et al., 2007). A review of studies by Bazarian (2009) concluded that there is sufficient evidence to link moderate or severe TBI and PD.

There is some debate about whether this increased risk reflects a causal relationship versus the manifestation of prodromal movement disorder symptoms resulting in falls and subsequent TBI. In a case-control study of 93 twin pairs discordant for PD, a prior mTBI with either posttraumatic amnesia or a loss of consciousness was associated with a 3.8 times increased risk of PD (Goldman et al., 2006). On average, injuries occurred 30 years before the PD diagnosis and thus prodromal PD symptoms cannot account for the increased rates of head injury in this study. In contrast, Rugbjerg, Ritz, Korb, Martinussen, and Olsen (2008) examined hospital records and found that although hospital contact for head injury was associated with an increased risk of a PD diagnosis, this was primarily due to injuries sustained in the 3 months prior to the diagnosis. The overall risk decreased with increasing time between injury and PD diagnosis with no significant risk when these events were separated by 10 or more years.

Thus, although it is unclear to what extent a single, mTBI increases the risk for PD, some research has suggested that TBI associated with loss of consciousness or of moderate to severe severity confers an increased risk. Multiple TBIs may also increase risk, although more evidence is needed. However, TBI alone is not the sole determinant of subsequent PD pathology. For example, Lee, Bordelon, Bronstein, and Ritz (2012) examined 357 cases of PD and found a twofold increase in risk of PD for individuals with a history of head injury. A history of TBI in addition to herbicide exposure raised this to a threefold increased risk. Other factors that can affect risk of PD in addition to TBI include psychopharmacologic drug use, pesticide exposure, and family history (Dick et al., 2007).

HEALTH AND MEDICAL OUTCOMES

TBI has been associated with a variety of negative medical outcomes including metabolic and endocrine changes (e.g., pituitary dysregulation, reduced amino acid levels), incontinence, diabetes, chronic pain, dysarthria, spasticity, swallowing problems, mobility, metabolic syndrome, deep vein thrombosis, and reflux (Agha et al., 2004; Bazarian et al., 2009; Børsheim, Bui, & Wolfe, 2007; Leal-Cerro et al., 2005; Murphy & Carmine, 2012; Safaz, Alaca, Yasar, Tok, & Yilmaz, 2008). For example, a recent study examining a large, retrospective cohort of more than 1 million admissions to the emergency room or hospital for TBI versus non-TBI trauma suggested that TBI was independently associated with an increased risk of subsequent ischemic stroke (hazard ratio, 1.31) at a median of 28-month follow-up (Burke et al., 2013).

Ishibe, Wlordarczyk, and Fulco (2009) reviewed TBI research from 1960 until 2008 to examine whether TBI (of all severity levels) is associated with specific long-term health outcomes. They found that moderate and severe TBIs were associated with a variety of negative health outcomes including endocrine dysfunction, growth hormone insufficiency, parkinsonism, AD, and adverse functional outcomes. Penetrating TBI was associated with premature mortality and long-term unemployment. Nevertheless, this may not be a simple unidirectional relationship; there may be other shared etiologies (e.g., a risk-taking personality, substance use) that lead to an increased risk for both TBI and also comorbid health conditions. The review by Ishibe et al. found limited or inadequate evidence to suggest that mTBI is associated with any long-term health outcomes.

A variety of studies have also demonstrated a small but significant association between TBI and reduced long-term survival, even in mTBI (Brown et al., 2004). For example, the 10-year mortality rate in survivors of TBI was significantly increased compared to expectation; however, the mortality rate was still low at only 2.6% in a sample of 790 individuals (Flaada et al., 2007). The reason for this increased mortality is unclear. Although it is not likely related to acute injury mechanisms, it may be associated with the multitude of associated health effects as noted. For example, survivors of moderate to severe TBI are 49 times more likely to die of aspiration pneumonia, 37 times more likely to die from seizures, 12 times more likely to die from septicemia, 49 times more likely to die of aspiration pneumonia, and 2.5 times more likely to die of digestive disorders (Harrison-Felix et al., 2009; Harrison-Felix, Whiteneck, DeVivo, Hammond, & Jha, 2004; Harrison-Felix, Whiteneck, Devivo, Hammond, & Jha, 2006; see Masel & DeWitt, 2010 for review). Overall, a history of moderate to severe TBI reduced life expectancy by 7 years. Nevertheless, it needs to be kept in mind that TBI and other life-shortening conditions are frequently comorbid and correlated and that a cause-effect relationship between TBI and reduced life expectancy has not been established.

These negative health outcomes can have a significant impact on healthcare use. In a previous study, we examined healthcare use over an 11-year period in 1,565 veterans with a history of TBI and an age- and gender-matched control group (Drag, Renninger, King, & Hoblyn, 2013). As a group, individuals with TBI used almost four times as many outpatient services and were almost nine times more likely to be hospitalized (this relationship was most striking for medical hospitalizations) compared to the control group. This increased use could not be attributed solely to increased rates of comorbid psychiatric conditions or to the effects of the injury itself.

FUNCTIONAL AND PSYCHOSOCIAL OUTCOMES

TBI can have a significant and lasting impact on functional abilities. It has been estimated that 43% of patients hospitalized for TBI go on to develop a disability by 1 year postdischarge (Selassie et al., 2008). The annual direct and indirect (e.g., loss of productivity) costs total around $60 billion in the United States alone (Finkelstein & Corso, 2006).

One study followed 86 patients who initially presented to the emergency room with an mTBI (defined as a GCS score higher than 13; Zumstein et al., 2011). At 10-year follow-up, 37% of patients reported a reduced quality of life and as a group, quality of life was reported to decrease since the 1-year follow-up period. The percentage of patients complaining of memory and concentration impairments rose from 11% at 1 year to 52% after 10 years. Not surprisingly, increased quality of life complaints were associated with depressed mood.

Colantonio and colleagues (2004) examined 306 patients with moderate to severe TBI an average of 14 years after injury and found that approximately one-quarter of the patients were dependent in instrumental activities of daily living, such as shopping, managing money, and getting places. Dependence in instrumental activities of daily living was associated with performance on the Trail Making Test. Other studies have similarly shown that cognitive functioning, including working memory, processing speed, and executive control, is a predictor of long-term outcomes, such as community integration, satisfaction with life, and disability levels (Williams, Rapport, Hanks, Millis, & Greene, 2013; Wood & Rutterford, 2006).

Not surprisingly, injury severity has been associated with functional outcome with more severe injuries leading to reduced life satisfaction, lower perceived health, and greater dependence in daily activities (Colantonio et al., 2004; Wood & Rutterford, 2006). However, some studies have failed to find a relationship between injury severity and functional outcomes, suggesting that indirect, secondary effects of TBI (e.g., depression) are contributing to negative outcomes more so than injury factors themselves (Testa, Malec, Moessner, & Brown, 2005). In addition, this decrease in functioning cannot be fully attributed to sustaining a physical injury in general, as patients with TBI show decreased functional independence even when compared to patients with orthopedic injuries.

With regard to long-term social effects of TBI, the literature is fairly clear that those individuals with histories of moderate to severe TBI tend to have problems with multiple aspects of social functioning (Jorge et al., 2004). These individuals tend to report having fewer friends, marital disruption, and overall poor social outcomes (Seibert et al., 2002; Temkin, Corrigan, Dikmen, & Machamer, 2009). Established relationships tend to become strained, leisure activities diminish, and opportunities to meet new potential friends are less frequent (Burleigh, Farber, & Mawr, 1998; Koskinen, 1998; Morton & Wehman, 1995). Those with reduced social interactions tend to report reduced satisfaction with life decades after their head injury, with community and social integration decreasing over time (Burleigh et al., 1998). Recently, Gross, Schüepp, Attenberger, Pargger, and Amsler (2012) found that individuals with severe TBIs 2.5 years prior showed reduced independent living and greater unemployment than non-TBI injured control subjects.

MENTAL HEALTH OUTCOMES

Correlations are well-established between head injury and mental health symptoms; however, establishing causation is much more tenuous. Adequately addressing the issue of whether the sundry of chronic mental health problems that are associated with TBI are the result of the injury itself requires careful consideration of scientific research methodology. There are several methodologic issues when trying to examine the long-term mental health outcomes associated with TBI. First, consideration of preinjury functioning is essential when evaluating the unique contribution of TBI. The presence of a substance use disorder, for example, could result from efforts to self-medicate emotional pain. Just as likely, however, substance abuse could be viewed as a predisposing risk factor for TBI. An adequate control sample is also a necessary part of research. Many studies cite the elevated prevalence of mental health symptoms among those with histories of TBI, relative to estimates in the population in general, as evidence that TBI contributes to poor mental health. This approach provides preliminary data, but an evaluation of the characteristics of head-injured samples requires demographically matched control subjects. Additionally, as head injuries are not usually sustained in the absence of other injuries, a distinction should be made between which mental health problems are due to a TBI and which problems are due to having suffered any injury. Ideally, control participants have sustained nonhead injuries (e.g., orthopedic injuries) and are matched to their head-injured counterparts on the basis of overall injury severity.

Premorbid Factors

In understanding long-term mental health outcomes of TBI, particularly mTBI, an understanding of preinjury functioning is essential. It is not an uncommon mistake for clinicians and researchers to assume that outcomes following TBI were caused by the head injury. It is now becoming clear that contextual and individual variables play a large role in the course of TBI. For example, preinjury life stress, history of previous TBI, and low IQ increase the risk of post-TBI psychopathology (Gale, Deary, & Boyle, 2013; van Veldhoven et al., 2011; Zamek, Farion, Sampson, & McGahern, 2013). Among those with histories of moderate and severe TBI, alcohol and other substance abuse is common (Corrigan & Hammond, 2013) and Tsaousides, Cantor, and Gordon (2011) found that the presence of preinjury alcohol and substance abuse to elevate the risk of post-TBI suicidal ideation.

Pre-TBI psychiatric features also have a strong influence on post-TBI outcome. Diagnoses of depression and anxiety disorders following TBI are much more common if individuals had depression, anxiety, and unemployment preinjury (Jorge et al., 2004). Depression following moderate and severe TBI is usually most apparent acutely and postacutely, but among those with mTBI, depression persisted mostly in those with preinjury psychopathology (Fann et al., 2004). Preexisting psychiatric status and personality variables not only affect the odds of developing a post-TBI psychiatric condition (Fann et al., 2004), but such a history also modifies post-TBI outcome in more nuanced ways. Premorbid psychiatric problems often lead to post-TBI adjustment problems (Leininger, Strong, & Donders, 2014). Premorbid personality influences occupational outcome after TBI (Sela-Kaufman, Rassovsky, Agranov, Levi, & Vakil, 2013). Preinjury depression and poor resilience predicted postinjury anxiety and PCS (McCauley et al., 2013).

Coping style also modifies risk of post-TBI psychopathology. McCauley (2013) found that preinjury depression and poor resilience predicted postinjury anxiety and PCS. Similarly, Maestas et al. (2013) found that informant ratings of pre-TBI coping was predictive of 3-month psychiatric outcome, concluding that an avoidant coping style hindered recovery.

In sum, accumulating research suggests that long-term outcome following TBI is strongly influenced by preinjury factors, such as alcohol and substance abuse, psychiatric diagnoses and symptoms, personality characteristics, coping style, and other individual differences. These need to be considered in research studies as well as in clinical examination.

PTSD

With the growing number of TBIs in the military population, there is a rapidly growing literature examining the interactive effects of PTSD and TBI. This literature usually concerns mTBI in a military sample, which is the focus of this section. As with mTBI, the diagnostic procedures for determining PTSD vary across studies, which, in our experience, is consistent with the variability in diagnostic thresholds in clinical practice. PTSD is relatively common among individuals reporting TBI, which is not surprising because head injuries can often be sustained in traumatic circumstances (particularly for recent service members). Vasterling et al. (2012) found that among those screening positive for TBI, 18% screened positive for PTSD. This co-occurrence has raised the intriguing question of whether there is an interactive effect of the two conditions. In other words, does having both conditions lead to worse long-term outcome than having either condition? The emerging conclusion seems to be that PTSD, and not mTBI, is responsible for the bulk of the postdeployment maladjustment and psychopathology that cannot be explained by premorbid factors (Bryant et al., 2010; O'Neil et al., 2013; Polusny et al., 2011; Ragsdale, Neer, Beidel, Frueh, & Stout, 2013). This relationship is particularly apparent in studies in which those with invalid symptom reports or performances were excluded. Consideration of validity is important given that poor effort is particularly common among those reporting both PTSD and mTBI, compared to those reporting either condition (Campbell et al., 2009). This is not to imply conscious deception, however, as there are many reasons for invalid performances and/or symptom reports (Silver, 2012).

In a study comparing the cognitive performance of individuals with PTSD with and without mTBI, mTBI status did not influence cognitive performance (Soble, Spanierman, & Smith, 2013). Similarly, Vasterling et al. (2012) found that mTBI produced limited neuropsychological test performance impairments, but that any ill-effects months later were due to PTSD, and not mTBI. Shandera-Oschner (2012) also found that 2.5 years after injury, PTSD, and not mTBI, accounted for cognitive impairments. Notably, each of these studies excluded participants for poor effort. Overall, research has fairly consistently shown that TBI and PTSD are frequently comorbid in military populations. PTSD symptomatology makes significant contributions to postinjury functioning, generally with minimal unique contributions from the head injury itself.

Depression and Suicidality

Mood disorders are common among individuals with all severities of TBI (Iverson, Pogoda, Gradus, & Street, 2013; Jorge et al., 2004). For example, Vasterling et al. (2012) reported that among those service members screening for (mostly mild) TBI, 31% also reported significant depression. However, a review of recent studies has concluded that although the prevalence of psychiatric problems in individuals with mTBI is high, it is not higher than the rates found in other groups, such as deployed veterans (O'Neil et al., 2013). It has also been suggested that a preinjury history of psychiatric illness is common in individuals with persistent depression following TBI (Fann et al., 2004). The number of mTBIs incurred may also matter; a recent finding with football players indicated that a single concussion may not significantly increase the risk of depression, but multiple concussions can lead to a significant risk of depression (Kerr, Marshall, Harding, & Guskiewicz, 2012). In this study, 3% of those with no concussions had a 9-year risk of significant depression, whereas 27% of those with 10 or more concussions had significant depression.

Depression is a significant concern for individuals with histories of moderate and severe TBI and the rate of depression is higher among those with TBI than among injured control subjects (Jorge et al., 2004). Depression in the context of TBI is associated with decreased quality of life (von Steinbuechel et al., 2012) and deficits in social role and functional status (Hudak, 2012) months to years after injury. Fann et al. (2004) observed that, among those with more severe head injuries, depression tends to be apparent soon after injury. Douglas and Spellacy (2000) found that 3.5–10 years after severe TBI, 57% of individuals had significant depression. In this study, depression was related to level of social support, and interestingly 60% of their caretakers also had significant depression.

Suicidal ideation is common among those who previously sustained a TBI years earlier and has been associated with poor psychosocial functioning (Simpson & Tate, 2007; Tsaousides et al., 2011). For example, among convicted offenders, TBI is one of several risk factors for suicidal ideation and behavior (Gunter, Chibnall, Antoniak, Philibert, & Black, 2013). Suicidal risk is especially high if the head-injured individual also has significant alcohol or substance abuse (Silver, Kramer, Greenwald, & Weissman, 2001; Teasdale, 2001). A recent VA report on the state of research in the VA concluded that suicide is common among individuals with TBI, but that suicidal ideation and behaviors may not be any more common than among individuals without head injuries who are matched for demographic factors (O'Neil et al., 2013). Protective risk factors for suicidal ideation following TBI include adequate social support, sense of purpose/hope, religion, and psychiatric treatment (Tsaousides et al., 2011).

Overall, depression is common in TBI and can be accompanied by suicidality. Factors influencing the prevalence of postinjury mood symptoms include injury severity, preinjury mental health history, social support, and substance abuse.

Psychosis

Psychosis is not particularly common following TBI, affecting 14.5% of individuals with moderate and severe TBI, 3.9% of those with mTBI, and 2.7% of orthopedically injury controls (Fann et al., 2004). Risk factors include the severity of the injury, history of prior neuropathology, family history of psychosis, and possible low intelligence (Wolkin, Malaspina, Perrin, McAllister, & Corcoran, 2011). In general, prior psychiatric history is the major risk factor for post-TBI psychosis and a review of the literature generally concludes that there is insufficient evidence that the neuropathologic consequences of TBI play a significant role in the development psychiatric disorders (Rogers & Read, 2007; See Flashman, McAllister, & Ferrell, 2012 for review).

POSTCONCUSSION SYNDROME

Thus far, we have individually addressed the various domains of cognitive, psychological, and psychosocial functioning that can be impacted following TBI. However, some individuals experience a persistent constellation of symptoms across all of these domains and thus a brief foray into PCS is needed. PCS is a constellation of cognitive, physical, emotional, and behavioral symptoms that can persist following a TBI (most frequently mild in severity). Symptoms can include difficulty concentrating, memory problems, dizziness, headache, depression, anxiety, and irritability (Ryan & Warden, 2003). PCS is listed in the DSM-V and described as a "major or mild neurocognitive disorder due to traumatic brain injury." This diagnosis requires the symptoms to present immediately after the occurrence of the TBI (or after the recovery of consciousness) and to persist past the "acute post-injury period" (American Psychiatric Association, 2013). PCS is also an official International Classification of Diseases code, although this coding allows for the postconcussive disturbances to be late emerging. This disorder has been somewhat controversial with respect to etiology with many studies indicating a psychological mechanism for the genesis and/or persistence of this symptom constellation. Recent literature has provided increasing empirical support to the notion that premorbid psychopathology, PTSD, and preinjury history of substance abuse are more impactful than head injury proper in producing PCS (Ponsford et al., 2012). This finding is particularly salient in studies that exclude participants for invalid symptom reporting or test performance (Meares et al., 2011; Nelson et al., 2012).

There is a broad literature that indicates that most individuals experience positive outcomes following mTBI with full resolution of any symptoms within months (typically 3 months but as long as 1 year; Carroll et al., 2004). However, there has been some debate about whether these group findings have masked a subset of individuals who do experience cognitive sequelae from single or repetitive injuries (i.e., "the miserable minority," Rohling, Larrabee, & Millis, 2012). Despite the expectation for recovery, some individuals continue to report persistent symptoms and it has been suggested that this may be due to noninjury factors, such as emotional distress or litigation and compensation issues (Belanger, Kretzmer, Vanderploeg, & French, 2010; Carroll et al., 2004; Iverson, 2005). Female gender, older age, medical issues, psychiatric symptoms, substance use, lack of a support system, and litigation are all predictors of prolonged symptoms following mTBI (Iverson, 2005).

PCS is of significance to the military and VA systems given the number of returning service members with mTBI and there has been much focus in the past few years on PCS in active duty service members and veterans. The VA Health Services Research and Development Service report, described previously, concluded that although cognitive, physical, and mental health symptoms are frequently reported following mTBI, there is little evidence to suggest that these symptoms are more common in service members with mTBI compared to those without mTBI (O'Neil et al., 2013). Of note, only eight of the studies reported a follow-up longer than 1 year with the longest follow-up being approximately 3 years. However, it is likely that these findings would apply to longer time periods as there is no reason to believe that symptoms related to a TBI should appear or worsen over time (and this is actually contradictory to the DSM definition of PCS). Several individual studies have examined longer-term outcomes and have reached similar conclusions.

A diagnosis of PCS is predicated on reported symptomatology and use of such a symptom-based approach is fraught with difficulties. Using a concept of PCS implies that the constellations of problems and behaviors follow, and are presumably caused by, the concussion. This is problematic because such symptoms have a high base rate and are common among healthy individuals (Bryant, 2011), individuals with psychiatric disorders (Vanderploeg & Belanger, 2013), and those with injuries not involving the head (Meares et al., 2011). As a result, PCS represents a nonspecific mixture of various somatic complaints that traverse nosologic categories and one can legitimately raise the question as to whether PCS is indeed a genuine entity independent of other factors. For example, it has been suggested that PCS is more accounted for by psychological comorbidities rather than injury-related factors. A study of 345 veterans with mTBI seen in a VA polytrauma service on average 3 years postinjury found that posttraumatic stress symptoms accounted for between 5% and 43% of the variance in reported PCS symptoms (Benge, Pastorek, & Thornton, 2009). PTSD symptoms accounted for over 20% of the variance in PCS symptoms such as anxiety, depression, irritability, low frustration tolerance, difficulty falling asleep, cognitive difficulties, fatigue, and loss of appetite. A second study by Belanger (2010) used a nonmilitary sample of 134 individuals with mTBI and 91 individuals with moderate to severe TBI. Even though the mTBI sample had a longer time since injury compared to the moderate to severe group (703 days compared to 244 days), the mTBI group endorsed more postconcussive symptoms. However, this group difference was no longer significant after controlling for PTSD. This suggests that symptom complaints in mTBI may be mostly due to emotional distress. This is also consistent with previous findings that injury severity is not necessarily associated with PCS severity (Carroll et al., 2004; Drag, Spencer, Walker, Pangilinan, & Bieliauskas, 2012). Overall, the research has fairly consistently demonstrated that PCS symptoms are not specific to TBI and thus difficult to attribute to head injury mechanisms themselves. The general expectation following a mild injury is for full recovery of symptoms over time, with persisting symptoms usually assumed to be related to non–TBI-related factors. This finding can be viewed in a positive light, as relatively more treatment options exist for psychiatric symptoms compared to mTBI. A recent study by Ruff, Riechers, Wang, Piero, and Ruff (2012) concluded that PCS symptoms and cognitive abilities can improve after treatment for poor sleep and PTSD.

NEUROPATHOLOGY AND NEUROIMAGING

It is clear that TBI can have significant long-term consequences and these negative outcomes reflect more than just the persistence of acute injury sequelae. An important part of understanding and addressing these long-term outcomes is to identify the neuropathologic changes that underlie these outcomes. One of the difficulties in understanding the pathogenesis of TBI, however, is that the injuries themselves can be extremely variable (e.g., a severe penetrating head injury can have very different pathologic mechanisms than a mild closed head injury).

Neuroimaging has developed at a rapid pace and holds great promise for helping to elucidate the physiologic changes associated with TBI that may place the brain at increased risk for negative outcomes. Much of the neuroimaging research in TBI has focused on the ability to detect acute effects of injury, such as diffuse cerebral swelling, contusions, hemorrhage, and herniation (see Kou, 2010 for review). Less is known about long-term neuroimaging outcomes. Immediately following a TBI, acute changes can include increased intracranial pressure, edema, inflammation, apoptosis, excitotoxicity, and loss of synapses as well as reparative changes, such as synaptogenesis and production of nerve growth or neurotrophic factor (Kolb & Teskey, 2012). These acute processes can then give way to more chronic effects, such as changes in glucose metabolism, white matter degeneration, and changes to the blood-brain barrier. Pop and Badaut (2012) hypothesized that abnormal permeability of the blood-brain barrier underlies much of the long-term dysfunction seen in TBI. This compromised neurovascular system can be chronic and affect protein clearance and lead to accelerated brain aging and disease pathophysiology.

Cross-sectional Studies

Cross-sectional designs have examined neuroimaging findings in individuals who sustained a TBI years to decades earlier. Levine and colleagues (2008) examined structural magnetic resonance imaging in 69 TBI patients (with varying severity levels) approximately 1 to 2 years postinjury. Compared to control subjects, the TBI group showed volume loss in frontal, temporal, and temporal cingulate regions. There was a dose-response relationship in that moderate to severe TBI was associated with greater volume loss compared to mTBI. Tate, Khedraki, Neeley, Ryser, and Bigler (2011) examined 65 patients (also of varying TBI severity) who completed inpatient rehabilitation on average 34 months postinjury. They did not have a control group with which to compare brain volumes but did find that within their sample, global brain volume was associated with immediate and delayed recall on the Rey Auditory Verbal Learning Test and time to completion on Trails A.

White matter changes have also been a focus of much research. Acceleration-deceleration injuries can lead to stretching and tearing of axons resulting in diffuse axonal injury. Diffuse axonal injury is not readily identifiable using traditional neuroimaging methods, such as magnetic resonance imaging and computed tomography but diffusion tensor imaging has been successful in identifying these white matter changes in TBI patients. Diffuse axonal injury can include axonal disconnection and degenerative axonal pathology, resulting in progressive white matter atrophy. A postmortem study of 23 cases of fatal head injury found widespread axonal pathology including axonal swelling and degeneration up to 3 years postinjury (Chen, Johnson, Uryu, Trojanowski, & Smit, 2009). No beta-amyloid plaques were found in the brains of the subset of long-term survivors (range, 27 days to 3 years). This was one of the first studies to show that axonal pathology can persist for a substantial period of time following TBI. Similarly, another postmortem study by Johnson and colleagues (2013) found evidence of white matter pathology in a subset of individuals with a history of a single TBI (severity not reported). Of these 25 individuals (on average 10 years postinjury; range, 1–47), 23 showed moderate to extensive regions of persistent inflammation and/or axonal pathology. Kennedy and colleagues examined magnetic resonance imaging and computed tomography in patients with severe TBI with an average postinjury period of 7 years. Compared to control subjects, patients with TBI showed lower fractional anisotropy and higher mean diffusivity (indicative of reduced white matter integrity) in the centrum semiovale and superior frontal and inferior frontal regions (Kennedy et al., 2009). Time since injury was correlated with neuroimaging findings in the superior frontal region (i.e., a longer postinjury period was associated with increased white matter pathology), suggesting a progressive decline in white matter functioning over time. White matter pathology on diffusion tensor imaging has been associated with cognitive functioning across domains of executive functioning, attention, and memory (Kraus et al., 2007).

In a study using PET to examine microglial activation on average 6 years following moderate to severe TBI, increased activation was found in a variety of areas including the thalamus, putamen, occipital cortex, and internal capsule, suggestive of a chronic inflammatory response (Ramlackhansingh et al., 2011). Binding was associated with cognitive performance on tests of processing speed.

Although the previous studies have generally used samples with moderate to severe TBI, there is some indication that even mTBI can lead to long-lasting white matter changes. Niogi et al. (2008) reported that 43 patients with mTBI (defined as a GCS score between 13 and 15) showed reduced fractional anisotropy (FA) in the uncinate fasciulus compared to control subjects and these low FA scores were correlated to memory performance. Tremblay (Tremblay et al., 2013) examined 15 former athletes older than age 50 with a history of sports-related concussion over three decades prior. Compared to a control group of nonconcussed athletes, the TBI group showed abnormal enlargement of the lateral ventricles, and cortical thinning in frontal, temporal, and parietal regions. There was an age-by-group interaction for ventricular enlargement and cortical thickness leading the authors to conclude that TBI exacerbates these normal aging-related changes. Reduced delayed recall and recognition on a complex figure test and reduced verbal fluency were also found and these cognitive deficits correlated with neuroimaging findings. In patients with mTBI, Kraus et al. (2007) also found decreased FA in certain areas including the longitudinal fasciulus and sagittal stratum, although not in all of the areas found in more severe injuries. They concluded that although mild injuries can affect axonal integrity, only more severe injuries affect both myelin and axons.

Longitudinal Studies

Neuroimaging studies using repeated-measures designs have documented progressive changes over time, further discrediting the misconception that improvement and/or stabilization is invariable following TBI. Using a repeated-measures design, Ng et al. (2008) examined 14 patients with moderate to severe TBI scanned at 4.5 months and 2.5 years following injury. Ten of the 14 patients showed visible atrophy over time along with increased cerebrospinal fluid volume and decreased hippocampal volumes. Similarly, Sidaros et al. (2009) scanned 24 patients with severe TBI at 8 weeks and again at 12 months postinjury with findings of continued atrophy in all 24 patients (a mean change of 4.0% compared to −0.18% in control subjects). Atrophy was correlated with posttraumatic amnesia and duration of coma, which further supports a dose-response relationship between TBI severity and neuroimaging findings.

Diffusion tensor imaging has also been used to monitor white matter changes over time with findings variable but generally indicative of both improvement and decline in certain brain regions. Greenberg, Mikulis, Ng, DeSouza, and Green (2008) examined FA in a sample of 13 patients with moderate or severe TBI at 4.5 months and again at 29 months. Although there were no differences in FA in the corpus callosum, FA in the frontal and temporal lobe decreased. Sidaros (Sidaros et al., 2008) found variable white matter changes in 22 patients with severe TBI. Although FA was reduced at the 8 weeks (initial scan) in the TBI group, at 12 months FA values had returned to normal levels in some areas (internal capsule, centrum semiovale) but decreased further in others (posterior corpus callosum). Farbota et al. (2012) also found evidence of improvements in white matter integrity in a sample of 12 patients with moderate to severe TBI. They examined diffusion tensor imaging TI at three time points over a 4-year period and found an increase in FA in the bilateral superior longitudinal fasciculus and the optic radiation. This increased FA was associated with improvements on Trail Making performance. Consistent with Sidaros et al., Farbota et al. also found evidence of reduced FA in the corpus callosum. Thus, it appears that both positive and negative white matter changes can occur in the several years following injury.

In sum, mTBI may result in subtle neuropathologic changes over time, although the clinical significance of these changes is unclear. In moderate and severe injuries, there are changes in both structural volume and white matter integrity with evidence of both improvement and decline over time.

MODERATORS OF LONG-TERM OUTCOMES

As we previously noted, not every individual who experiences a TBI goes on to develop a mood disorder, dementia, or disability. There are many factors that can affect outcomes of TBI, some of which have been addressed. We briefly discuss three moderating factors that have been a focus in recent research: (1) ApoE, (2) age, and (3) cognitive reserve. ApoE is a protein important for cholesterol and lipid transport and has been thought to play a role in the central nervous system's response to injury (for review, see Blennow 2012). The ApoE gene has three alleles (2, 3, and 4) with e3 being the most common. The e4 allele is associated with a variety of negative outcomes, including the beta-amyloid deposition and plaque formations that are the hallmark of AD. It has been hypothesized that ApoE status may moderate the association between TBI and AD, suggesting a possible synergistic effect between e4 status and TBI. In one study, Mayeux et al. (1995) found that although a history of TBI alone was not associated with an increased risk of AD, an e4 allele and TBI combined resulted in a 10-fold increased risk of AD. However, a close examination of the study numbers suggests that this ratio may be inflated. In looking at the sample, there were only seven AD patients (out of 113) and one control (i.e., non-AD) participant (out of 123) that had both TBI and an e4 allele. These small numbers reduce the reliability of these odds ratios. For example, if there were just one more control participant with e4 status and a history of TBI (making a total of two in this group), the odds ratio would be reduced by half to five. By adding two more control participants to this group (making a total of three in this group) the odds ratio would no longer be significant. Thus, although a 10-fold increased risk certainly sounds alarming, the small number of cases calls into question the significance of these findings.

Several studies have looked at more general long-term outcomes using the Glasgow Outcome Scale, a measure of functional outcomes and disability, and show associations between e4 status and negative outcomes. Ponsford et al. (2011) found that in a sample of 648 patients ranging in TBI severity, e4 status was associated with poorer functioning on the Glasgow Outcome Scale on average 2 years after injury. Similarly, Millar et al. (2003) examined 6-month and 18-year outcomes in 396 individuals with a history of severe TBI and found a trend for e4 carriers to be less likely to have good outcomes than noncarriers (22% compared to 31% of the sample). No differences were found in neuropsychological functioning. A meta-analysis of 14 studies encompassing 2,527 patients found that at 6 months after injury, e4 status was associated with a poor outcome (relative risk, 1.36; Zhou et al., 2008). A longitudinal study by Alexander et al. (2007) followed 123 patients with severe TBI over 24 months and found that although e4 was not associated with lower outcomes at any single time point, individuals with an e4 allele had a slower recovery rate over the 2-year time period. Thus, e4 status in individuals with TBI, although not convincingly related to AD, may confer an increased risk of negative outcomes in general.

It has also generally been accepted that age at injury affects outcomes with increasing age associated with poorer outcomes (e.g., Corkin et al., 1989; Himanen et al., 2006; Senathi-Raja et al., 2010). One study found that every 10 years of age was associated with an odds ratio of 1.47 for death and 1.48 for unfavorable outcomes at 6 months following severe TBI (Hukkelhoven et al., 2003). Marquez de la Plata et al. (2008) examined disability outcomes in the TBI Model Systems data and found that over a 5-year postinjury period, the most improvements on disability ratings were seen in the youngest group (ages 16–26) and the greatest declines were seen in the older groups (defined as 27 years and older). Although age had a significant overall effect on disability ratings over the 5-year period, this effect was small—age accounted for only 4% of variance in scores. Millis et al. (2001) also examined TBI patients (ranging from complicated mild to severe injuries) 5 years postinjury and found that increasing age was associated with a decline in cognitive functioning over this time period. This supports previous findings by Corkin et al. (1989) that also found greater decline in intellectual functioning and visuospatial functioning in older adults between 10 and 30 years postinjury. However, the findings of negative outcomes in older patients are not entirely consistent. For example, Ponsford, Draper, and Schönberger (2008) examined a sample of patients ranging in injury severity and found that approximately 10 years after injury, age was not associated with disability outcome.

Finally, cognitive reserve can affect outcomes following TBI. Kessler et al. (2007) found that larger premorbid brain volumes and higher levels of education may decrease vulnerability to the cognitive effects of TBI. However, this study of 25 patients with a range of injury severities failed to find an association between premorbid intelligence on cognitive outcomes. In contrast, Raymont et al. (2008) found that in Vietnam veterans with penetrating head injury, preinjury intelligence was the most consistent predictor of outcomes over a 30-year period. It has been suggested that TBI and normal aging may interact in that brain damage from TBI may lower cognitive reserve (or the ability to withstand the normal aging process), thus increasing vulnerability to other pathologic processes (Lye & Shores, 2000; Moretti et al., 2012). Thus, although an intact brain may be sufficiently resistant to age-related change, an injured brain may be significantly impacted by the aging process, particularly in the presence of other moderating factors (e.g., inflammatory disease).

CONCLUSIONS

We have reviewed the recent literature on the effects of TBI on a range of long-term cognitive, psychological, and medical outcomes and addressed some of the inconsistencies in the literature. A primary conclusion that can be drawn from the review is that head injury severity significantly moderates outcomes with minimal evidence of negative long-term outcomes following an isolated mTBI. Persistence of symptoms in these cases is often attributable to psychiatric or other noninjury factors. There is no convincing evidence at this time that blast injuries (compared to blunt-force injuries) result in worse outcomes if psychiatric symptoms are taken into account. There has been some suggestion that multiple mTBIs can have mild, if any effects, although more research is needed. With regard to CTE, there may be enough recent evidence to warrant large, prospective studies; however, there is a pressing need for more methodologically sound research in this area before any conclusions can be drawn. CTE has been identified in only a subset of individuals who sustain a TBI and it is unclear to what extent the neuropathology and cognitive and behavioral symptoms associated CTE are specific to CTE as a diagnostic entity.

Moderate to severe injuries have consistently been demonstrated to increase the risk for adverse outcomes, which can include AD, posttraumatic epilepsy, possibly PD, reduced life expectancy, and negative health outcomes. Not surprisingly, these injuries can have significant cognitive effects and cognitive functioning can change over time, improving in some individuals but declining or remaining stable in others. Changes in brain volume and white matter integrity over time (possibly even in mTBI) have also been demonstrated and have been correlated with cognitive functioning.

Psychological comorbidities are common in TBI (but perhaps not more so than in other populations) and can account for a variety of negative outcomes. For example, it has been consistently demonstrated that in individuals with PTSD and TBI, PTSD symptoms alone can account for PCS and other symptoms. A premorbid history of psychological symptoms also places individuals at greater risk for adverse outcomes.

It is also important to note that although TBI can have negative long-term effects in some individuals, there is a wide range of outcomes across individuals who sustain head injuries. In addition to injury variables, there are a host of other premorbid (e.g., cognitive reserve, genetic factors, psychological symptoms) and postinjury (e.g., substance use, environmental stress, psychological symptoms) factors that can contribute to long-term functioning (likely more so than the injury itself in many cases) as well as moderate the effects of the TBI. Not all individuals who sustain a TBI go on to develop negative outcomes and not all individuals who experience negative outcomes have sustained a head injury. Individuals with TBI are more different than alike and these individual factors need to be taken into account in both research and clinical settings.

REFERENCES

Agha, A., Rogers, B., Sherlock, M., O'Kelly, P., Tormey, W., Phillips, J., & Thompson, C. J. (2004). Anterior pituitary dysfunction in survivors of traumatic brain injury. *The Journal of Clinical Endocrinology and Metabolism, 89*(10), 4929–4936. doi:10.1210/jc.2004-0511

Alexander, S., Kerr, M. E., Kim, Y., Kamboh, M. I., Beers, S. R., & Conley, Y. P. (2007). Apolipoprotein E4 allele presence and functional outcome after severe traumatic brain injury. *Journal of Neurotrauma, 24*(5), 790–797. doi:10.1089/neu.2006.0133

American Psychiatric Association. (2013). *Diagnostic and Statistical Manual of Mental Disorders.* (W. DC, Ed.) (5th edition). Washington, DC: American Psychiatric Association.

Annegers, J., Hauser, W., Coan, S., & Rocca, W. (1998). A population-based study of seizures after traumatic brain injuries. *New England Journal of Medicine, 338*, 20–24.

Asikainen, I., Kaste, M., & Sarna, S. (1999). Early and late posttraumatic seizures in traumatic brain injury rehabilitation patients: Brain injury factors causing late seizures and influence of seizures on long-term outcome. *Epilepsia, 40*(5), 584–589. Retrieved from http://www.ncbi.nlm.nih.gov/pubmed/10386527

Baugh, C. M., Stamm, J. M., Riley, D. O., Gavett, B. E., Shenton, M. E., Lin, A.,... Stern, R. A. (2012). Chronic traumatic encephalopathy: Neurodegeneration following repetitive concussive and subconcussive brain trauma. *Brain Imaging and Behavior, 6*(2), 244–254. doi:10.1007/s11682-012-9164-5

Bazarian, J. J., Cernak, I., Noble-Haeusslein, L., Potolicchio, S., & Temkin, N. (2009). Long-term neurologic outcomes after traumatic brain injury. *The Journal of Head Trauma Rehabilitation, 24*(6), 439–451. doi:10.1097/HTR.0b013e3181c15600

Belanger, H. G., Kretzmer, T., Vanderploeg, R. D., & French, L. M. (2010a). Symptom complaints following combat-related traumatic brain injury: Relationship to traumatic brain injury severity and posttraumatic stress disorder. *Journal of the International Neuropsychological Society, 16*(1), 194–199. doi:10.1017/S1355617709990841

Belanger, H. G., Spiegel, E., & Vanderploeg, R. D. (2010b). Neuropsychological performance following a history of multiple self-reported concussions: A meta-analysis. *Journal of the International Neuropsychological Society, 16*(2), 262–267. doi:10.1017/S1355617709991287

Bendlin, B. B., Ries, M. L., Lazar, M., Alexander, A. L., Dempsey, R. J., Rowley, H. A, . . . Johnson, S. C. (2008). Longitudinal changes in patients with traumatic brain injury assessed with diffusion-tensor and volumetric imaging. *NeuroImage, 42*(2), 503–514. doi:10.1016/j.neuroimage.2008.04.254

Benge, J. F., Pastorek, N. J., & Thornton, G. M. (2009). Postconcussive symptoms in OEF-OIF veterans: Factor structure and impact of posttraumatic stress. *Rehabilitation Psychology, 54*(3), 270–278. doi:10.1037/a0016736

Binder, L. M. (1997). A review of mild head trauma. Part II: Clinical implications. *Journal of Clinical and Experimental Neuropsychology, 19*(3), 432–457. doi:10.1080/01688639708403871

Blennow, K., Hardy, J., & Zetterberg, H. (2012). The neuropathology and neurobiology of traumatic brain injury. *Neuron, 76*(5), 886–899. doi:10.1016/j.neuron.2012.11.021

Børsheim, E., Bui, Q. U. T., & Wolfe, R. R. (2007). Plasma amino acid concentrations during late rehabilitation in patients with traumatic brain injury. *Archives of Physical Medicine and Rehabilitation, 88*(2), 234–238. doi:10.1016/j.apmr.2006.11.003

Bouix, S., Pasternak, O., Rathi, Y., Pelavin, P. E., Zafonte, R., & Shenton, M. E. (2013). Increased gray matter diffusion anisotropy in patients with persistent post-concussive symptoms following mild traumatic brain injury. *PloS one, 8*(6), e66205. doi:10.1371/journal.pone.0066205

Bower, J. H., Maraganore, D. M., Peterson, B. J., McDonnell, S. K., Ahlskog, J. E., & Rocca, W. A. (2003). Head trauma preceding PD: A case-control study. *Neurology, 60*(10), 1610–1615. doi:10.1212/01.WNL.0000068008.78394.2C

Brown, A. W., Leibson, C. L., Malec, J. F., Perkins, P. K., Diehl, N. N., & Larson, D. R. (2004). Long-term survival after traumatic brain injury: A population-based analysis. *NeuroRehabilitation, 19*(1), 37–43. Retrieved from http://www.ncbi.nlm.nih.gov/pubmed/14988586

Bryant, R. (2011). Post-traumatic stress disorder vs traumatic brain injury. *Dialogues in Clincial Neuroscience, 13,* 251–262.

Bryant, R., O'Donnell, M. L., Creamer, M., McFarlane, A. C., Clark, C. R., & Silove, D. (2010). The psychiatric sequelae of traumatic injury. *The American Journal of Psychiatry, 167*(3), 312–320. doi:10.1176/appi.ajp.2009.09050617

BU Center for the Study of Traumatic Encephalopathy: Case Studies. (n.d.). Retrieved from http://www.bu.edu/cste/case-studies/

Burke, J. F., Stulc, J. L., Skolarus, L. E., Sears, E. D., Zahuranec, D. B., & Morgenstern, L. B. (2013). Traumatic brain injury may be an independent risk factor for stroke. *Neurology, 81*(1), 33–39. doi:10.1212/WNL.0b013e318297eecf

Burleigh, S. A., Farber, R. S., & Mawr, B. (1998). Community integration and life satisfaction after traumatic brain injury: Long-term findings. *American Journal of Occupational Therapy, 52,* 45–52.

Campbell, T., Nelson, L., Lumpkin, R., Yoash-Gantz, R., Pickett, T., & McCormick, C. (2009). Neuropsychological measures of processing speed and executive functioning in combat veterans with PTSD, TBI, and comorbid TBI/PTSD. *Psychiatric Annals, 39,* 796.

Carroll, L. J., Cassidy, J. D., Peloso, P. M., Holst, H. Von, Holm, L., Paniak, C., & Pe, M. (2004). Prognosis for mild traumatic brain injury: Results of the WHO Collaborating Centre Task Force on Mild Traumatic Brain Injury. *Journal of Rehabilitation Medicine, 43,* 84–105. doi:10.1080/16501960410023859

Cassidy, J. D., Carroll, L., Peloso, P., Borg, J., von Holst, H., Holm, L., . . . Coronado, V. (2004). Incidence, risk factors and prevention of mild traumatic brain injury: Results of the WHO Collaborating Centre Task Force on Mild Traumatic Brain Injury. *Journal of Rehabilitation Medicine, 36,* 28–60. doi:10.1080/16501960410023732

Chen, H., Richard, M., Sandler, D. P., Umbach, D. M., & Kamel, F. (2007). Head injury and amyotrophic lateral sclerosis. *American Journal of Epidemiology, 166*(7), 810–816. doi:10.1093/aje/kwm153

Chen, X., Johnson, V. E., Uryu, K., Trojanowski, J. Q., & Smit, D. H. (2009). A lack of amyloid β plaques despite persistent accumulation of amyloid β in axons of long-term survivors of traumatic brain injury. *Brain Pathology, 19*(2), 214–223. doi:10.1111/j.1750-3639.2008.00176.x.A

Chio, A., Benzi, G., Dossena, M., Mutani, R., & Mora, G. (2005). Severely increased risk of amyotrophic lateral sclerosis among Italian professional football players. *Brain, 128,* 472–476.

Colantonio, A., Ratcliff, G., Chase, S., Kelsey, S., Escobar, M., & Vernich, L. (2004). Long-term outcomes after moderate to severe traumatic brain injury. *Disability and Rehabilitation, 26*(5), 253–261. doi:10.1080/09638280310001639722

Corkin, S., Rosen, T. J., Sullivan, E. V., & Clegg, R. A. (1989). Penetrating head injury in young adulthood decline in later years exacerbates cognitive. *The Journal of Neuroscience, 9*(11), 3876–3883.

Corrigan, J. D., & Hammond, F. M. (2013). Traumatic brain injury as a chronic health condition. *Archives of Physical Medicine and Rehabilitation, 94*(6), 1199–1201. doi:10.1016/j.apmr.2013.01.023

Costanza, A., Weber, K., & Gandy, S. (2011). Contact sport-related chronic traumatic encephalopathy in the elderly: Clinical expression and structural substrates. *Neuropathology and Applied Neurobiology, 37*(6), 570–584. doi:10.1111/j.1365-2990.2011.01186.x.Contact

Crisco, J. J., Fiore, R., Beckwith, J. G., Chu, J. J., Brolinson, P. G., Duma, S., . . . Greenwald, R. M. (2010). Frequency and location of head impact exposures in individual collegiate football players. *Journal of Athletic Training, 45*(6), 549–559. doi:10.4085/1062-6050-45.6.549

Dashnaw, M., Petraglia, A., & Bailes, J. (2012). An overview of the basic science of concussion and subconcussion: Where are we and where are we going. *Neurosurgical Focus, 33,* 1–9.

Dick, F. D., De Palma, G., Ahmadi, A., Scott, N. W., Prescott, G. J., Bennett, J., . . . Felice, A. (2007). Environmental risk factors for Parkinson's disease and parkinsonism: The Geoparkinson study. *Occupational and Environmental Medicine, 64*(10), 666–672. doi:10.1136/oem.2006.027003

Dijkers, M. P., Harrison-Felix, C., & Marwitz, J. H. (2010). The traumatic brain injury model systems: History and contributions to clinical service and research. *The Journal of Head Trauma Rehabilitation, 25*(2), 81–91. doi:10.1097/HTR.0b013e3181cd3528

Douglas, J. M., & Spellacy, F. J. (2000). Correlates of depression in adults with severe traumatic brain injury and their carers. *Brain Injury*, *14*(1), 71–88. Retrieved from http://www.ncbi.nlm.nih.gov/pubmed/10670663

Draper, K., & Ponsford J. (2009). Long-term outcome following traumatic brain injury: A comparison of subjective reports by those injured and their relatives. *Neuropsychological Rehabilitation*, *19*(5), 645–646.

Drag, L., Renninger, C., King, R., & Hoblyn, J. (2013). Predictors of inpatient and outpatient healthcare utilization in veterans with traumatic brain injury. *The Journal of Head Trauma Rehabilitation*, *28*(1), 39–47. doi:10.1097/HTR.0b013e318263bb61

Drag, L. L., & Bieliauskas, L. A. (2010). Contemporary review 2009: Cognitive aging. *Journal of Geriatric Psychiatry and Neurology*, *23*(2), 75–93. doi:10.1177/0891988709358590

Drag, L. L., Spencer, R. J., Walker, S. J., Pangilinan, P. H., & Bieliauskas, L. A. (2012). The contributions of self-reported injury characteristics and psychiatric symptoms to cognitive functioning in OEF/OIF veterans with mild traumatic brain injury. *Journal of the International Neuropsychological Society*, *18*(3), 576–584. doi:10.1017/S1355617712000203

Eskridge, S., Macera, C., Galarneau, M., Holbrook, T., Woodruff, S., MacGregor, A. J., . . . Shaffer, R. (2013). Influence of combat blast-related mild traumatic brain injury acute symptoms on mental health and service discharge outcomes. *Journal of Neurotrauma*, *30*(16), 1391–1397.

Ettenhofer, M. L., & Abeles, N. (2009). The significance of mild traumatic brain injury to cognition and self-reported symptoms in long-term recovery from injury. *Journal of Clinical and Experimental Neuropsychology*, *31*(3), 363–372. doi:10.1080/13803390802175270

Fann, J. R., Burington, B., Leonetti, A., Jaffe, K., Katon, W. J., & Thompson, R. S. (2004). Psychiatric illness following traumatic brain injury in an adult health maintenance organization population. *Archives of General Psychiatry*, *61*(1), 53–61. doi:10.1001/archpsyc.61.1.53

Farbota, K. D., Bendlin, B. B., Alexander, A. L., Rowley, H. A., Dempsey, R. J., & Johnson, S. C. (2012). Longitudinal diffusion tensor imaging and neuropsychological correlates in traumatic brain injury patients. *Frontiers in Human Neuroscience*, *6*(June), 160. doi:10.3389/fnhum.2012.00160

Faul, M., Xu, L., Wald, M., & Coronado, V. (2010). *Traumatic brain injury in the United States: Emergency department visits, hospitalizations and deaths 2002–2006*. Atlanta, GA: Center for Disease Control and Prevention.

Finkelstein E. A., Corso P. S., & Miller, T. R. (2006). *The incidence and economic burden of injuries in the United States*. New York: Oxford University Press.

Flaada, J. T., Leibson, C. L., Mandrekar, J. N., Diehl, N., Perkins, P. K., Brown, A. W., & Malec, J. F. (2007). Relative risk of mortality after traumatic brain injury: A population-based study of the role of age and injury severity. *Journal of Neurotrauma*, *24*(3), 435–445. doi:10.1089/neu.2006.0119

Flashman, L. A., McAllister, T., & Ferrell, R. (2012). Traumatic brain injury and schizophrenia. In B. A. Marcopulos & M. M. Kurtz (Eds.), *Clinical neuropsychological foundations of schizophrenia*. New York: AACN/Psychology Press.

Fleminger, S. (2003). Head injury as a risk factor for Alzheimer's disease: The evidence 10 years on; a partial replication. *Journal of Neurology, Neurosurgery & Psychiatry*, *74*(7), 857–862. doi:10.1136/jnnp.74.7.857

Gale, C. R., Deary, I. J., & Boyle, S. H. (2013). Cognitive ability in early adulthood and risk of 5 specific psychiatric disorders in middle age. *JAMA Psychiatry*, *65*(12), 1410–1418.

Gavett, B. E., Cantu, R. C., Shenton, M., Lin, A. P., Nowinski, C. J., McKee, A. C., & Stern, R. A. (2011). Clinical appraisal of chronic traumatic encephalopathy: Current perspectives and future directions. *Current Opinion in Neurology, 24*(6), 525–531. doi:10.1097/WCO.0b013e32834cd477

Gavett, B. E., Stern, R. A, & McKee, A. C. (2011). Chronic traumatic encephalopathy: A potential late effect of sport-related concussive and subconcussive head trauma. *Clinics in Sports Medicine, 30*(1), 179–188, xi. doi:10.1016/j.csm.2010.09.007

Goldacre, M., Abisgold, J., Yeates, D., & Seagroatt, V. (2006). Risk of multiple sclerosis after head injury: Record linkage study. *Journal of Neurology, Neurosurgery & Psychiatry2, 77,* 351–353.

Goldman, S. M., Tanner, C. M., Oakes, D., Bhudhikanok, G. S., Gupta, A., & Langston, J. W. (2006). Head injury and Parkinson's disease risk in twins. *Annals of Neurology, 60*(1), 65–72. doi:10.1002/ana.20882

Goldstein, L. E., Fisher, A. M., Tagge, C. A, Zhang, X.-L., Velisek, L., Sullivan, J. A., . . . McKee, A. C. (2012). Chronic traumatic encephalopathy in blast-exposed military veterans and a blast neurotrauma mouse model. *Science Translational Medicine, 4*(134), 134ra60. doi:10.1126/scitranslmed.3003716

Goodin, D. S., Ebers, G. C., Johnson, K. P., Rodriguez, M., Sibley, W. A., & Wolinsky, J. S. (1999). The relationship of MS to phsyical trauma and psychological stress. *Neurology, 52,* 1737-1745.

Greenberg, G., Mikulis, D. J., Ng, K., DeSouza, D., & Green, R. E. (2008). Use of diffusion tensor imaging to examine subacute white matter injury progression in moderate to severe traumatic brain injury. *Archives of Physical Medicine and Rehabilitation, 89*(12 Suppl), S45–S50. doi:10.1016/j.apmr.2008.08.211

Gross, T., Schüepp, M., Attenberger, C., Pargger, H., & Amsler, F. (2012). Outcome in polytraumatized patients with and without brain injury. *Acta anaesthesiologica Scandinavica, 56*(9), 1163–1174. doi:10.1111/j.1399-6576.2012.02724.x

Gunter, T. D., Chibnall, J. T., Antoniak, S. K., Philibert, R. A., & Black, D. W. (2013). Childhood trauma, traumatic brain injury, and mental health disorders associated with suicidal ideation and suicide-related behavior in a community corrections sample. *The Journal of the American Academy of Psychiatry and the Law, 41*(2), 245–255. Retrieved from http://www.ncbi.nlm.nih.gov/pubmed/23771938

Guskiewicz, K. M., Marshall, S. W., Bailes, J., McCrea, M., Cantu, R. C., Randolph, C., & Jordan, B. D. (2005). Association between recurrent concussion and late-life cognitive impairment in retired professional football players. *Neurosurgery, 57*(4), 719–726. doi:10.1227/01.NEU.0000175725.75780.DD

Guskiewicz, K. M., Mihalik, J., Shankar, V., Marshall, S. W., Crowell, D., Oliaro, S., . . . Hooker, D. (2007). Measurement of head impacts in collegiate football players; Relationship between head imact biomechanics and acute clinical outcome after concussion. *Neurosurgery, 61*(6), 1244–1253. doi:10.1227/01.NEU.0000280146.37163.79

Harris, M. A., Shen, H., Marion, S. A., Tsui, J. K. C., & Teschke, K. (2013). Head injuries and Parkinson's disease in a case-control study. *Occupational and Environmental Medicine, oemed-2013.* doi:10.1136/oemed-2013-101444

Harrison-Felix, C. L., Whiteneck, G. G., Jha, A., DeVivo, M. J., Hammond, F. M., & Hart, D. M. (2009). Mortality over four decades after traumatic brain injury rehabilitation: A retrospective cohort study. *Archives of Physical Medicine and Rehabilitation, 90*(9), 1506–1513. doi:10.1016/j.apmr.2009.03.015

Harrison-Felix, C., Whiteneck, G., DeVivo, M., Hammond, F. M., & Jha, A. (2004). Mortality following rehabilitation in the Traumatic Brain Injury Model Systems of Care. *NeuroRehabilitation, 19*(1), 45–54. Retrieved from http://www.ncbi.nlm.nih.gov/pubmed/14988587

Harrison-Felix, C., Whiteneck, G., Devivo, M. J., Hammond, F. M., & Jha, A. (2006). Causes of death following 1 year postinjury among individuals with traumatic brain injury. *The Journal of Head Trauma Rehabilitation, 21*(1), 22–33. Retrieved from http://www.ncbi.nlm.nih.gov/pubmed/16456389

Hart, J., Kraut, M. A, Womack, K. B., Strain, J., Didehbani, N., Bartz, E., . . . Cullum, C. M. (2013). Neuroimaging of cognitive dysfunction and depression in aging retired National Football League players: A cross-sectional study. *JAMA Neurology, 70*(3), 326–335. doi:10.1001/2013.jamaneurol.340

Heilbronner, R. L., Bush, S. S., Ravdin, L. D., Barth, J. T., Iverson, G. L., Ruff, R. M., . . . Broshek, D. K. (2009). Neuropsychological consequences of boxing and recommendations to improve safety: A National Academy of Neuropsychology education paper. *Archives of Clinical Neuropsychology, 24*(1), 11–19. doi:10.1093/arclin/acp005

Herman, S. (2002). Epilepsy after brain insult: Targeting epileptogenesis. *Neurology, 59*, S21–S26.

Himanen, L., Portin, R., Isoniemi, H., Helenius, H., Kurki, T., & Tenovuo, O. (2006). Longitudinal cognitive changes in traumatic brain injury: A 30-year follow-up study. *Neurology, 66*(2), 187–192. doi:10.1212/01.wnl.0000194264.60150.d3

Hudak, A. M., Hynan, L. S., Harper, C. R., & Diaz-Arrastia, R. (2012). Association of depressive symptoms with functional outcome after traumatic brain injury. *Journal of Head Trauma Rehabilitation, 27*, 87–98.

Hukkelhoven, C. W. P. M., Steyerberg, E. W., Rampen, A. J. J., Farace, E., Habbema, J. D. F., Marshall, L. F., . . . Maas, A. I. R. (2003). Patient age and outcome following severe traumatic brain injury: An analysis of 5600 patients. *Journal of Neurosurgery, 99*(4), 666–673. doi:10.3171/jns.2003.99.4.0666

Ikonomovic, M. D., Uryu, K., Abrahamson, E. E., Ciallella, J. R., Trojanowski, J. Q., Lee, V. M.-Y., . . . DeKosky, S. T. (2004). Alzheimer's pathology in human temporal cortex surgically excised after severe brain injury. *Experimental Neurology, 190*(1), 192–203. doi:10.1016/j.expneurol.2004.06.011

Institute of Medicine Committee on Gulf War and Health: Brain Injury in Veterans and Long-Term Health Outcomes (2009). *Gulf War and Health, Volume 7: Long-Term Consequences of Traumatic Brain Injury.* Washington, DC: The National Academies Press.

Irwin, D. J., & Trojanowski, J. Q. (2013). Many roads to Parkinson's disease neurodegeneration: Head trauma-a road more traveled than we know? *Movement Disorders, 28*(9), 1167–1170. doi:10.1002/mds.25551

Ishibe, N., Wlordarczyk, R. C., & Fulco, C. (2009). Overview of the Institute of Medicine's Committee search strategy and review process for Gulf War and Health: Long-term Consequences of Traumatic Brain Injury. *Journal of Head Trauma Rehabilitation, 24*(6), 424–429.

Iverson, G. L. (2005). Outcome from mild traumatic brain injury. *Current Opinion in Psychiatry, 18*(3), 301–317.

Iverson, K. M., Pogoda, T. K., Gradus, J. L., & Street, A. E. (2013). Deployment-related traumatic brain injury among Operation Enduring Freedom/Operation Iraqi Freedom veterans: Associations with mental and physical health by gender. *Journal of Women's Health (2002)*, *22*(3), 267–275. doi:10.1089/jwh.2012.3755

Jafari, S., Etminan, M., Aminzadeh, F., & Samii, A. (2013). Head injury and risk of Parkinson disease: A systematic review and meta-analysis. *Movement Disorders*, *28*(9), 1222–1229. doi:10.1002/mds.25458

Johnson, V. E., Stewart, J. E., Begbie, F. D., Trojanowski, J. Q., Smith, D. H., & Stewart, W. (2013). Inflammation and white matter degeneration persist for years after a single traumatic brain injury. *Brain*, *136*(Pt 1), 28–42. doi:10.1093/brain/aws322

Johnson, V. E., Stewart, W., & Smith, D. H. (2010). Traumatic brain injury and amyloid-β pathology : A link to Alzheimer's disease. *Nature Reviews and Neuroscience*, *11*, 361–370.

Johnson, V. E., Stewart, W., & Smith, D. H. (2012). Widespread τ and amyloid-β pathology many years after a single traumatic brain injury in humans. *Brain Pathology*, *22*(2), 142–149. doi:10.1111/j.1750-3639.2011.00513.x

Jorge, R. E., Robinson, R. G., Moser, D., Tateno, A., Crespo-Facorro, B., & Arndt, S. (2004). Major depression following traumatic brain injury. *Archives of General Psychiatry*, *61*(1), 42–50. doi:10.1001/archpsyc.61.1.42

Kang, J.-H., & Lin, H.-C. (2012). Increased risk of multiple sclerosis after traumatic brain injury: A nationwide population-based study. *Journal of Neurotrauma*, *29*(1), 90–95. doi:10.1089/neu.2011.1936

Kay, T., Harrington, D., Adams, R., Anderson, T., Berrol, S., Cicerone, K., . . . Dahlberg, C. (1993). Definition of mild traumatic brain injury. *Journal of Head Trauma Rehabilitation*, *8*(3), 86–87.

Kennedy, M. R. T., Wozniak, J. R., Muetzel, R. L., Mueller, B. A., Pantekoek, K., & Lim, K. O. (2009). White matter and neurocognitive changes in adults with chronic traumatic brain injury. *Journal of the International Neuropsychological Society*, *15*(1), 130–136. doi:10.1017/S1355617708090024.White

Kerr, Z. Y., Marshall, S. W., Harding, H. P., & Guskiewicz, K. M. (2012). Nine-year risk of depression diagnosis increases with increasing self-reported concussions in retired professional football players. *The American Journal of Sports Medicine*, *40*(10), 2206–2212. doi:10.1177/0363546512456193

Kessler, R. C., Angermeyer, M., Anthony, J. C., De Graaf, R., Demyttenaere, K., Gasquet, I., . . . Ustün, T. B. (2007). Lifetime prevalence and age-of-onset distributions of mental disorders in the World Health Organization's World Mental Health Survey Initiative. *World Psychiatry*, *6*(3), 168–176. Retrieved from http://www.pubmedcentral.nih.gov/articlerender.fcgi?artid=2174588&tool=pmcentrez&rendertype=abstract

Kolb, B., & Teskey, G. C. (2012). Age, experience, injury, and the changing brain. *Developmental Psychobiology*, *54*(3), 311–325. doi:10.1002/dev.20515

Koskinen, S. (1998). Quality of life 10 years after a very severe traumatic brain injury (TBI): The perspective of the injured and the closest relative. *Brain Injury*, *12*(8), 631–648. Retrieved from http://www.ncbi.nlm.nih.gov/pubmed/9724835

Kou, Z., Wu, Z., Tong, K. A., Holshouser, B., Benson, R. R., Hu, J., & Haacke, E. M. (2010). The role of advanced MR imaging findings as biomarkers of traumatic brain injury. *The Journal of Head Trauma Rehabilitation*, *25*(4), 267–282. doi:10.1097/HTR.0b013e3181e54793

Kraus, M. F., Susmaras, T., Caughlin, B. P., Walker, C. J., Sweeney, J. A., & Little, D. M. (2007). White matter integrity and cognition in chronic traumatic brain injury: A diffusion tensor imaging study. *Brain*, *130*(Pt 10), 2508–2519. doi:10.1093/brain/awm216

Lange, R. T., Pancholi, S., Brickell, T. A., Sakura, S., Bhagwat, A., Merritt, V., & French, L. M. (2012). Neuropsychological outcome from blast versus non-blast: Mild traumatic brain injury in U.S. military service members. *Journal of the International Neuropsychological Society, 18*(3), 595–605. doi:10.1017/S1355617712000239

Larrabee, G. J., Binder, L. M., Rohling, M. L., & Ploetz, D. M. (2013). Meta-Analytic Methods and the importance of non-TBI factors related to outcome in mild traumatic brain injury: Response to Bigler et al. (2013). *The Clinical Neuropsychologist, 27*(2), 215–237.

Leal-Cerro, A., Flores, J. M., Rincon, M., Murillo, F., Pujol, M., Garcia-Pesquera, F., . . . Casanueva, F. F. (2005). Prevalence of hypopituitarism and growth hormone deficiency in adults long-term after severe traumatic brain injury. *Clinical Endocrinology, 62*(5), 525–532. doi:10.1111/j.1365-2265.2005.02250.x

Lee, P.-C., Bordelon, Y., Bronstein, J., & Ritz, B. (2012). Traumatic brain injury, paraquat exposure, and their relationship to Parkinson disease. *Neurology, 79*(20), 2061–206. doi:10.1212/WNL.0b013e3182749f28

Leininger, S., Strong, C.-A. H., & Donders, J. (2014). Predictors of outcome after treatment of mild traumatic brain injury: A pilot study. *The Journal of Head Trauma Rehabilitation. 29*, 109–116.

Levine, B., Kovacevic, N., Nica, E. I., Cheung, G., Gao, F., Schwartz, M. L., & Black, S. E. (2008). The Toronto Traumatic Brain Injury Study: Injury severity and quantified MRI. *Neurology, 70*(10), 771–778. doi:10.1212/01.wnl.0000304108.32283.aa

Lowenstein, D. H. (2009). Epilepsy after head injury: an overview. *Epilepsia, 50*(Suppl 2), 4–9. doi:10.1111/j.1528-1167.2008.02004.x

Luethcke, C. A, Bryan, C. J., Morrow, C. E., & Isler, W. C. (2011). Comparison of concussive symptoms, cognitive performance, and psychological symptoms between acute blast-versus nonblast-induced mild traumatic brain injury. *Journal of the International Neuropsychological Society, 17*(1), 36–45. doi:10.1017/S1355617710001207

Luoto, T. M., Tenovuo, O., Kataja, A., Brander, A., Öhman, J., & Iverson, G. L. (2013). Who gets recruited in mild traumatic brain injury research? *Journal of Neurotrauma, 30*(1), 11–6. doi:10.1089/neu.2012.2611

Lye, T. C., & Shores, E. A. (2000). Traumatic brain injury as a risk factor for Alzheimer's disease: A review. *Neuropsychology Review, 10*(2), 115–129.

Macera, C. A, Aralis, H. J., Rauh, M. J., & MacGregor, A. J. (2013). Do sleep problems mediate the relationship between traumatic brain injury and development of mental health symptoms after deployment? *Sleep, 36*(1), 83–90. doi:10.5665/sleep.2306

Maestas, K. L., Sander, A. M., Clark, A. N., van Veldhoven, L. M., Struchen, M. A, Sherer, M., & Hannay, H. J. (2013). Preinjury coping, emotional functioning, and quality of life following uncomplicated and complicated mild traumatic brain injury. *The Journal of Head Trauma Rehabilitation, 28*, 12–17. doi:10.1097/HTR.0b013e31828654b4

Marquez de la Plata, C. D., Hart, T., Hammond, F. M., Frol, A. B., Hudak, A., Harper, C. R., . . . Diaz-Arrastia, R. (2008). Impact of age on long-term recovery from traumatic brain injury. *Archives of Physical Medicine and Rehabilitation, 89*(5), 896–903. doi:10.1016/j.apmr.2007.12.030

Martland, H. (1928). Punch drunk. *The Journal of the American Medical Association, 91*(15), 1103–1107.

Masel, B. E., & DeWitt, D. S. (2010). Traumatic brain injury: A disease process, not an event. *Journal of Neurotrauma, 27*(8), 1529–1540. doi:10.1089/neu.2010.1358

Mawdsley, C., & Ferguson, F. (1963). Neurological disease in boxers. *The Lancet, 2*, 799–801.

Mayeux, R., Ottman, R., Maestre, G., Ngai, C., Tang, M.-X., Ginsberg, H., . . . Shelanski, M. (1995). Synergistic effects of traumatic head injury and apolipoprotein-epsilon4 in patients with Alzheimer's disease. *Neurology, 45*(3), 555–557. doi:10.1212/WNL.45.3.555

McCauley, S. R., Wilde, E. A., Miller, E. R., Frisby, M. L., Garza, H. M., Varghese, R., . . . McCarthy, J. J. (2013). Preinjury resilience and mood as predictors of early outcome following mild traumatic brain injury. *Journal of Neurotrauma, 30*(8), 642–652. doi:10.1089/neu.2012.2393

McCrea, M., Iverson, G. L., McAllister, T. W., Hammeke, T. A., Powell, M. R., Barr, W. B., & Kelly, J. P. (2009). An integrated review of recovery after mild traumatic brain injury (MTBI): Implications for clinical management. *The Clinical Neuropsychologist, 23*(8), 1368–1390. doi:10.1080/13854040903074652

McCrory, P., Meeuwisse, W., Kutcher, J., Jordan, B., & Gardner, A. (2013). What is the evidence for chronic concussion-related changes in retired atheletes: Behavioural, pathological and clinical outcomes? *British Journal of Sports Medicine, 47*, 327–330.

McKee, A. C., Cantu, R. C., Nowinski, C. J., Hedley-whyte, T., Gavett, B. E., Budson, A. E., . . . Stern, R. A. (2009). Chronic traumatic encephalopathy in athletes: Progrsesive tauopathy following repetitive head injury. *Journal of Neuropathology and Experimental Neurology, 68*(7), 709–735. doi:10.1097/NEN.0b013e3181a9d503.Chronic

McKee, A. C., Stein, T. D., Nowinski, C. J., Stern, R. A., Daneshvar, D. H., Alvarez, V. E., . . . Cantu, R. C. (2013). The spectrum of disease in chronic traumatic encephalopathy. *Brain, 136*(Pt 1), 43–64. doi:10.1093/brain/aws307

Meares, S., Shores, E. A., Taylor, A. J., Batchelor, J., Bryant, R. A., Baguley, I. J., . . . Marosszeky, J. E. (2011). The prospective course of postconcussion syndrome: The role of mild traumatic brain injury. *Neuropsychology, 25*(4), 454–465. doi:10.1037/a0022580

Millar, K., Nicoll, J. R., Thornhill, S., Murray, G. D., & Teasdale, G. M. (2003). Long term neuropsychological outcome after head injury: Relation to APOE genotype. *Journal of Neurology, Neurosurgery, and Psychiatry, 74*(8), 1047–1052. Retrieved from http://www.pubmedcentral.nih.gov/articlerender.fcgi?artid=1738588&tool=pmcentrez&rendertype=abstract

Millis, S. R., Rosenthal, M., Novack, T., Sherer, M., Nick, T., Kreutzer, J., . . . Ricker, J. (2001). Long-term neuropsychological outcome after traumatic brain injury. *Journal of Head Trauma Rehabilitation, 16*(4), 343–355.

Moretti, L., Cristofori, I., Weaver, S. M., Chau, A., Portelli, J. N., & Grafman, J. (2012). Cognitive decline in older adults with a history of traumatic brain injury. *Lancet Neurology, 11*(12), 1103–1112. doi:10.1016/S1474-4422(12)70226-0

Mortimer, J., van Duijn, C., Chandra, V., Fratiglioni, L., Graves, A., Heyman, A., . . . Rocca, W. (1991). Head trauma as a risk factor for Alzheimer's disease: A collaborative re-analysis of case-control studies. EURODEM Risk Factors Research Group. *International Journal of Epidemiology, 20*, S28–S35.

Morton, M. V., & Wehman, P. (1995). Psychosocial and emotional sequelae of individuals with traumatic brain injury: A literature review and recommendations. *Brain injury, 9*(1), 81–92. Retrieved from http://www.ncbi.nlm.nih.gov/pubmed/7874099

Murphy, M. P., & Carmine, H. (2012). Long-term health implications of individuals with TBI: A rehabilitation perspective. *NeuroRehabilitation, 31*(1), 85–94. doi:10.3233/NRE-2012-0777

Nelson, N. W., Hoelzle, J. B., Doane, B. M., McGuire, K. A., Ferrier-Auerbach, A. G., Charlesworth, M. J., . . . Sponheim, S. R. (2012). Neuropsychological outcomes of U.S. Veterans with report of remote blast-related concussion and current psychopathology.

Journal of the International Neuropsychological Society, 18(5), 845–855. doi:10.1017/ S1355617712000616

Ng, K., Mikulis, D. J., Glazer, J., Kabani, N., Till, C., Greenberg, G., . . . Green, R. E. (2008). Magnetic resonance imaging evidence of progression of subacute brain atrophy in moderate to severe traumatic brain injury. *Archives of Physical Medicine and Rehabilitation, 89*(12 Suppl), S35–44. doi:10.1016/j.apmr.2008.07.006

Niogi, S. N., Mukherjee, P., Ghajar, J., Johnson, C. E., Kolster, R., Lee, H., . . . McCandliss, B. D. (2008). Structural dissociation of attentional control and memory in adults with and without mild traumatic brain injury. *Brain, 131*(Pt 12), 3209–3221. doi:10.1093/brain/ awn247

O'Neil, M., Carlson, K., Storzbach, D., Brenner, L., Freeman, M., Quinones, A., . . . Kansagara, D. (2013). *Complications of Mild Traumatic Brain Injury in Veterans and Military Personnel: A Systematic Review.* Washington, DC: Department of Veterans Affairs Health Servicse Research and Development Service.

Omalu, B., DeKosky, S., Hamilton, R., Minster, R., Kamboh, M., Shakir, A. M., & Wecht, C. (2006). Chronic traumatic encephalopathy in a national football league player: Part II. *Neurosurgery, 59*(5), 1086–1092; discussion 1092–1093. doi:10.1227/01. NEU.0000245601.69451.27

Omalu, B., Hammers, J. L., Bailes, J., Hamilton, R. L., Kamboh, M. I., Webster, G., & Fitzsimmons, R. P. (2011). Chronic traumatic encephalopathy in an Iraqi war veteran with posttraumatic stress disorder who committed suicide. *Neurosurgical Focus, 31*(5), E3. doi:10.3171/2011.9.FOCUS11178

Omalu, B. I., DeKosky, S. T., Minster, R. L., Kamboh, M. I., Hamilton, R. L., & Wecht, C. H. (2005). Chronic traumatic encephalopathy in a National Football League player. *Neurosurgery, 57*(1), 128–134. doi:10.1227/01.NEU.0000163407.92769.ED

Omalu, B. I., Hamilton, R. L., Kamboh, M. I., DeKosky, S. T., & Bailes, J. (2010). Chronic traumatic encephalopathy (CTE) in a National Football League player: Case report and emerging medicolegal practice questions. *Journal of Forensic Nursing, 6*(1), 40–46. doi:10.1111/j.1939-3938.2009.01064.x

Peters, T. L., Fang, F., Weibull, C. E., Sandler, D. P., Kamel, F., & Ye, W. (2013, May). Severe head injury and amyotrophic lateral sclerosis. *Amyotrophic Lateral Sclerosis & Frontotemporal Degeneration, 14,* 267–272.

Pfleger, C., Koch-Henriksen, N., Stenager, E., Flachs, E., & Johansen, C. (2009). Head injury is not a risk factor for multiple sclerosis: A prospective cohort study. *Multiple Sclerosis, 15,* 294–298.

Plassman, B. L., Havlik, R. J., Steffens, D. C., Helms, M. J., Newman, T. N., Drosdick, D., . . . Breitner, J. C. S. (2000). Documented head injury in early adulthood and risk of Alzheimer's disease and other dementias. *Neurology, 55*(8), 1158–1166. doi:10.1212/ WNL.55.8.1158

Polusny, M. A., Kehle, S. M., Nelson, N. W., Erbes, C. R., Arbisi, P. A., & Thuras, P. (2011). Longitudinal effects of mild traumatic brain injury and posttraumatic stress disorder comorbidity on postdeployment outcomes in national guard soldiers deployed to Iraq. *Archives of General Psychiatry, 68*(1), 79–89. doi:10.1001/ archgenpsychiatry.2010.172

Ponsford, J., Cameron, P., Fitzgerald, M., Grant, M., & Mikocka-Walus, A. (2011). Long-term outcomes after uncomplicated mild traumatic brain injury: A comparison with trauma controls. *Journal of Neurotrauma, 28*(6), 937–946. doi:10.1089/neu.2010.1516

Ponsford, J., Cameron, P., Fitzgerald, M., Grant, M., Mikocka-Walus, A., & Schönberger, M. (2012). Predictors of postconcussive symptoms 3 months after mild traumatic brain injury. *Neuropsychology, 26*(3), 304–313. doi:10.1037/a0027888

Ponsford, J., Draper, K., & Schönberger, M. (2008). Functional outcome 10 years after traumatic brain injury: Its relationship with demographic, injury severity, and cognitive and emotional status. *Journal of the International Neuropsychological Society, 14*(2), 233–242. doi:10.1017/S1355617708080272

Pop, V., & Badaut, J. (2012). A neurovascular perspective for long-term chagnes after brain trauma. *Translational Stroke Research, 2*(4), 533–545. doi:10.1007/s12975-011-0126-9.A

Porter, M., & Fricker, P. (1996). Controlled prospective neuropsychological assessment of active experienced amateur boxers. *Clinical Journal of Sport Medicine, 6*(2), 90–96.

Ragsdale, K. A., Neer, S. M., Beidel, D. C., Frueh, B. C., & Stout, J. W. (2013). Posttraumatic stress disorder in OEF/OIF veterans with and without traumatic brain injury. *Journal of Anxiety Disorders, 27*(4), 420–426. doi:10.1016/j.janxdis.2013.04.003

Ramlackhansingh, A. F., Brooks, D. J., Greenwood, R. J., Bose, S. K., Turkheimer, F. E., Kinnunen, K. M., . . . Sharp, D. J. (2011). Inflammation after trauma: Microglial activation and traumatic brain injury. *Annals of Neurology, 70*(3), 374–383. doi:10.1002/ana.22455

Raymont, V., Salazar, A. M., Lipsky, R., Goldman, D., Tasick, G., & Grafman, J. (2010). Correlates of posttraumatic epilepsy 35 years following combat brain injury. *Neurology, 75*(3), 224–229. doi:10.1212/WNL.0b013e3181e8e6d0

Raymont, V., Greathouse, A., Reding, K., Lipsky, R., Salazar, A., & Grafman, J. (2008). Demographic, structural and genetic predictors of late cognitive decline after penetrating head injury. *Brain, 131*(Pt 2), 543–558. doi:10.1093/brain/awm300

Rogers, J. M., & Read, C. A. (2007). Psychiatric comorbidity following traumatic brain injury. *Brain Injury, 21*(13-14), 1321–1333. doi:10.1080/02699050701765700

Rohling, M. L., Binder, L. M., Demakis, G. J., Larrabee, G. J., Ploetz, D. M., & Langhinrichsen-Rohling, J. (2011). A meta-analysis of neuropsychological outcome after mild traumatic brain injury: Re-analyses and reconsiderations of Binder et al. (1997), Frencham et al. (2005), and Pertab et al. (2009). *The Clinical Neuropsychologist, 25*(4), 608–623. doi:10.1080/13854046.2011.565076

Rohling, M. L., Larrabee, G. J., & Millis, S. R. (2012). The "miserable minority" following mild traumatic brain injury: Who are they and do meta-analyses hide them? *The Clinical Neuropsychologist, 26*(2), 197–213. doi:10.1080/13854046.2011.647085

Ruff, R., Riechers, R. 2nd, Wang, X., Piero, T., & Ruff, S. (2012). For veterans with mild traumatic brain injury, improved posttraumatic stress disorder severity and sleep correlated with symptomatic improvement. *Journal of Rehabilitation Research & Development, 49*, 1305–1320.

Rugbjerg, K., Ritz, B., Korb, L., Martinussen, N., & Olsen, J. (2008). Risk of Parkinson's disease after hospital contact for head injury: Population based case-control study. *BMJ, 337*, 1–6. doi:10.1136/bmj.a2494

Ryan, L. M., & Warden, D. L. (2003). Post concussion syndrome. *International Review of Psychiatry, 15*(4), 310–316. doi:10.1080/09540260310001606692

Safaz, I., Alaca, R., Yasar, E., Tok, F., & Yilmaz, B. (2008). Medical complications, physical function and communication skills in patients with traumatic brain injury: A single centre 5-year experience. *Brain Injury, 22*(10), 733–739. doi:10.1080/02699050802304714

Salazar, A., Jabbari, B., Vance, S., Grafman, J., Amin, D., & Dillon, J. (1985). Epilepsy after penetrating head injury. I: Clinical correlates—a report of the Vietnam Head Injury Study. *Neurology, 35,* 1406–1414.

Savica, R., Parisi, J. E., Wold, L. E., Josephs, K. A., & Ahlskog, J. E. (2012). High school football and risk of neurodegeneration: A community-based study. *Mayo Clinic Proceedings, 87*(4), 335–340. doi:10.1016/j.mayocp.2011.12.016

Sayed, N., Culver, C., Dams-O'Connor, K., Hammond, F., & Diaz-Arrastia, R. (2013). Clinical phenotype of dementia after traumatic brain injury. *Journal of Neurotrauma, 30*(13), 1117–1122. doi:10.1089/neu.2012.2638

Schmidt, S., Kwee, L. C., Allen, K. D., & Oddone, E. Z. (2010). Association of ALS with head injury, cigarette smoking and APOE genotypes. *Journal of the Neurological Sciences, 291*(1–2), 22–29. doi:10.1016/j.jns.2010.01.011

Schnebel, B., Gwin, J. T., Anderson, S., & Gatlin, R. (2007). In vivo study of head impacts in football: A comparison of National Collegiate Athletic Association Division I versus high school impacts. *Neurosurgery, 60*(3), 490–495; discussion 495–6. doi:10.1227/01. NEU.0000249286.92255.7F

Seibert, P. S., Reedy, D. P., Hash, J., Webb, A., Stridh-Igo, P., Basom, J., & Zimmerman, C. G. (2002). Brain injury: Quality of life's greatest challenge. *Brain Injury, 16*(10), 837–848. doi:10.1080/02699050210131939

Sela-Kaufman, M., Rassovsky, Y., Agranov, E., Levi, Y., & Vakil, E. (2013). Premorbid personality characteristics and attachment style moderate the effect of injury severity on occupational outcome in traumatic brain injury: Another aspect of reserve. *Journal of Clinical and Experimental Neuropsychology, 35*(6), 584–595. doi:10.1080/13803395.2013 .799123

Selassie, A. W., Zaloshnja, E., Langlois, J., Miller, T., Jones, P., & Steiner, C. (2008). Incidence of long-term disability following traumatic brain injury hospitalization, United States, 2003. *Journal of Head Trauma Rehabilitation, 23,* 123–131.

Senathi-Raja, D., Ponsford, J., & Schönberger, M. (2010). Impact of age on long-term cognitive function after traumatic brain injury. *Neuropsychology, 24*(3), 336–344. doi:10.1037/ a0018239

Shandera-Ochsner, A. (2012). *Outcome following concussion and psychological trauma: An investigation of long-term cognitive and emotional functioning in veterans with PTSD* (Unpublished doctoral dissertation, University of Kenturcky, Lexington, KY).

Shively, S., Scher, A. I., Perl, D. P., & Diaz-Arrastia, R. (2012). Dementia resulting from traumatic brain injury: What is the pathology? *Archives of Neurology, 69*(10), 1245–1251. doi:10.1001/archneurol.2011.3747

Sidaros, A., Engberg, A. W., Sidaros, K., Liptrot, M. G., Herning, M., Petersen, P., . . . Rostrup, E. (2008). Diffusion tensor imaging during recovery from severe traumatic brain injury and relation to clinical outcome: A longitudinal study. *Brain, 131*(Pt 2), 559–572. doi:10.1093/brain/awm294

Sidaros, A., Skimminge, A., Liptrot, M. G., Sidaros, K., Engberg, A. W., Herning, M., . . . Rostrup, E. (2009). Long-term global and regional brain volume changes following severe traumatic brain injury: A longitudinal study with clinical correlates. *NeuroImage, 44*(1), 1–8. doi:10.1016/j.neuroimage.2008.08.030

Silver, J. M. (2012). Effort, exaggeration and malingering after concussion. *Journal of Neurology, Neurosurgery, and Psychiatry, 83*(8), 836–841. doi:10.1136/ jnnp-2011-302078

Silver, J. M., Kramer, R., Greenwald, S., & Weissman, M. (2001). The association between head injuries and psychiatric disorders: Findings from the New Haven NIMH Epidemiologic Catchment Area Study. *Brain injury*, *15*(11), 935–945. doi:10.1080/02699050110065295

Silverberg, N., Lange, R., Millis, S., Rose, A., Hopp, G., Leach, S., & Iverson, G. (2013). Post-concussion symptom reporting following multiple mild traumatic brain injuries. *Journal of Neurotrauma*, *30*, 1398–1404.

Simpson, G., & Tate, R. (2007). Suicidality in people surviving a traumatic brain injury: Prevalence, risk factors and implications for clinical management. *Brain Injury*, *21*(13-14), 1335–1351. doi:10.1080/02699050701785542

Siva, A., Radhakrishnan, K., Kurland, L., O'Brien, P., Swanson, J., & Rodriguez, M. (1993). Trauma and multiple sclerosis. *Neurology*, *43*, 1871–1874.

Small, G. W., Kepe, V., Siddarth, P., Ercoli, L. M., Merrill, D. A., Donoghue, N., . . . (2013). PET scanning of brain tau in retired national football league players: preliminary findings. *American Journal of Geriatric Psychiatry*, *2*, 138–144.

Soble, J. R., Spanierman, L. B., & Smith, J. F. (2013). Neuropsychological functioning of combat veterans with posttraumatic stress disorder and mild traumatic brain injury. *Journal of Clinical and Experimental Neuropsychology*, (*35*), 551–561.

Spencer, R. J., Drag, L. L., Walker, S. J., & Bieliauskas, L. A. (2010). Self-reported cognitive symptoms following mild traumatic brain injury are poorly associated with neuropsychological performance in OIF/OEF veterans. *The Journal of Rehabilitation Research and Development*, *47*(6), 521. doi:10.1682/JRRD.2009.11.0181

Stanford Epilepsy Center (2013). Retrieved from http://neurology.stanford.edu/epilepsy/patientcare/videos/e_12.html

Starkstein, S. E., & Jorge, R. (2005). Dementia after traumatic brain injury. *International Psychogeriatrics*, *17*(S1), S93. doi:10.1017/S1041610205001973

Stern, R. A., Riley, D. O., Daneshvar, D. H., Nowinski, C. J., Cantu, R. C., & McKee, A. C. (2011). Long-term consequences of repetitive brain trauma: Chronic traumatic encephalopathy. *PM & R : The Journal of Injury, Function, and Rehabilitation*, *3*(10 Suppl 2), S460–467. doi:10.1016/j.pmrj.2011.08.008

Tate, D. F., Khedraki, R., Neeley, E. S., Ryser, D. K., & Bigler, E. D. (2011). Cerebral volume loss, cognitive deficit, and neuropsychological performance: Comparative measures of brain atrophy: II. Traumatic brain injury. *Journal of the International Neuropsychological Society : JINS*, *17*(2), 308–316. doi:10.1017/S1355617710001670

Teasdale, T. W. (2001). Suicide after traumatic brain injury: A population study. *Journal of Neurology, Neurosurgery & Psychiatry*, *71*(4), 436–440. doi:10.1136/jnnp.71.4.436

Temkin, N. R., Corrigan, J. D., Dikmen, S. S., & Machamer, J. (2009). Social functioning after traumatic brain injury. *The Journal of Head Trauma Rehabilitation*, *24*(6), 460–467. doi:10.1097/HTR.0b013e3181c13413

Testa, J. A., Malec, J. F., Moessner, A. M., & Brown, A. W. (2005). Outcome after traumatic brain injury: Effects of aging on recovery. *Archives of Physical Medicine and Rehabilitation*, *86*(9), 1815–1823. doi:10.1016/j.apmr.2005.03.010

Tremblay, S., De Beaumont, L., Henry, L. C., Boulanger, Y., Evans, A. C., Bourgouin, P., . . . Lassonde, M. (2013). Sports concussions and aging: A neuroimaging investigation. *Cerebral Cortex*, *23*(5), 1159–1166. doi:10.1093/cercor/bhs102

Tsaousides, T., Cantor, J. B., & Gordon, W. A. (2011). Suicidal ideation following traumatic brain injury: Prevalence rates and correlates in adults living in the community. *The Journal of Head Trauma Rehabilitation, 26*(4), 265–275. doi:10.1097/HTR.0b013e3182225271

Turner, R. C., Lucke-Wold, B. P., Robson, M. J., Omalu, B. I., Petraglia, A. L., & Bailes, J. E. (2012). Repetitive traumatic brain injury and development of chronic traumatic encephalopathy: A potential role for biomarkers in diagnosis, prognosis, and treatment? *Frontiers in Neurology, 3*(January), 186. doi:10.3389/fneur.2012.00186

US Department of Defense. (2013). DOD establishes first brain tissue bank to study traumatic brain injury in service members. Retrieved from http://www.defense.gov/releases/release.aspx?releaseid=16094

Van Veldhoven, L. M., Sander, A. M., Struchen, M. A., Sherer, M., Clark, A. N., Hudnall, G. E., & Hannay, H. J. (2011). Predictive ability of preinjury stressful life events and post-traumatic stress symptoms for outcomes following mild traumatic brain injury: Analysis in a prospective emergency room sample. *Journal of Neurology, Neurosurgery, and Psychiatry, 82*(7), 782–787. doi:10.1136/jnnp.2010.228254

Vanderploeg, R. D., & Belanger, H. G. (2013). Screening for a remote history of mild traumatic brain injury: When a good idea is bad. *The Journal of Head Trauma Rehabilitation, 28*(3), 211–218. doi:10.1097/HTR.0b013e31828b50db

Vanderploeg, R. D., Curtiss, G., & Belanger, H. G. (2005). Long-term neuropsychological outcomes following mild traumatic brain injury. *Journal of the International Neuropsychological Society, 11*(3), 228–236. doi:10.1017/S1355617705050289

Vasterling, J. J., Brailey, K., Proctor, S. P., Kane, R., Heeren, T., & Franz, M. (2012). Neuropsychological outcomes of mild traumatic brain injury, post-traumatic stress disorder and depression in Iraq-deployed US Army soldiers. *The British Journal of Psychiatry: The Journal of Mental Science, 201*(3), 186–192. doi:10.1192/bjp.bp.111.096461

Von Steinbuechel, N., Wilson, L., Gibbons, H., Muehlan, H., Schmidt, H., Schmidt, S., . . . Truelle, J.-L. (2012). QOLIBRI overall scale: A brief index of health-related quality of life after traumatic brain injury. *Journal of Neurology, Neurosurgery, and Psychiatry, 83*(11), 1041–1047. doi:10.1136/jnnp-2012-302361

Wall, S. E., Williams, W. H., Cartwright-Hatton, S., Kelly, T. P., Murray, J., Murray, M., . . . Turner, M. (2006). Neuropsychological dysfunction following repeat concussions in jockeys. *Journal of Neurology, Neurosurgery, and Psychiatry, 77*(4), 518–520. doi:10.1136/jnnp.2004.061044

Williams, M. W., Rapport, L. J., Hanks, R. A., Millis, S. R., & Greene, H. A. (2013). Incremental validity of neuropsychological evaluations to computed tomography in predicting long-term outcomes after traumatic brain injury. *The Clinical Neuropsychologist, 27*(3), 356–375. doi:10.1080/13854046.2013.765507

Wolkin, A., Malaspina, D., Perrin, M., McAllister, T., & Corcoran, C. (2011). Psychotic disorders. In J. Silver, T. W. McAllister, & S. Yudofsky (Eds.), *Textbook of Traumatic Brain Injury, Second Edition* (pp. 189–197). Washington, DC: American Psychiatric Publishing.

Wood, R. L., & Rutterford, N. A. (2006). Demographic and cognitive predictors of long-term psychosocial outcome following traumatic brain injury. *Journal of the International Neuropsychological Society, 12*(3), 350–358. Retrieved from http://www.ncbi.nlm.nih.gov/pubmed/16903127

Yeh, C.-C., Chen, T.-L., Hu, C.-J., Chiu, W.-T., & Liao, C.-C. (2013). Risk of epilepsy after traumatic brain injury: A retrospective population-based cohort study. *Journal of Neurology, Neurosurgery, and Psychiatry, 84*(4), 441–445. doi:10.1136/jnnp-2012-302547

Zaloshnja, E., Miller, T., Langlois, J. A., & Selassie, A. W. (2008). Prevalence of long-term disability from traumatic brain injury in the civilian population of the United States, 2005. *The Journal of Head Trauma Rehabilitation, 23*(6), 394–400. doi:10.1097/01.HTR.0000341435.52004.ac

Zamek, R., Farion, K., Sampson, M., & McGahern, C. (2013). Prognosticators of persistent symptoms following pediatric concussion: A systematic review. *JAMA pediatrics, 167*(3), 259–265.

Zhou, W., Xu, D., Peng, X., Zhang, Q., Jia, J., & Crutcher, K. A. (2008). Meta-analysis of APOE4 allele and outcome after traumatic brain injury. *Journal of Neurotrauma, 25*(4), 279–290. doi:10.1089/neu.2007.0489

Zumstein, M. A., Moser, M., Mottini, M., Ott, S. R., Sadowski-Cron, C., Radanov, B. P., . . . Exadaktylos, A. (2011). Long-term outcome in patients with mild traumatic brain injury: A prospective observational study. *The Journal of Trauma, 71*(1), 120–127. doi:10.1097/TA.0b013e3181f2d670

3

FORENSIC NEUROPSYCHOLOGY

Annual Review

Jerry J. Sweet and Daniel J. Goldman

For at least the last two decades, forensic neuropsychology has been prominent in the professional practice literature. More specifically, the publication of peer-reviewed literature related to forensic neuropsychology grew dramatically in the 1990s (Sweet, King, Malina, Bergman, & Simmons, 2002) and continued to grow proportional to other practice topics in the 2000s (Sweet & Guidotti Breting, 2012). For example, the latter authors found that between 2001 and 2010, two popular clinical neuropsychology journals (*Archives of Clinical Neuropsychology* and *The Clinical Neuropsychologist*) published far more peer-reviewed studies on a forensic topic (i.e., malingering) than on Alzheimer disease, stroke and cerebrovascular disease, mild cognitive impairment, and Parkinson disease, *combined*. Previously, by examining national neuropsychology conference programs, Sweet et al. (2002) had shown that forensic neuropsychology was also prominent at major professional meetings, which provide continuing education for practitioners. The combination of a voluminous peer review literature and visible presence within continuing education programs likely is responsible for the American Academy of Clinical Neuropsychology having sponsored a consensus conference related to forensic neuropsychology (Heilbronner et al., 2009). Similarly, the popularity of this general subject area is evident in the publication frequency of entire textbooks addressing a full range of forensic neuropsychology topics (e.g., Boone, 2013; Larrabee, 2012b; Sherman & Brooks, 2012).

In this chapter we review recent and current literature that has the potential to influence forensic neuropsychology. Operationally, most of the literature cited is within the range of 2011–2013. By the nature of this textbook, unless necessary to discuss a current topic, we do not include citations prior to 2010. Our approach to selecting literature for this review was purely rational (i.e., not quantitative or systematic). Although informed by the contents of recent textbooks relevant to forensic neuropsychology, as well as recent review papers, we relied on a past very detailed inventory of papers published in clinical neuropsychology journals (Sweet et al., 2002) only as a crude guide to begin the online search process undertaken in *LexusNexus Academic, MedLine,* and *PsychInfo*. Because our goal was to identify potentially influential publications, our approach to filtering the voluminous literature about forensic neuropsychology was admittedly subjective: personal judgment based on professional experience and practice. For example, it is indisputable that the topic of response bias (e.g., insufficient effort, symptom overreporting, detection of malingering) is regularly predominant in the forensic neuropsychology literature. Yet, not many of these response bias articles are truly influential, because they simply reinforce previous findings. This is especially true when compared to a single court ruling or precedent-setting legal case outcome, which have the potential to change subsequent evidentiary standards, or, as a more specific example, a single definitive scientific paper that may change the way neuropsychologists evaluate claimants, change the way test data are interpreted with regard to particular symptoms, change the admissibility of brain imaging as evidence, or otherwise broadly affect neuropsychological testimony in civil or criminal trials. This is the broader perspective from which we emphasize recent meaningful literature contributions that seem to have potential for affecting neuropsychology's testifying experts.

INFLUENCE OF NEW TECHNOLOGIES IN COURTROOMS

Medical and scientific technologies relevant to direct evaluation of the brain have been viewed by some as holding great potential for addressing topics that presently fall within the purview of clinical neuropsychologists. As interest rises, a growing literature of legal treatises authored by attorneys has developed. These legal treatises debate the implications for the courtroom of advances in neuroscience.

An online search of "law reviews" in LexisNexis Academic on January 14, 2013, using the key word "neuroscience" returned over 400 items in the previous 2 years. Many of these involved narrow reference to the need to reconsider definitions and implications of addictions based on neuroscience developments. To narrow down the pool of items, the terms "neuropsychology OR neuropsychologist OR neuropsychological" were searched for the time interval of the previous 2 years. This resulted in 16 citations, four of which are relevant to the broader topic of general aspects of neuroscience admissibility in the courtroom.

The general tenor of legal treatises pertaining to developing neurotechnologies is well reflected in a law review quote by Eggen and Laury (2011). These attorney authors state, "The 'neuroscience revolution' has now gained the attention of legal thinkers and is poised to be the catalyst for significant changes in society and the law" (p. 4). A reasonable point of discussion among legal scholars has been whether advances in brain assessment technologies may force a change in views regarding what is defined as "brain damage" and whether the presence of newly identified molecular and neurophysiologic brain abnormalities can be conceptualized as a determinant of behavior that was previously viewed as volitional or caused by a psychological state, which now may be viewed as disease- or injury-related. To use language provided by Eggen and Laury, legal scholars have begun to discuss whether neuroscience evidence, if admitted, would "effectively transform a mental disability into a physical disability" (p. 70). An example provided in the Eggen and Laury review is that of a recent US Supreme Court decision (*Brown v. Entertainment Merchants Association*, 2011) in which the dissenting opinion regarding the relationship between video games and real world violence included reference to neuroscience research.

Whereas neuroscience advances may improve accuracy of clinical and legal decision-making, there are negative aspects that require careful consideration. In sharp contrast to proponents, there is a belief among some legal thinkers that the near-term influence of neuroscience is limited. In that vein, Morse (2011) has commented, "At most, in the near to intermediate term, neuroscience may make modest contributions to legal policy and case adjudication." Borrowing a term popularized by the former Federal Reserve chairman Alan Greenspan, Morse views the opinions of neuroscience advocates as "irrational exuberance" (p. 838). Morse's arguments against broad admissibility of neuroscience primarily address the imagined effects on criminal proceedings, while ignoring civil law implications. Morse posits that a primary motivation for those most enthusiastic about neuroscience is a stealth search for mitigation evidence that may excuse criminal behavior. In constructing his argument to lower expectations regarding neuroscience's influence, Morse points out the well-known fact of at best a modest correlation between scores on executive-cognitive tasks and real world behavior, and yet functional imaging studies rely on the same imperfect cognitive measures. Hence, this limits the technologic contributions of functional imaging in understanding real-world behavior.

From a different perspective, and perhaps discomforting to those who fear neuroscience information will have undue influence on triers-of-fact, Weisberg, Keil, Goodstein, Rawson, and Gray (2008) performed decision-making experiments with naive adults, neuroscience students, and neuroscience experts who were supplied information that varied in "good" versus "bad" logic, either with or without neuroscience information. Whereas participants in all three groups judged the good logic information as more satisfying, the neuroscience information was described as having a striking effect on the nonexperts' judgments, in terms of masking the quality of the bad logic. In the words of these authors, ". . . people seem all too ready to accept explanations that allude to neuroscience, even if they are not accurate reflections of the scientific data, and even if they would otherwise be seen as far less satisfying" (p. 477).

Nevertheless, there are legal experts who believe that the contributions of neuroscience technologies are likely to be limited. For example, Roth (2012) has argued that criminal sentencing is the area most likely to be influenced. That is, evidence for brain abnormalities should only be introduced during the sentencing phase, as a mitigating factor, among other such factors.

Lie detection technologies have been researched for decades and debated for just as many years. Subsequent to the *Frye v. United States* (1923) ruling, they have routinely been excluded from court proceedings. Nevertheless, neuroscience research, primarily related to functional neuroimaging (e.g., functional magnetic resonance imaging [fMRI]), has caused some to consider the possibility that this scenario may change. Thus far, the prevailing opinion appears to be that procedures such as fMRI are not ready for court admission as evidence. For example, Law (2011) argued that "fMRI-based lie detection is not ready for evidentiary admissibility at this point in time, simply because it cannot be shown reliably and validly to prove or disprove any fact" (p. 23). Law opines that courts need to consider new technologies, such as fMRI, in light of Federal Rule of Evidence 702 and the 1993 Supreme Court Daubert ruling for admissibility of evidence. Law argues for a particularly exacting scrutiny, for example not only the fMRI error rate, but also the error rate for the underlying cognitive task used to activate the brain while in the scanner. As a further example of greater exactness, Law (2011) proposed that beyond the expectation of simple peer review publication, secondary publications of replication should be evaluated, and a determination should be made regarding whether graduate-level textbooks have adopted support for the new technologies.

Suggesting that triers-of-fact can limit or assign weight appropriately to neuroscience evidence in individual cases, Eggen and Laury (2011) have offered the following:

> Some might argue that this would produce a counter-effect in that juries would give undue weight to neuroscience in making their decisions. But the same has been said of most kinds of scientific and technical evidence, and such evidence appears regularly in the courtroom. The attorneys, through appropriate cross-examination, and the court, through careful jury instructions, must address neuroscience as they do the other expert evidence. This could mean sometimes preventing the jury from hearing the evidence at all. (p. 27–28)

Clinical Status of Imaging

Beyond the influence of neuroscience information in general, there has been concern whether colorful brain images have undue influence on triers-of-fact. For example, McCabe and Castel (2008) demonstrated that brain images greatly affect judgment of the scientific merit of published studies, even when compared to other visual images, such as graphs. These authors contend that providing a concrete physical anchor for what is otherwise a cognitive construct is persuasive.

Fortunately, courts increasingly base their admissibility rules on science. Therefore, reviews of scientific studies in the professional literature have an impact on discussions among legal scholars and eventual rulings on admissibility made in courtrooms. Various technologies, including functional imaging and structural imaging of the brain have been considered, with specific regard to whether they are appropriate as evidence in the courtroom. No change in the general tenor of these scientific reviews has occurred in recent years. For example, consider the sentiment of Khoshbin and Khoshbin (2007), as they conclude their review:

> The risks of the misuse of brain imaging in the courtroom are undeniable. We have strongly recommended that even structural brain images be used only for the purpose of linking a structural abnormality or injury to a specific deficit and then to be used only as a tool for interpretation by the expert witness to assess its clinical significance. Furthermore, we have recommended that functional brain

images not be used for the purpose of linking a particular functional change in a modular fashion in the brain to assess motivation, propensity, or responsibility for a complex behavior or an inability to inhibit it (very similar to the inadequacies of polygraphs currently used for lie-detection). (p. 191–192)

The previous view is comparable to Moriarty's (2008) negative view. Moriarty discussed the problems with neuroscience methodologies predating fMRI, such as single-photon emission computed tomography (SPECT) and positron emission tomography (PET), when used to inform legal decisions, such as death sentence rulings. This appears to be a point on which legal and clinical authorities are beginning to agree (Rushing & Langleben, 2011).

In civil proceedings, the most common point of contention for neuropsychologists is the existence of brain dysfunction in cases where traumatic brain injury (TBI) is alleged. Often, the issue at hand involves mild TBI (mTBI). A relevant review by Wortzel, Filley, Anderson, Oster, and Arciniegas (2008) specifically addressed whether SPECT should be admissible in litigated mTBI cases. Noting that neuropsychological impairments and neuropsychiatric symptoms did not have a consistent relationship to SPECT findings, these authors also noted that positive SPECT findings are not specific and therefore are not diagnostic of mTBI. The conclusion of Wortzel et al. was that SPECT should not be considered as "stand-alone" evidence when giving expert testimony on mTBI. There appears to have been no substantial change in scientific or clinical guidance to date on the use of SPECT for evaluating TBI. Specifically, the American College of Radiology "Appropriateness Criteria" (Davis et al., 2012) continue to rate both SPECT and PET a "1" on a scale of 1–9, in which 1 signifies least appropriate usage, for the entire severity range of TBI, regardless of complications, such as skull fracture or bleeding. The single exception is noted as "Variant 5 Subacute or chronic closed head injury with cognitive and/or neurologic deficit(s)," for which a rating of 4 is given for SPECT and PET (p. 5). This rating indicates that the procedures *may* be appropriate for select cases. In no instance do the usage criteria assign SPECT or PET a rating that would be consistent with "usually appropriate," which includes ratings of 7, 8, and 9, a category that may be more consistent with evidentiary standards. Given that the American College of Radiology criteria represent the current clinical guidance for the medical specialty that is devoted to imaging of the brain, there seems little clinical support, and therefore limited opportunity, in the near term for functional imaging such as SPECT or PET to have widespread admissibility in US courtrooms.

Newer structural imaging procedures also appear to have relatively slow acceptance in courtrooms, which again can be tied to lack of sufficient clinical scientific support. For example, diffusion tensor imaging (DTI) has been suggested by some clinical researchers as having potential as a biomarker for mTBI (Aoki, Inokuchi, Gunshin, Yahagi, & Suwa, 2012). On the basis of meta-analytic results from 13 published studies, Aoki et al. (2012) concluded that there was "potential utility in clinical settings" for using DTI to identify microstructural brain damage after mTBI (p. 875).

However, this view stands in contrast to Larrabee, Binder, Rohling, and Ploetz (2013), who criticized the methodology of Aoki et al., and whose critique of the underlying studies and meta-analytic results brought them to the opposite conclusion. In any event, with even the most positive viewpoint of Aoki et al. (2012), admissibility in courtrooms is not based on "potential." For the present, there appears to be no reason to disagree with the viewpoint of Wortzel, Kraus, Filley, Anderson, and Arciniegas (2011), whose review of clinical studies concluded that although DTI is a "promising emerging neuroimaging technique," it will seldom be appropriate for expert witnesses to use DTI as a basis for opinions in mTBI forensic cases (p. 522). In greater detail, based on their conclusion that DTI findings are not specific to such disorders as mTBI, Wortzel et al. state:

> Experts must be discouraged from claiming too much for this technology, using it to form opinions in isolation of or in conflict with other diagnostic data, or making bold cause- and-effect claims between mild TBI and white matter integrity findings. (p. 522)

As expressed by Ricker (2012) after detailed review of various neuroimaging literatures, such as fMRI and SPECT, there is not a sufficient basis for the results of these techniques to be admitted into evidence at present. In Ricker's opinion, it will take years of additional systematic research, including extensive comparisons between clinical and forensic samples, before the potential to make a clear contribution in forensic settings can be realized. Until that time arrives, when individual courts allow new imaging techniques as evidence, there may be comfort in the findings that the feared undue influence on triers-of-fact has not been found in some of the carefully designed judgment and decision-making research that has examined the impact of using brain images on jury outcomes (cf. Roskies, Schweitzer, & Saks, 2013).

Returning to the implicit question from the technology section (i.e., whether the contribution of neuropsychological assessments will be altered or marginalized by medical technological assessments), the recent study by Williams, Rapport, Hanks, Millis, and Greene (2013) offers relevant information. These clinical researchers compared computerized tomography of the brain, initial injury variables, demographic variables, and neuropsychological data in predicting TBI outcomes. Results demonstrated that initial inpatient neuropsychological data contributed unique variance in predicting functional disability at 1 and 2 years postinjury, whereas computerized tomography findings did not predict functional outcomes.

COURT RULINGS AND ACCEPTANCE OF NEUROPSYCHOLOGISTS AS EXPERTS

Forensic neuropsychology has become prominent within clinical neuropsychology, such that textbooks entirely devoted to related subject matter continue to appear annually (Boone, 2013; Larrabee, 2012b). In addition, clinical neuropsychologists are widely accepted in legal proceedings as expert witnesses (Rushing & Langleben, 2011;

Sweet & Westerveld, 2012). These two facts explain why attorneys continue to seek out basic information regarding related practice specifics and concepts (Liefland, 2012), and why lawyers and psychology practitioners continue to seek out detailed information pertaining to specific forensic proceedings, such as those associated with an Atkins hearing (Fabian, Thompson IV, & Lazarus, 2011). The degree of common acceptance in a wide range of forensic proceedings is impressive, and has withstood changes in evidentiary standards that have moved over time toward greater scientific bases and more extensive judicial scrutiny (Kaufmann, 2012).

There have not been any major court rulings or changes in evidentiary standards in recent years that have affected general admissibility of neuropsychological evidence or, more generally, neuropsychologists qualifying as experts (Kaufmann, 2012; Sweet, Ecklund-Johnson, & Malina, 2008). As is true of any expert, including physicians, on a case-by-case basis an individual neuropsychologist may be excluded from testifying in a specific forensic proceeding (1) when straying from mainstream practice, (2) when offering opinions that have no solid basis, or (3) when offering opinions that are inappropriate in terms of scope of practice or in terms of crossing legal boundaries assigned to experts.

As an example of the latter, the appeal of a criminal defendant's conviction contended that a neuropsychologist was erroneously excluded from mentioning past specific traumas that were deemed by the trial judge to be more prejudicial than probative (*Le v. Barnes*, 2012). The appeal was denied by District Court. The appeal decision reflects that at times an expert's testimony can be forcibly limited on legal grounds that have nothing to do with the expert's qualifications or the basis of the expert's opinions. Importantly, the neuropsychologist and other psychologists involved in this particular case were allowed to address a variety of neurologic and psychiatric topics relevant to the case. Only the topic thought to be prejudicial was excluded from testimony. The point is that exclusion is most often limited to one part of testimony; it is rare for neuropsychologists to be barred from testifying at all.

Again, there does not appear to be a trend of exclusions of neuropsychologists as experts or of exclusions of neuropsychological evidence. In fact, there have been instances of resentencing appeals being granted in criminal cases in which evidence of a neuropsychological nature should have been, but was not, presented during the original defense of the case, including an instance in which a death sentence was vacated specifically because the defense attorney "failed to consult a neurologist, neuropsychologist or neuropsychiatrist" (*Hernandez v. Martel*, 2011, cited in Rushing and Langleben, 2011, p. 584).

POSTTRAUMATIC STRESS DISORDER, MTBI, AND COMORBIDITY

Within the last several years the most widely covered health topics in the popular press have been posttraumatic stress disorder (PTSD) and mTBI. Understandably, the interest level on these two topics has been generated from concerns regarding war zone military personnel who have increasingly been found to suffer from one or both conditions (cf. Vasterling, Bryant, & Keane, 2012), and athletes engaged in contact sports, who have increasingly been found to suffer from the latter condition (Herring et al., 2011). Neuropsychologists' involvement in the evaluation process has been stated with authority, for both the military context (McCrea et al., 2008) and the civilian sports context (Echemendia et al., 2011). Both contexts often have forensic implications, given the military's service-connected benefits status and the potential for litigation claims related to amateur and professional sports (e.g., National Football League litigation and settlement; football helmet industry litigation).

Progress in Quantifying mTBI and PTSD During and After Military Service

The accurate diagnosis of mTBI is challenging if attempted in retrospect (cf. Ruff et al., 2009), when the diagnostic process is by necessity based on the vagaries of self-report and less than complete or even absent documentation of potential injury events. Review of records closest to the injury date, such as emergency room triage notes, is indispensable for answering the crucial question of whether there was, in fact, a historical TBI, particularly when analyzing the self-report of a self-interested party. Self-report is unreliable, and decades of research has shown that when primarily relied upon, it is a particularly poor means of diagnosing retrospective TBI and other disorders (Barsky, 2002; Barth, 2009; Don & Carragee, 2009; Iverson, 2006; Iverson, Lange, Brooks, & Rennison, 2010; Marino et al., 2009; Wang, Chan, & Deng, 2006).

The comorbidity of mTBI and PTSD among combat-exposed active military and veterans has received increased attention (cf. Vasterling et al., 2012). Betthauser, Bahraini, Krengel, and Brenner (2012) reviewed the literature related to using self-report measures to identify mTBI and PTSD symptoms in military service veterans. Acknowledging the reliability and validity constraints, and noting that self-report should not be used as a sole basis for diagnosis, the Betthauser et al. review nevertheless identified some interesting findings. Specifically, there have been repeated studies demonstrating a strong relationship between the association of emotional symptoms (i.e., PTSD, depression) as well as pain and headache symptoms with greater endorsement of postconcussive symptoms, findings that have been well documented for years in civilian samples (Ponsford et al., 2012; Ponsford et al., 2000).

Therefore, it is important that research continue the measurement of the acute effects of TBI. For example, Kelly, Coldren, Parish, Dretsch, and Russell (2012) found that assessment within 72 hours of battlefield concussion using the brief computerized test battery known as Automated Neuropsychological Assessment Metrics was clinically useful in documenting initial effects and in discriminating concussed soldiers from healthy control subjects and nonconcussed injury control subjects.

Acute assessment of concussion in the military has also been found to have discriminative value in establishing prognosis (i.e., identifying those who will recover faster, and perhaps those who will be able to return to duty). Interestingly, Kennedy et al. (2012) assessed acute battlefield concussion using the Military Acute Concussion

Evaluation and found that loss of consciousness and initial cognitive scores did not predict recovery speed or return to duty, whereas age, headache severity, and presence or absence of combat stress reaction discriminated the groups.

A reasonable question receiving attention from clinical researchers is, "Is the neuropsychology of blast-related TBI different from the neuropsychology of nonblast TBI?" If the two are not different in terms of neuropsychological outcomes, then much of the information already learned in decades of research may be directly applicable to blast TBI. Belanger et al. (2011) studied symptoms reported by active-duty or veteran military personnel who experienced blast-related or nonblast TBI. Of 18 postconcussive symptoms, only hearing distinguished the groups, with the blast-related TBI group reporting more hearing disturbance. The group with the greatest amount of PTSD symptoms also reported significantly greater postconcussive symptoms. Similarly, other neuropsychological researchers have reported that mTBI caused by blast did not produce longstanding cognitive impairment; instead, later subtle findings were likely related to factors, such as depression or PTSD (Nelson et al., 2012). Such findings related to blast injury appear comparable to civilian findings that postconcussion syndrome symptoms can be predicted by preinjury psychiatric anxiety or depression and by postinjury acute stress, but not by mTBI (Meares et al., 2011).

Findings related to response bias also appear to be comparable. For example, Sollman and Berry (2011) provided an updated meta-analysis of peer-reviewed studies pertaining to the use of stand-alone performance validity tests (PVTs). In this meta-analytic study of such measures as the Test of Memory Malingering (TOMM), Word Memory Test (WMT), and Medical Symptom Validity Test (MSVT), it remains clear that numerous studies continue to find that a compensation-seeking context is consistently associated with risk of invalid performance. Similar concerns regarding the military context of compensation- or benefit-seeking have been expressed (Hoge, Goldberg, & Castro, 2009), and appear to be supported by studies, such as that of Armistead-Jehle and Buican (2012), who found that a disability evaluation context in a military sample produced a significantly greater number of stand-alone PVT failures than a sample seen for clinical evaluation services.

Progress in Quantifying Sports Concussion Initially and Remotely

A striking degree of concern regarding sports-related concussion is evident throughout American society. Media coverage of concussion in sports at all levels of play from young athletes (e.g., Pop Warner Football) to high school and college-level athletes and professional sports (e.g., National Football League) is a daily occurrence. Although the bulk of attention has been on football, such sports as ice hockey, soccer, basketball, and others have also received attention (Harmon et al., 2013). Several professional organizations have issued position statements on best practices, based on the latest scientific research. The use of cognitive testing and psychometric approaches to evaluate sports-related concussion has been supported by the American Academy of Neurology (Giza et al., 2013), American College of Sports Medicine, American

Academy of Family Physicians, American Academy of Orthopaedic Surgeons, American Medical Society for Sports Medicine, American Orthopaedic Society for Sports Medicine, and American Osteopathic Academy of Sports Medicine (Herring et al., 2011), and the Fourth International Conference on Concussion, held in Zurich (Echemendia et al., 2013; Giza et al., 2013; Harmon et al., 2013; McCrory et al., 2013), among other organizations. In particular, some experts have taken a more definitive position that brief cognitive screenings, which may be useful initially, are not a substitute for more thorough neuropsychological evaluations (Echemendia et al., 2013). Moreover, many of the professional organization statements make it clear that neuropsychologists play a key role in the multidisciplinary treatment of a team's management of sports-related concussion (Echemendia et al., 2011; McCrory et al., 2013).

DISCRIMINATING BETWEEN TYPES OF RESPONSE VALIDITY

Historically, the forensic neuropsychology literature has characterized response bias measures that identify invalid performance and those that identify invalid symptom reporting with the same terminology: "symptom validity testing" (SVT). Recently, beginning with Larrabee (2012a), researchers are applying more precise terminology, using *performance validity test* for a measure that can identify suspicious underperformance on ability tests, and restricting the term *symptom validity test* to measures that identify suspicious verbal behavior (overreporting or underreporting of symptoms). To be clear, it has been evident for years that the two types of measures can reflect separate, and yet at times correlated, examinee biases, and that both are needed to evaluate response validity (Nelson et al., 2007; Smart et al., 2008; Van Dyke, Millis, Axelrod, & Hanks, 2013). However, as research continues, the more precise terminology will better convey to practitioners specific findings related to each type of response bias. In other respects, as noted previously in this chapter, the annual high-frequency contribution of new PVT and SVT studies pertaining to neuropsychological response bias continues, and is simply too vast to describe in detail here (see Greve, Curtis, & Bianchini, 2013 for a recent review).

MULTIPLE RESPONSE BIAS MEASURES IN A SINGLE EVALUATION

For many years, guidance to practitioners has been clear and strong with regard to the need to prospectively evaluate response bias when evaluating individuals in a forensic context (American Academy of Clinical Neuropsychology, 2007; Bush & NAN Policy & Planning Committee, 2005; Bush et al., 2005). With the inclusion of SVTs and PVTs now accepted as necessary, the question of how much is sufficient has been a major discussion point in the literature. Few true experts would disagree with the general observation that assuring the validity of all test results is essential. The need for continuous assessment of response bias throughout an evaluation has been stressed (Boone, 2009). Related, a conclusion regarding response bias being present is viewed as strengthened as "the number and extent of findings consistent with the absence or presence of response bias increases" (Heilbronner et al., 2009, p. 1107).

Apart from acceptance of practitioner guidance, empirical questions pertaining to the use and effectiveness of multiple measures continue to be addressed. Given that effort can vary across an evaluation and also knowing that PVTs do not have the same sensitivity, it is not surprising that clinical researchers, such as Greve, Binder, and Bianchini (2009), found better classification rates of malingering using multiple PVTs (e.g., Portland Digit Recognition Test, TOMM, and WMT) versus any of the PVTs individually.

Similarly, among TBI litigants and disability claimants, performances on multiple embedded performance validity indicators have been shown to have a significant relationship to ability test scores (Davis, Axelrod, McHugh, Hanks, & Millis, 2013). In this latter study, forensic examinees that passed all eight embedded performance validity indicators had significantly better performances on ability tests than those who failed two or more indicators. Previously, Victor, Boone, Serpa, Buehler, and Ziegler (2009) had shown that among credible examinees (i.e., those with no incentive to perform poorly, who also produced credible stand-alone PVT performances) failure rate on four embedded PVTs rarely exceeded one. However, from a purely statistical perspective, practitioners must consider that the risk of false-positive results rises as more PVTs are administered (cf. Berthelson, Mulchan, Odland, Miller, & Mittenberg, 2013). Ultimately, concluding that an examinee's presentation represents response bias, rather than genuine disorder, remains a "big picture" determination that is not based on test scores alone. Rather, this broader conclusion requires consideration of multiple types and sources of information, minimally including consideration of initial injury characteristics, known injury outcomes, and dose-response relationships in nonlitigants (Sweet, Goldman, & Guidotti Breting, 2013).

PEDIATRIC TOPICS

Pediatric neuropsychology continues to develop as a subspecialty within clinical neuropsychology, and in 2013 was voted to move forward by the American Board of Professional Psychology as its first ever "subspecialty" designation. The pediatric neuropsychology literature with forensic applications is relatively limited, but continues to grow. Indeed, the first book dedicated specifically to pediatric forensic neuropsychology was published in 2012 (Sherman & Brooks, 2012), and covers a range of topics, including theoretical, conceptual, and psychometric issues, as well as applied clinical issues. Peer-reviewed journal articles discussed in this review predominantly addressed assessment of TBI in children and adolescents, as well as measurement of performance validity, test effort, and motivation.

TBI in Children

Assessment of TBI in pediatric samples, including in forensic settings, is a growing area of interest. Yet, the literature using forensic samples remains small. As with all neuropsychological evaluations, knowledge of base rates is critical in assessing symptoms of mTBI and in differential diagnosis (cf. Sweet et al., 2013). Because many symptoms of mTBI are nonspecific, relevant base rate information includes the prevalence of common mTBI symptoms in noninjured individuals. Couch and Leathem (2011) examined the prevalence of such symptoms over the previous year in 124 children aged 11–13. Results demonstrated high base rates (over 70%) for symptoms, such as feeling "grumpy/cross," experiencing "frustration," and feeling mental or physical fatigue. Additionally, five or more symptoms (predominantly behavioral and emotional) were experienced on a daily or weekly basis by 20% of these authors' non–brain-injured sample. The authors conclude that caution is warranted in interpretation of such common symptoms in neuropsychological evaluations of children with mTBI, as their true significance for differential diagnosis is uncertain. Similarly, McNally et al. (2013) examined the relative contributions of injury characteristics and noninjury child and family variables in predicting postconcussive symptoms. The authors found that in the first few months following a TBI, injury characteristics significantly predicted postconcussive symptoms. However, the contribution of injury characteristics decreased over time, whereas noninjury variables (e.g., demographic factors and premorbid child factors) were more consistently predictive of persistent postconcussive symptoms.

The much larger literature regarding general clinical assessment of TBI in children is indirectly related to the forensic arena, but is not addressed here in detail. In order to empirically support test selection and diagnostic conclusions, neuropsychologists working as forensic experts should remain aware of such work. For example, several recent empirical studies investigate the utility of commonly used tests in assessing and differentially diagnosing TBI versus other common conditions, such as attention-deficit/hyperactivity disorder (e.g., Allen, Thaler, Ringdahl, Barney, & Mayfield, 2012). Similarly, recent research (e.g., Barney et al., 2011) continues to bolster the conclusion that results of neuropsychological tests of attention used to assess children with TBI are often discrepant from parent ratings of inattention and hyperactivity.

Motivation, Test Effort, and Performance Validity

Consistent with the adult forensic neuropsychology literature, the largest topic area within the pediatric literature concerns assessment of effort and performance validity. As the specialty practice of pediatric forensic neuropsychology grows, ability to accurately assess performance validity will be critical. Several recent studies provide evidence that helps to validate embedded PVTs for children, such as the Digit Span subtest of the Wechsler Intelligence Scale for Children-Fourth Edition (e.g., Kirkwood, Hargrave, & Kirk, 2011; Loughan, Perna, & Hertza, 2012). Other recent evidence indicates that, just as in adult populations, children who fail stand-alone PVTs (e.g., the Medical Symptom Validity Test) perform significantly worse on neuropsychological tests across a number of domains, even when secondary gain factors are not apparent (Kirkwood, Yeates, Randolph, & Kirk, 2012).

The Victoria Symptom Validity Test has shown good potential to assess performance validity in children and adolescents, including those with known neurologic disorders (Brooks, 2012).

Assessment of Psychopathology

Questions regarding the presence and impact of psychopathology are commonly asked of pediatric clinical neuropsychologists in forensic settings, yet the recent literature specific to forensic populations is also small. Often, information regarding symptoms is predominantly obtained via self-report of the child and his or her caregivers, which can result in significant discrepancies for a variety of reasons. Forensically relevant variables have been found to moderate informant agreement regarding symptoms of psychopathology in adolescents charged with crimes, including offense category, level of psychopathic traits, and socially desirable response bias (Penney & Skilling, 2012). When conducting evaluations of adolescents in a forensic context, recent evidence demonstrates the importance of using response bias measures and taking into consideration personality traits and offense categories.

Special Education

Pediatric neuropsychologists are increasingly involved in special education. Because of the potential for litigation when expected accommodations are not granted or expensive expert services not paid by a school district, the area can be viewed as a forensic context (Hurewitz & Kerr, 2011). Neuropsychologists provide evaluations and reports that can be used in school programming, treatment, and/or legal disputes. The published literature in this area is quite small, but will likely grow as neuropsychologists become more involved in special education. Hurewitz and Kerr (2011) published an important article that walks through the unique issues and topics within special education. The paper discusses the ways in which a neuropsychologist may become involved in the special education system, as well as the possible roles a neuropsychologist may fill, including as a member of the Individualized Education Plan team, as an independent educational evaluator, and as an expert witness in due process hearings. For clinical neuropsychologists unfamiliar with special education, Hurewitz and Kerr provide an excellent and accessible guide to the topics that must be considered.

Although not technically a pediatric population, neuropsychologists are also increasingly asked to evaluate college students seeking academic accommodations and/or stimulant medications. Assessment of performance validity is particularly important in the context of such a clear primary gain. Recent work has demonstrated the effectiveness of embedded and stand-alone measures in differentiating genuine impairment from feigned mental retardation (Musso, Barker, Jones, Roid, & Gouvier, 2011), dyslexia (Lindstrom, Coleman, Thomassin, Southall, & Lindstrom, 2011), and attention-deficit/hyperactivity disorder (Jasinski et al., 2011), especially when students are overtly seeking an evaluation for accommodations and/or medications (Pella, Hill, Shelton, Elliott, & Gouvier, 2012).

PERSONALITY TESTS

Personality tests, such as the Minnesota Multiphasic Personality Inventory-2nd Edition (MMPI-2), MMPI-2 Restructured Form (MMPI-2-RF), and the Personality Assessment Inventory (PAI), continue to be used frequently in forensic neuropsychological evaluations. Personality tests such as these are valuable because they provide objective clinical symptom data and measures of response bias (e.g., symptom overreporting and underreporting). Indeed, the MMPI-2 has been the measure of personality and emotional functioning most commonly used by neuropsychologists (cf. Rabin, Barr, & Burton, 2005), largely due to its extensive validity scales and the immense empirical literature devoted to it. Recent literature most relevant to forensic practice primarily addresses the MMPI-2 and MMPI-2-RF validity scales and their applications in a variety of forensic situations. This literature reflects a shift toward the MMPI-2-RF from the MMPI-2, with a substantially greater number of articles addressing the MMPI-2-RF than the MMPI-2. Forensically relevant literature on the PAI, although much smaller, also primarily addresses issues of profile validity and feigning.

MMPI-2

Recent publications addressing the MMPI-2 validity scales have continued to broadly support their effectiveness in detecting various aspects of response bias and malingering. For example, the symptom validity scale (MMPI-2 Fake Bad Scale, commonly called "the FBS") has been criticized for gender bias, with some studies suggesting that the scale may overidentify women as noncredible responders as compared to men (e.g., Butcher, Gass, Cumella, Kally, & Williams, 2008). However, Lee, Graham, Sellbom, and Gervais (2012) found no evidence of gender bias in FBS for a large sample of individuals undergoing medicolegal evaluations. Another recent paper examined the relative predictive power of five MMPI-2 validity scales (Infrequency or F, Infrequency Psychopathology or Fp, FBS, Response Bias Scale or RBS, and the Henry-Heilbronner Index) to discriminate between individuals who were neuropsychologically evaluated in a clinical context versus those involved in litigation and/or the pursuit of financial compensation. Several statistical approaches suggested RBS was the best of the five for identifying individuals in litigation (Tsushima, Geling, & Fabrigas, 2011). The same research group found RBS to also be the most accurate validity scale in differentiating TBI litigants with valid versus invalid test cognitive test effort (Tsushima, Geling, & Woo, 2013). Similarly, using an analog simulation design, Sullivan and Elliott (2012) found RBS to be the strongest MMPI-2 validity scale predictor of feigned memory impairment, outperforming FBS, F, and K. Peck et al (2013) investigated the ability of FBS and RBS to identify poor effort in a forensic sample of TBI claimants and a clinical sample with nonepileptic seizures. FBS and RBS, alone and in combination, effectively distinguished between individuals who met criteria for malingering and those who did not; when used in combination, no members of the TBI group or nonepileptic seizure group with good effort were misclassified.

MMPI-2 and MMPI-2-RF

Several recent studies investigate both MMPI-2 and MMPI-2-RF validity scales, all of which support their use in detecting response bias. For an excellent updated review of the validity scales in MMPI-2 and MMPI-2-RF, including the empirical basis for their use in forensic settings, see Hoelzle, Nelson, and Arbisi (2012). Jones and Ingram (2011) compared original MMPI-2 validity scales to new scales developed for the MMPI-2/RF. These authors found that the new scales (HHI, RBS, FBS, and FBS-r) outperformed the original F-family of scales in classifying active duty military personnel who passed versus failed a PVT. Related, Archer, Hagan, Mason, Handel, and Archer (2012) compared L and K from the MMPI-2 to L-r and K-r from the MMPI-2-RF in a sample of custody evaluation litigants and found substantial consistency between the test versions. An archival study by Dragon, Ben-Porath, and Handel (2012) demonstrated that unscorable MMPI-2 and MMPI-2-RF responses occur in a high proportion most commonly in forensic samples. Bolstering the case for their use in forensic contexts, these authors demonstrated that Revised Clinical scale scores are robust to a high proportion of unscorable responses in terms of both validity and interpretability.

MMPI-2-RF

As the newest version of the MMPI, the MMPI-2-RF continues to face questions regarding the validity of its results and its application in forensic settings. Ben-Porath (2012) comprehensively addresses challenges to MMPI-2-RF–based testimony, including issues related to Daubert standards and the growing empirical basis for the new version. The studies described in the present review, as well as many others published since the MMPI-2-RF was released in 2008, continue to expand the empirical basis for using the MMPI-2-RF in forensic neuropsychological assessment, particularly for detecting response bias and malingering. For example, recent validation studies have suggested optimal cutoff scores for both the overreporting and underreporting validity scales in a variety of clinical and forensic populations (e.g., Schroeder et al., 2012). The validity scales are very effective in classifying those who are feigning cognitive impairment, as indicated by PVT failure, in both military (Jones, Ingram, & Ben-Porath, 2012) and non–head injury disability claimants (Tarescavage, Wygant, Gervais, & Ben-Porath, 2013). In a military sample, FBS/FBS-r and RBS have been shown to differentiate among those with and without pending disability claims (e.g., Nelson et al., 2011). The MMPI-2-RF validity scales, particularly Fs and Fp-r, also have excellent utility in distinguishing between noncredible somatic complaints and genuine medical illness (Sellbom, Wygant, & Bagby, 2012).

Several articles pertaining to the clinical validity of MMPI-2-RF results bear mentioning. First, it is important to note that rates of elevated scales in the normative sample are remarkably consistent with epidemiologic data, providing critical base-rate information for interpreting scale elevations appropriately (Tarescavage, Marek, et al., 2013). Second, the instrument shows good diagnostic construct validity (Sellbom, Bagby, Kushner, Quilty, & Ayearst, 2012), including evidence of a profile associated with PTSD in a forensic disability sample (Sellbom, Lee, Ben-Porath, Arbisi, & Gervais, 2012). Third, invalid profiles of disability claimants, as determined by validity scale elevations, are associated with attenuated extratest criterion validity and with significantly greater elevations on all of the Restructured Clinical scales as compared to profiles without elevated validity scales (Wiggins, Wygant, Hoelzle, & Gervais, 2012). A similar result was obtained in a combined sample of college students, male prisoners, and male psychiatric outpatients from a Veterans Administration facility (Forbey, Lee, Ben-Porath, Arbisi, & Gartland, 2013). Specifically, scores on MMPI-2-RF substantive scales and collateral measures were significantly affected in the expected direction when the MMPI-2-RF validity scales indicated overreporting or underreporting response styles.

PAI

In contrast to the MMPI family of tests, relevant literature on the PAI continues to grow at a more limited pace. Gaines, Giles, and Morgan (2013) developed a new index of symptom exaggeration termed the Multiscale Feigning Index. Validated on a sample of male inmates on an inpatient psychiatric unit and using Structured Interview of Reported Symptoms as the feigning criterion, regression analyses indicated that the Multiscale Feigning Index was a stronger predictor of feigning than traditional PAI validity indicators.

Other recent articles examine the PAI profiles specific to diagnoses of mTBI and PTSD. One new study examined PAI profile differences between patients with mTBI who are and are not compensation seeking (Whiteside, Galbreath, Brown, & Turnbull, 2012). The authors found significant group differences, with the compensation-seeking patients demonstrating greater negative response bias and higher scores on scales related to somatic and internalizing symptoms. Similarly, two recent papers demonstrated that the PAI's validity scales are generally effective in distinguishing feigned from genuine PTSD (Rogers, Gillard, Wooley, & Ross, 2012; Thomas, Hopwood, Orlando, Weathers, & McDevitt-Murphy, 2011), suggesting the instrument's viability for use in forensic settings.

FORENSIC NEUROPSYCHOLOGICAL ASSESSMENT OF PAIN

Because pain and cognitive complaints often co-occur among those seeking personal injury treatment and compensation, the evaluation of pain has proven a growing area of interest for neuropsychologists. *The Clinical Neuropsychologist* recently published a special issue on pain psychology (for an introduction to the issue, see Greiffenstein & Bianchini [2013]). Additionally, recent evidence has continued to replicate the finding that among injured individuals who are eventually considered "disabled," the largest amount of variance at 12 months postinjury is accounted for by psychiatric, rather than physical, factors (O'Donnell et al., 2013). This is not the first study to draw such conclusions; see the discussion in Block, Ben-Porath, and Marek (2013) of decades of outcome studies showing psychosocial factors as predictors of poor surgical outcomes.

As is true in any forensic evaluation, assessing performance validity and response bias is critical. Greiffenstein, Gervais, Baker, Artiola, and Smith (2013) examined individuals with complex regional pain syndrome-type I (formerly termed "reflex sympathetic dystrophy") who were in the process of seeking disability. Failure rates on PVTs were high, ranging from 23% on the Test of Memory Malingering to 50% on Reliable Digit Span. Similarly, validity of symptom reporting on the MMPI-2 or MMPI-2-RF was also problematic, ranging from 15% to 50% of subsamples with compromised validity. Such findings clearly demonstrate that individuals who report pain in a secondary gain context may exaggerate their related disability, not only by *reporting* an exaggerated degree of discomfort and disability, but also by *behaving* as though basic cognitive processes are disrupted.

Some years earlier, published studies such as Greiffenstein et al. (2013) led clinical researchers to define *malingered pain-related disability* as "intentional exaggeration or fabrication of cognitive, emotional, behavioral, or physical dysfunction attributed to pain for the purposes of obtaining financial gain, to avoid work, or obtain drugs" (Bianchini, Greve, & Glynn, 2005, p. 407). More recently, two of these authors provided an overview of pain assessment from a psychological perspective (Greve, Bianchini, & Brewer, 2013), noting the direct applicability in a secondary gain context of PVTs (e.g., TOMM, WMT) and SVTs (validity scales from MMPI-2 and MMPI-2-RF) commonly used to evaluate response validity in cases alleging neuropsychological dysfunction to the evaluation of cases alleging chronic disabling pain. Greve, Bianchini, et al. (2013) provide multiple data classification tables showing score frequency differences between individuals with no incentive versus those with incentive to appear disabled by pain and convincingly argue that both PVTs and SVTs are needed to ensure accurate discrimination of credible versus exaggerated presentations of pain. In this regard, forensic evaluation of pain appears comparable to forensic evaluation of other disorders, such as TBI and PTSD, in terms of requiring attention to evaluating response validity broadly (Elhai, Sweet, Guidotti Breting, & Kaloupek, 2012).

SUMMARY

The clinical research literature related to forensic neuropsychology continues to expand at an impressive rate. There are too many topics and publications on even the most important forensic topic to provide comprehensive coverage in a single chapter. Developing neuroscience technologies, such as those involving neuroimaging, are increasingly considered for inclusion in courtroom proceedings, but as yet have not made significant inroads. The potential for admission of new neuroscience technologies has raised concern among both legal scholars and behavioral experts. Although the science behind these technologies will continue to improve, it is not clear that any yet identified techniques will prove truly informative on matters that are ultimately more within the purview of behavioral experts, such as neuropsychologists. Clinical judgment, meaning the reasoning and multimethod integrative ability of trained professional neuropsychologists, remains the glue that ties data together in order to answer psycholegal questions. Related to the increasing reliance on clinical neuropsychologists as testifying experts, there are no systemic evidentiary problems for our specialty. The occasional exclusion of specific experts or specific tests in unique jurisdictions is expected, does not form a worrisome pattern, and merely illustrates the highly individualistic nature of trials.

Related to world events and associated media coverage, such topics as mTBI and concussion in civilian life and mTBI, concussion, and PTSD in military life have increasingly been topics addressed in the professional literatures of numerous disciplines. As these can relate to legal and administrative proceedings, it has been informative to see the growth of peer-reviewed research that provides guidance, especially in bringing the decades of prior research to bear in creating expectations regarding natural outcomes and response to treatment.

As specific forensic literature continues to be published, there will surely be additional studies confirming the need to evaluate the different forms that response bias can take. There will undoubtedly continue to be discussion regarding the need to use multiple validity indicators, and in doing so being mindful of, and responsive to, concerns regarding the issue of false-positives. Specific populations, such as children and adolescents, as well as individuals reporting chronic pain, will likely continue to receive increased attention in the forensic literature.

As detailed in the introduction to this chapter, the topic of malingering has been very prominent in the clinical neuropsychology literature for decades, and remains so. Our specialty has effectively invested considerable time and energy into developing relevant methods because the failure to identify malingering is costly to society. Examples include media coverage of a billion dollars lost by the Railroad Retirement Board to fraudulent disability (e.g., Rashbaum, 2012), more than a million dollars lost in a single fraudulent personal injury claim (Chapman, 2011), and estimates in the multi-billions of dollars lost to feigned disability in the Social Security system (Chafetz & Underhill, 2013). With limited societal resources at hand for those who are legitimately injured or ill, such data ensure that malingering will remain the most prominent topic in forensic neuropsychology in years to come.

REFERENCES

Allen, D. N., Thaler, N. S., Ringdahl, E. N., Barney, S. J., & Mayfield, J. (2012). Comprehensive Trail Making Test performance in children and adolescents with traumatic brain injury. *Psychological Assessment, 24*(3), 556–564. doi:10.1037/a0026263

American Academy of Clinical Neuropsychology. (2007). American Academy of Clinical Neuropsychology (AACN) practice guidelines for neuropsychological assessment and consultation. *The Clinical Neuropsychologist, 21*(2), 209–231. doi:10.1080/13825580601025932

Aoki, Y., Inokuchi, R., Gunshin, M., Yahagi, N., & Suwa, H. (2012). Diffusion tensor imaging studies of mild traumatic brain injury: A meta-analysis. *J Neurol Neurosurg Psychiatry, 83*(9), 870–876. doi:10.1136/jnnp-2012-302742

Archer, E. M., Hagan, L. D., Mason, J., Handel, R., & Archer, R. P. (2012). MMPI-2-RF characteristics of custody evaluation litigants. *Assessment, 19*(1), 14–20. doi:10.1177/1073191110397469

Armistead-Jehle, P., & Buican, B. (2012). Evaluation context and Symptom Validity Test performances in a U.S. Military sample. *Archives of Clinical Neuropsychology, 27*(8), 828–839. doi:10.1093/arclin/acs086

Barney, S. J., Allen, D. N., Thaler, N. S., Park, B. S., Strauss, G. P., & Mayfield, J. (2011). Neuropsychological and behavioral measures of attention assess different constructs in children with traumatic brain injury. *The Clinical Neuropsychologist, 25*(7), 1145–1157. doi:10.1080/13854046.2011.595956

Barsky, A. J. (2002). Forgetting, fabricating, and telescoping: The instability of the medical history. *Archives of Internal Medicine, 162*, 981–984.

Barth, R. J. (2009). Examinee-reported history is not a credible basis for clinical or administrative decision making. *AMA Guides Newsletter.*

Belanger, H. G., Proctor-Weber, Z., Kretzmer, T., Kim, M., French, L. M., & Vanderploeg, R. D. (2011). Symptom complaints following reports of blast versus non-blast mild TBI: Does mechanism of injury matter? *The Clinical Neuropsychologist, 25*(5), 702–715. doi:10.1080/13854046.2011.566892

Ben-Porath, Y. S. (2012). Addressing challenges to MMPI-2-RF-based testimony: Questions and answers. *Archives of Clinical Neuropsychology, 27*(7), 691–705. doi:10.1093/arclin/acs083

Berthelson, L., Mulchan, S. S., Odland, A. P., Miller, L. J., & Mittenberg, W. (2013). False positive diagnosis of malingering due to the use of multiple effort tests. *Brain Injury, 27*(7-8), 909–916. doi:10.3109/02699052.2013.793400

Betthauser, L. M., Bahraini, N., Krengel, M. H., & Brenner, L. A. (2012). Self-report measures to identify post traumatic stress disorder and/or mild traumatic brain injury and associated symptoms in military veterans of Operation Enduring Freedom (OEF)/Operation Iraqi Freedom (OIF). *Neuropsychol Rev, 22*(1), 35–53. doi:10.1007/s11065-012-9191-4

Bianchini, K. J., Greve, K. W., & Glynn, G. (2005). On the diagnosis of malingered pain-related disability: Lessons from cognitive malingering research. *The Spine Journal, 5*(4), 404–417. doi:10.1016/j.spinee.2004.11.016

Block, A. R., Ben-Porath, Y. S., & Marek, R. J. (2013). Psychological risk factors for poor outcome of spine surgery and spinal cord stimulator implant: A review of the literature and their assessment with the MMPI-2-RF. *The Clinical Neuropsychologist, 27*(1), 81–107. doi:10.1080/13854046.2012.721007

Boone, K. B. (2009). The need for continuous and comprehensive sampling of effort/response bias during neuropsychological examinations. *The Clinical Neuropsychologist, 23*(4), 729–741. doi:10.1080/13854040802427803

Boone, K. B. (2013). *Clinical practice of forensic neuropsychology: An evidence-based approach.* New York: Guilford Press.

Brooks, B. L. (2012). Victoria Symptom Validity Test performance in children and adolescents with neurological disorders. *Archives of Clinical Neuropsychology, 27*(8), 858–868. doi:10.1093/arclin/acs087

Brown v. Entertainment Merchants Association, No. 08-1448, 131 2729 (Supreme Court 2011).

Bush, S. S., & NAN Policy & Planning Committee. (2005). Independent and court-ordered forensic neuropsychological examinations: Official statement of the National Academy of Neuropsychology. *Archives of Clinical Neuropsychology, 20*(8), 997–1007. doi:10.1016/j.acn.2005.06.003

Bush, S. S., Ruff, R. M., Troster, A. I., Barth, J. T., Koffler, S. P., Pliskin, N. H., . . . Silver, C. H. (2005). Symptom validity assessment: Practice issues and medical necessity NAN policy & planning committee. *Archives of Clinical Neuropsychology, 20*(4), 419–426. doi:10.1016/j.acn.2005.02.002

Butcher, J. N., Gass, C. S., Cumella, E., Kally, Z., & Williams, C. L. (2008). Potential for bias in MMPI-2 assessments using the Fake Bad Scale (FBS). *Psychological Injury and Law, 1*(3), 191–209.

Chafetz, M., & Underhill, J. (2013). Estimated costs of malingered disability. *Archives of Clinical Neuropsychology, 28*(7), 633–639. Chapman, E. (2011). Fraud—July 2011. *Weightmans Newsletter.* Retrieved from http://www.weightmans.com/library/newsletters/fraud_-_july_2011/contempt_of_court.aspx

Couch, C. M., & Leathem, J. M. (2011). An initial study to establish symptom base rates of traumatic brain injury in children. *Archives of Clinical Neuropsychology, 26*(4), 349–355. doi:10.1093/arclin/acr028

Davis, J. J., Axelrod, B. N., McHugh, T. S., Hanks, R. A., & Millis, S. R. (2013). Number of impaired scores as a performance validity indicator. *J Clin Exp Neuropsychol, 35*(4), 413–420. doi:10.1080/13803395.2013.781134

Davis, P. C., Wippold, F. J., Cornelius, R. S., Aiken, A. H., Angtuaco, E. J., Berger, K. L., . . . Douglas, A. C. (2012). ACR Appropriateness Criteria Head Trauma. Retrieved from http://www.acr.org/Quality-Safety/Appropriateness-Criteria

Don, A. S., & Carragee, E. J. (2009). Is the self-reported history accurate in patients with persistent axial pain after a motor vehicle accident? *The Spine Journal, 9*(1), 4–12. doi:10.1016/j.spinee.2008.11.002

Dragon, W. R., Ben-Porath, Y. S., & Handel, R. W. (2012). Examining the impact of unscorable item responses on the validity and interpretability of MMPI-2/MMPI-2-RF Restructured Clinical (RC) Scale scores. *Assessment, 19*(1), 101–113. doi:10.1177/1073191111415362

Echemendia, R. J., Iverson, G. L., McCrea, M., Broshek, D. K., Gioia, G. A., Sautter, S. W., . . . Barr, W. B. (2011). Role of neuropsychologists in the evaluation and management of sport-related concussion: An inter-organization position statement. *The Clinical Neuropsychologist, 25*(8), 1289–1294. doi:10.1080/13854046.2011.618466

Echemendia, R. J., Iverson, G. L., McCrea, M., Macciocchi, S. N., Gioia, G. A., Putukian, M., & Comper, P. (2013). Advances in neuropsychological assessment of sport-related concussion. *British Journal of Sports Medicine, 47*(5), 294–298. doi:10.1136/bjsports-2013-092186

Eggen, J. M., & Laury, E. J. (2011). Toward a neuroscience model of tort law: How functional neuroimaging will transform tort doctrine. *Columbia Science and Technology Law Review, 1*, 1–92.

Elhai, J. D., Sweet, J., Guidotti Breting, L. M., & Kaloupek, D. G. (2012). Assessment contexts that threaten response validity. In J. J. Vasterling, A. Bryant, & T. M. Keane (Eds.), *PTSD and mild traumatic brain injury* (pp. 174–200). New York: Guilford Press.

Fabian, J. M., Thompson IV, W. W., & Lazarus, J. B. (2011). Life, death, and IQ: It's much more than just a score: Understanding and utilizing forensic psychological and neuropsychological evaluations in Atkins Intellectual Disability/Mental Retardation cases. *Cleveland State Law Review, 59,* 399–430.

Forbey, J. D., Lee, T. T., Ben-Porath, Y. S., Arbisi, P. A., & Gartland, D. (2013). Associations between MMPI-2-RF validity scale scores and extra-test measures of personality and psychopathology. *Assessment, 20*(4), 448–461. doi:10.1177/1073191113478154

Frye v. United States, 293 F. 1013 (D.C. Cir. 1923).

Gaines, M. V., Giles, C. L., & Morgan, R. D. (2013). The detection of feigning using multiple PAI scale elevations: A new index. *Assessment, 20*(4), 437–447. doi:10.1177/1073191112458146

Giza, C. C., Kutcher, J. S., Ashwal, S., Barth, J., Getchius, T. S., Gioia, G. A., . . . Zafonte, R. (2013). Summary of evidence-based guideline update: Evaluation and management of concussion in sports: report of the Guideline Development Subcommittee of the American Academy of Neurology. *Neurology, 80*(24), 2250–2257. doi:10.1212/WNL.0b013e31828d57dd

Greiffenstein, M. F., & Bianchini, K. J. (2013). Introduction to pain psychology special issue. *The Clinical Neuropsychologist, 27*(1), 14–16. doi:10.1080/13854046.2012.739645

Greiffenstein, M. F., Gervais, R., Baker, W. J., Artiola, L., & Smith, H. (2013). Symptom validity testing in medically unexplained pain: A chronic regional pain syndrome type 1 case series. *The Clinical Neuropsychologist, 27*(1), 138–147. doi:10.1080/13854046.2012.722686

Greve, K. W., Bianchini, K. J., & Brewer, S. T. (2013). The assessment of performance and self-report validity in persons claiming pain-related disability. *The Clinical Neuropsychologist, 27*(1), 108–137. doi:10.1080/13854046.2012.739646

Greve, K. W., Binder, L. M., & Bianchini, K. J. (2009). Rates of below-chance performance in forced-choice symptom validity tests. *The Clinical Neuropsychologist, 23*(3), 534–544. doi:10.1080/13854040802232690

Greve, K. W., Curtis, K. L., & Bianchini, K. J. (2013). Symptom validity testing: A summary of current research. In S. Koffler, J. Morgan, I. Baron, & M. Greiffenstein (Eds.), *Neuropsychology science & practice* (Vol. 1, pp. 61–94). New York: Oxford University Press.

Harmon, K. G., Drezner, J. A., Gammons, M., Guskiewicz, K. M., Halstead, M., Herring, S. A., . . . Roberts, W. O. (2013). American Medical Society for Sports Medicine position statement: Concussion in sport. *British Journal of Sports Medicine, 47*(1), 15–26. doi:10.1136/bjsports-2012-091941

Heilbronner, R. L., Sweet, J., Morgan, J. E., Larrabee, G. J., Millis, S. R., & Conference Participants. (2009). American Academy of Clinical Neuropsychology consensus conference statement on the neuropsychological assessment of effort, response bias, and malingering. *The Clinical Neuropsychologist, 23*(7), 1093–1129. doi:10.1080/13854040903155063

Herring, S. A., Cantu, R. C., Guskiewicz, K. M., Putukian, M., Kibler, W. B., Bergfeld, J. A., . . . American College of Sports Medicine. (2011). Concussion (mild traumatic brain injury) and the team physician: A consensus statement—2011 update. *Med Sci Sports Exerc, 43*(12), 2412–2422. doi:10.1249/MSS.0b013e3182342e64

Hoelzle, J. B., Nelson, N. W., & Arbisi, P. A. (2012). MMPI-2 and MMPI-2-Restructured Form validity scales: Complementary approaches to evaluate response validity. *Psychological Injury and Law, 5*(3-4), 174–191. doi:10.1007/s12207-012-9139-2

Hoge, C. W., Goldberg, H. M., & Castro, C. A. (2009). Care of war veterans with mild traumatic brain injury—flawed perspectives. *New England Journal of Medicine, 360*(16), 1588–1591.

Hurewitz, F., & Kerr, S. (2011). The role of the independent neuropsychologist in special education. *The Clinical Neuropsychologist, 25*(6), 1058–1074. doi:10.1080/13854046.2011.565077

Iverson, G. L. (2006). Misdiagnosis of the persistent postconcussion syndrome in patients with depression. *Archives of Clinical Neuropsychology, 21*(4), 303–310. doi:10.1016/j.acn.2005.12.008

Iverson, G. L., Lange, R. T., Brooks, B. L., & Rennison, V. L. (2010). "Good old days" bias following mild traumatic brain injury. *The Clinical Neuropsychologist, 24*(1), 17–37. doi:10.1080/13854040903190797

Jasinski, L. J., Harp, J. P., Berry, D. T., Shandera-Ochsner, A. L., Mason, L. H., & Ranseen, J. D. (2011). Using symptom validity tests to detect malingered ADHD in college students. *The Clinical Neuropsychologist, 25*(8), 1415–1428. doi:10.1080/13854046.2011.630024

Jones, A., & Ingram, M. V. (2011). A comparison of selected MMPI-2 and MMPI-2-RF validity scales in assessing effort on cognitive tests in a military sample. *The Clinical Neuropsychologist, 25*(7), 1207–1227. doi:10.1080/13854046.2011.600726

Jones, A., Ingram, M. V., & Ben-Porath, Y. S. (2012). Scores on the MMPI-2-RF scales as a function of increasing levels of failure on cognitive symptom validity tests in a military sample. *The Clinical Neuropsychologist, 26*(5), 790–815. doi:10.1080/13854046.2012.693202

Kaufmann, P. M. (2012). Admissibility of expert opinions based on neuropsychological evidence. In G. Larrabee (Ed.), *Forensic neuropsychology: A scientific approach* (2nd ed.) (pp. 70–100). New York: Oxford University Press.

Kelly, M. P., Coldren, R. L., Parish, R. V., Dretsch, M. N., & Russell, M. L. (2012). Assessment of acute concussion in the combat environment. *Archives of Clinical Neuropsychology, 27*(4), 375–388. doi:10.1093/arclin/acs036

Kennedy, C. H., Porter Evans, J., Chee, S., Moore, J. L., Barth, J. T., & Stuessi, K. A. (2012). Return to combat duty after concussive blast injury. *Archives of Clinical Neuropsychology, 27*(8), 817–827. doi:10.1093/arclin/acs092

Khoshbin, L. S., & Khoshbin, S. (2007). Imaging the mind, minding the image: An historical introduction to brain imaging and the law. *American Journal of Law & Medicine, 33*, 171–192.

Kirkwood, M. W., Hargrave, D. D., & Kirk, J. W. (2011). The value of the WISC-IV Digit Span subtest in detecting noncredible performance during pediatric neuropsychological examinations. *Archives of Clinical Neuropsychology, 26*(5), 377–384. doi:10.1093/arclin/acr040

Kirkwood, M. W., Yeates, K. O., Randolph, C., & Kirk, J. W. (2012). The implications of symptom validity test failure for ability-based test performance in a pediatric sample. *Psychological Assessment, 24*(1), 36–45. doi:10.1037/a0024628

Larrabee, G. J. (2012a). Performance validity and symptom validity in neuropsychological assessment. *Journal of the International Neuropsychological Society, 18*(04), 625–631. doi:10.1017/s1355617712000240

Larrabee, G. J. (Ed.). (2012b). *Forensic neuropsychology: A scientific approach* (2nd ed.). New York: Oxford University Press.

Larrabee, G. J., Binder, L. M., Rohling, M. L., & Ploetz, D. M. (2013). Meta-analytic methods and the importance of non-TBI factors related to outcome in mild traumatic brain injury: Response to Bigler et al. (2013). *The Clinical Neuropsychologist, 27*(2), 215–237. doi:10.1080/13854046.2013.769634

Law, J. (2011). Cherry-picking memories: Why neuroimaging-based lie detection requires a new framework for the admissibility of scientific evidence under FRE 702 and Daubert. *Yale Journal of Law & Technology, 14*, 1.

Le v. Barnes, No. SACV 12-393-DSF(CW), LEXIS, 175559 (U.S. Dist. 2012).

Lee, T. T., Graham, J. R., Sellbom, M., & Gervais, R. O. (2012). Examining the potential for gender bias in the prediction of symptom validity test failure by MMPI-2 symptom validity scale scores. *Psychological Assessment, 24*(3), 618–627. doi:10.1037/a0026458

Liefland, L. (2012). Psych testing 101: A lawyer's guide to psychological reports. *The Champion, 36*, 40–42.

Lindstrom, W., Coleman, C., Thomassin, K., Southall, C. M., & Lindstrom, J. H. (2011). Simulated dyslexia in postsecondary students: Description and detection using embedded validity indicators. *The Clinical Neuropsychologist, 25*(2), 302–322. doi:10.1080/13854046.2010.537280

Loughan, A. R., Perna, R., & Hertza, J. (2012). The value of the wechsler intelligence scale for children-fourth edition digit span as an embedded measure of effort: An investigation into children with dual diagnoses. *Archives of Clinical Neuropsychology, 27*(7), 716–724. doi:10.1093/arclin/acs072

Marino, S. E., Meador, K. J., Loring, D. W., Okun, M. S., Fernandez, H. H., Fessler, A. J., . . . Werz, M. A. (2009). Subjective perception of cognition is related to mood and not performance. *Epilepsy & Behavior, 14*(3), 459–464. doi:10.1016/j.yebeh.2008.12.007

McCabe, D. P., & Castel, A. D. (2008). Seeing is believing: The effect of brain images on judgments of scientific reasoning. *Cognition, 107*(1), 343–352.

McCrea, M., Pliskin, N., Barth, J., Cox, D., Fink, J., French, L., . . . Yoash-Gantz, R. (2008). Official position of the military TBI task force on the role of neuropsychology and rehabilitation psychology in the evaluation, management, and research of military veterans with traumatic brain injury. *The Clinical Neuropsychologist, 22*(1), 10–26. doi:10.1080/13854040701760981

McCrory, P., Meeuwisse, W. H., Echemendia, R. J., Iverson, G. L., Dvorak, J., & Kutcher, J. S. (2013). What is the lowest threshold to make a diagnosis of concussion? *British Journal of Sports Medicine, 47*(5), 268–271. doi:10.1136/bjsports-2013-092247

McNally, K. A., Bangert, B., Dietrich, A., Nuss, K., Rusin, J., Wright, M., . . . Yeates, K. O. (2013). Injury versus noninjury factors as predictors of postconcussive symptoms following mild traumatic brain injury in children. *Neuropsychology, 27*(1), 1–12. doi:10.1037/a0031370

Meares, S., Shores, E. A., Taylor, A. J., Batchelor, J., Bryant, R. A., Baguley, I. J., . . . Marosszeky, J. E. (2011). The prospective course of postconcussion syndrome: The role of mild traumatic brain injury. *Neuropsychology, 25*(4), 454–465. doi:10.1037/a0022580

Moriarty, J. C. (2008). Flickering admissibility: Neuroimaging evidence in the U.S. courts. *Behavioral Sciences & the Law, 26*(1), 29–49. doi:10.1002/bsl.795

Morse, S. (2011). Avoiding irrational NeuroLaw exuberance: A plea for neuromodesty. *Law, Innovation and Technology, 3*(2), 209–228.

Musso, M. W., Barker, A. A., Jones, G. N., Roid, G. H., & Gouvier, W. D. (2011). Development and validation of the Stanford Binet-5 Rarely Missed Items-Nonverbal index for the detection of malingered mental retardation. *Archives of Clinical Neuropsychology*, *26*(8), 756–767. doi:10.1093/arclin/acr078

Nelson, N. W., Hoelzle, J. B., Doane, B. M., McGuire, K. A., Ferrier-Auerbach, A. G., Charlesworth, M. J., . . . Sponheim, S. R. (2012). Neuropsychological outcomes of U.S. Veterans with report of remote blast-related concussion and current psychopathology. *Journal of the International Neuropsychological Society*, *18*(5), 845–855. doi:10.1017/S1355617712000616

Nelson, N. W., Hoelzle, J. B., McGuire, K. A., Sim, A. H., Goldman, D. J., Ferrier-Auerbach, A. G., . . . Sponheim, S. R. (2011). Self-report of psychological function among OEF/OIF personnel who also report combat-related concussion. *The Clinical Neuropsychologist*, *25*(5), 716–740. doi:10.1080/13854046.2011.579174

Nelson, N. W., Sweet, J. J., Berry, D. T., Bryant, F. B., Granacher, R. P., Arbisi, P., . . . Greve, K. (2007). Response validity in forensic neuropsychology: Exploratory factor analytic evidence of distinct cognitive and psychological constructs. *Journal of the International Neuropsychological Society*, *13*(3), 440–449.

O'Donnell, M. L., Varker, T., Holmes, A. C., Ellen, S., Wade, D., Creamer, M., . . . Forbes, D. (2013). Disability after injury: The cumulative burden of physical and mental health. *J Clin Psychiatry*, *74*(2), e137–143. doi:10.4088/JCP.12m08011

Peck, C. P., Schroeder, R. W., Heinrichs, R. J., Vondran, E. J., Brockman, C. J., Webster, B. K., & Baade, L. E. (2013). Differences in MMPI-2 FBS and RBS scores in brain injury, probable malingering, and conversion disorder groups: A preliminary study. *The Clinical Neuropsychologist*, *27*(4), 693–707. doi:10.1080/13854046.2013.779032

Pella, R. D., Hill, B. D., Shelton, J. T., Elliott, E., & Gouvier, W. D. (2012). Evaluation of embedded malingering indices in a non-litigating clinical sample using control, clinical, and derived groups. *Archives of Clinical Neuropsychology*, *27*(1), 45–57. doi:10.1093/arclin/acr090

Penney, S. R., & Skilling, T. A. (2012). Moderators of informant agreement in the assessment of adolescent psychopathology: Extension to a forensic sample. *Psychological Assessment*, *24*(2), 386–401. doi:10.1037/a0025693

Ponsford, J., Cameron, P., Fitzgerald, M., Grant, M., Mikocka-Walus, A., & Schonberger, M. (2012). Predictors of postconcussive symptoms 3 months after mild traumatic brain injury. *Neuropsychology*, *26*(3), 304–313. doi:10.1037/a0027888

Ponsford, J., Willmott, C., Rothwell, A., Cameron, P., Kelly, A., Nelms, R., . . . Ng, K. (2000). Factors influencing outcome following mild traumatic brain injury in adults. *Journal of the International Neuropsychological Society*, *6*(05), 568–579.

Rabin, L. A., Barr, W. B., & Burton, L. A. (2005). Assessment practices of clinical neuropsychologists in the United States and Canada: A survey of INS, NAN, and APA Division 40 members. *Archives of Clinical Neuropsychology*, *20*(1), 33–65. doi:10.1016/j.acn.2004.02.005

Rashbaum, W. K. (2012). More arrests of retirees in fraud case at L.I.R.R., *The New York Times*. Retrieved from http://www.nytimes.com/2012/09/13/nyregion/more-lirr-retirees-arrested-on-fraud-charges.html

Ricker, J. (2012). Functional neuroimaging in forensic neuropsychology. In G. Larrabee (Ed.), *Forensic neuropsychology: A scientific approach* (2nd ed.) (pp. 160–178). New York: Oxford University Press.

Rogers, R., Gillard, N. D., Wooley, C. N., & Ross, C. A. (2012). The detection of feigned disabilities: The effectiveness of the Personality Assessment Inventory in a traumatized inpatient sample. *Assessment*, *19*(1), 77–88. doi:10.1177/1073191111422031

Roskies, A. L., Schweitzer, N., & Saks, M. J. (2013). Neuroimages in court: Less biasing than feared. *Trends in Cognitive Sciences, 17*, 99–101.

Roth, S. B. (2012). The emergence of neuroscience evidence in Louisiana. *Tul. L. Rev., 87*, 197–197.

Ruff, R. M., Iverson, G. L., Barth, J. T., Bush, S. S., Broshek, D. K., Policy, N. A. N., & Planning, C. (2009). Recommendations for diagnosing a mild traumatic brain injury: A National Academy of Neuropsychology education paper. *Archives of Clinical Neuropsychology, 24*(1), 3–10. doi:10.1093/arclin/acp006

Rushing, S. E., & Langleben, D. D. (2011). Relative function: Nuclear brain imaging in United States courts. *Journal of Psychiatry & Law, 39*, 567–593.

Schroeder, R. W., Baade, L. E., Peck, C. P., VonDran, E. J., Brockman, C. J., Webster, B. K., & Heinrichs, R. J. (2012). Validation of MMPI-2-RF validity scales in criterion group neuropsychological samples. *The Clinical Neuropsychologist, 26*(1), 129–146. doi:10.1080/13854046.2011.639314

Sellbom, M., Bagby, R. M., Kushner, S., Quilty, L. C., & Ayearst, L. E. (2012). Diagnostic construct validity of MMPI-2 Restructured Form (MMPI-2-RF) scale scores. *Assessment, 19*(2), 176–186. doi:10.1177/1073191111428763

Sellbom, M., Lee, T. T., Ben-Porath, Y. S., Arbisi, P. A., & Gervais, R. O. (2012). Differentiating PTSD symptomatology with the MMPI-2-RF (Restructured Form) in a forensic disability sample. *Psychiatry Res, 197*(1-2), 172–179. doi:10.1016/j.psychres.2012.02.003

Sellbom, M., Wygant, D., & Bagby, M. (2012). Utility of the MMPI-2-RF in detecting non-credible somatic complaints. *Psychiatry Res, 197*(3), 295–301. doi:10.1016/j.psychres.2011.12.043

Sherman, E. M., & Brooks, B. L. (Eds.). (2012). *Pediatric forensic neuropsychology.* New York: Oxford University Press.

Smart, C. M., Nelson, N. W., Sweet, J. J., Bryant, F. B., Berry, D. T., Granacher, R. P., & Heilbronner, R. L. (2008). Use of MMPI-2 to predict cognitive effort: A hierarchically optimal classification tree analysis. *Journal of the International Neuropsychological Society, 14*(05), 842–852.

Sollman, M. J., & Berry, D. T. (2011). Detection of inadequate effort on neuropsychological testing: A meta-analytic update and extension. *Archives of Clinical Neuropsychology, 26*(8), 774–789. doi:10.1093/arclin/acr066

Sullivan, K. A., & Elliott, C. (2012). An investigation of the validity of the MMPI-2 response bias scale using an analog simulation design. *The Clinical Neuropsychologist, 26*(1), 160–176. doi:10.1080/13854046.2011.647084

Sweet, J., Ecklund-Johnson, E., & Malina, A. (2008). Forensic neuropsychology: an overview of issues and directions. In J. E. Morgan & J. Ricker (Eds.), *Textbook of clinical neuropsychology* (pp. 869–890). New York: Taylor & Francis.

Sweet, J., Goldman, D. J., & Guidotti Breting, L. M. (2013). Traumatic brain injury: Guidance in a forensic context from outcome, dose-response, and response bias research. *Behavioral Sciences & the Law, 31*, 756–788.

Sweet, J., & Guidotti Breting, L. (2012). Symptom validity test research: Status and clinical implications. *Journal of Experimental Psychopathology, 4*, 6–19.

Sweet, J., King, J. H., Malina, A. C., Bergman, M. A., & Simmons, A. (2002). Documenting the prominence of forensic neuropsychology at national meetings and in relevant professional journals from 1990 to 2000. *The Clinical Neuropsychologist, 16*(4), 481–494.

Sweet, J., & Westerveld, M. (2012). Pediatric neuropsychology in forensic proceedings: Roles and procedures in the courtroom and beyond. In E. M. Sherman & B. L. Brooks (Eds.) (pp. 3–23). *Pediatric forensic neuropsychology.* New York: Oxford University Press.

Tarescavage, A. M., Marek, R. J., Finn, J. A., Hicks, A., Rapier, J. L., & Ben-Porath, Y. S. (2013). Minnesota Multiphasic Personality Inventory-2-Restructured Form (MMPI-2-RF) normative elevation rates: Comparisons with epidemiological prevalence rates. *The Clinical Neuropsychologist, 27,* 1106–1120.

Tarescavage, A. M., Wygant, D. B., Gervais, R. O., & Ben-Porath, Y. S. (2013). Association between the MMPI-2 Restructured Form (MMPI-2-RF) and malingered neurocognitive dysfunction among non-head injury disability claimants. *The Clinical Neuropsychologist, 27*(2), 313–335. doi:10.1080/13854046.2012.744099

Thomas, K. M., Hopwood, C. J., Orlando, M. J., Weathers, F. W., & McDevitt-Murphy, M. E. (2011). Detecting feigned PTSD using the Personality Assessment Inventory. *Psychological Injury and Law, 5*(3-4), 192–201. doi:10.1007/s12207-011-9111-6

Tsushima, W. T., Geling, O., & Fabrigas, J. (2011). Comparison of MMPI-2 validity scale scores of personal injury litigants and disability claimants. *The Clinical Neuropsychologist, 25*(8), 1403–1414. doi:10.1080/13854046.2011.613854

Tsushima, W. T., Geling, O., & Woo, A. (2013). Comparison of four MMPI-2 validity scales in identifying invalid neurocognitive dysfunction in traumatic brain injury litigants. *Applied Neuropsychology: Adult, 20*(4), 263–271. doi:10.1080/09084282.2012.701679

Van Dyke, S. A., Millis, S. R., Axelrod, B. N., & Hanks, R. A. (2013). Assessing effort: Differentiating performance and symptom validity. *The Clinical Neuropsychologist, 27,* 1–13. doi:10.1080/13854046.2013.835447

Vasterling, J. J., Bryant, R. A., & Keane, T. M. (Eds.). (2012). *PTSD and mild traumatic brain injury:* New York: Guilford Press.

Victor, T. L., Boone, K. B., Serpa, J. G., Buehler, J., & Ziegler, E. A. (2009). Interpreting the meaning of multiple symptom validity test failure. *The Clinical Neuropsychologist, 23*(2), 297–313. doi:10.1080/13854040802232682

Wang, Y., Chan, R. C., & Deng, Y. (2006). Examination of postconcussion-like symptoms in healthy university students: Relationships to subjective and objective neuropsychological function performance. *Archives of Clinical Neuropsychology, 21*(4), 339–347. doi:10.1016/j.acn.2006.03.006

Weisberg, D. S., Keil, F. C., Goodstein, J., Rawson, E., & Gray, J. R. (2008). The seductive allure of neuroscience explanations. *Journal of Cognitive Neuroscience, 20*(3), 470–477.

Whiteside, D. M., Galbreath, J., Brown, M., & Turnbull, J. (2012). Differential response patterns on the Personality Assessment Inventory (PAI) in compensation-seeking and non-compensation-seeking mild traumatic brain injury patients. *J Clin Exp Neuropsychol, 34*(2), 172–182. doi:10.1080/13803395.2011.630648

Wiggins, C. W., Wygant, D. B., Hoelzle, J. B., & Gervais, R. O. (2012). The more you say the less it means: Overreporting and attenuated criterion validity in a forensic disability sample. *Psychological Injury and Law, 5*(3-4), 162–173. doi:10.1007/s12207-012-9137-4

Williams, M. W., Rapport, L. J., Hanks, R. A., Millis, S. R., & Greene, H. A. (2013). Incremental validity of neuropsychological evaluations to computed tomography in predicting long-term outcomes after traumatic brain injury. *The Clinical Neuropsychologist, 27*(3), 356–375. doi:10.1080/13854046.2013.765507

Wortzel, H. S., Filley, C. M., Anderson, C. A., Oster, T., & Arciniegas, D. B. (2008). Forensic applications of cerebral single photon emission computed tomography in mild traumatic brain injury. *Journal of the American Academy of Psychiatry and the Law Online, 36*(3), 310–322.

Wortzel, H. S., Kraus, M. F., Filley, C. M., Anderson, C. A., & Arciniegas, D. B. (2011). Diffusion tensor imaging in mild traumatic brain injury litigation. *Journal of the American Academy of Psychiatry and the Law Online, 39*(4), 511–523.

4

BLAST-RELATED TRAUMATIC BRAIN INJURY

Review and Update

Nathaniel W. Nelson and Peter T. Keenan

INTRODUCTION AND CONTEXT

Soldiers and other personnel who have served in support of the recent wars in Iraq (Operation Iraqi Freedom [OIF], now Operation New Dawn) and Afghanistan (Operation Enduring Freedom [OEF]) have confronted explosive blast at concerning (Eskridge et al., 2012; Hoge et al., 2008; Murray et al., 2005; Sayer et al., 2008; Schneiderman, Braver, & Kang, 2008; Terrio et al., 2009), if not unprecedented rates (McCrea et al., 2008; Owens et al., 2008). This is largely owing to the novel combat strategies that have been implemented on the part of insurgents. In a review of medical difficulties encountered in a sample of 4,831 US Army personnel who underwent care through an echelon II medical facility during OIF, Murray et al. (2005) found that improvised explosive devices (IEDs) and mortars caused 78% of wounded-in-action casualties. In a more recent review of the Joint Theater Trauma Registry from 2001 to 2011, Chan, Siller-Jackson, Verrett, Wu, and Hale (2012) found battle injuries to the head and neck to be present in more than 42% of those evacuated from the combat theater, with explosive devices, such as IED and rocket-propelled grenade, representing the most frequent sources of injury. In the latter study, blast accounted for a staggering 88.6% of all craniomaxillofacial injuries, a rate that was dramatically greater than alternate injury mechanisms, such as ballistics (7%) and motor vehicle collisions (2%).

In addition to traumatic brain injury (TBI), blast injures other body regions, particularly areas that are not well protected, such as the orbits and face (Cho, Bakken, Reynolds, Schlifka, & Powers, 2009; Ivanovic, Jovic, & Vukelic-Markovic, 1996). Other examples include traumatic amputations of limbs and fingers (Benfield et al., 2012; Ramasamy, Harrisson, Clasper, & Stewart, 2008), penetrating gluteal injury (Lesperance, Martin, Beekley, & Steele, 2008), ocular injuries and visual disruption (Cockerham, Lemke, Glynn-Milley, Zumhagen, & Cockerham, 2013; Petras, Bauman, & Elsayed, 1997; Weichel, Colyer, Bautista, Bower, & French, 2009), auditory and vestibular injuries (Lew, Jerger, Guillory, & Henry, 2007; Scherer & Schubert, 2009), spinal column injuries (Bell et al., 2009), and burn injuries (Mora, Ritenour, Wade, & Holcomb, 2009). Hence, "polytrauma" is an appropriate term to describe the various physical injuries that might arise as a result of blast exposure in OEF/OIF samples (Sayer et al., 2008).

Concussion (termed mild TBI [mTBI] by some) is among the most common physical injury reported in OEF/OIF samples (Eskridge et al., 2012; MacGregor, Dougherty, & Galarneau, 2011; McCrea et al., 2009). The term concussion is preferable because it refers to temporary cessation of mental function, without jumping to a misleading conclusion about physical brain damage. However, we will use mTBI to maintain continuity with other literature, with the understanding that this label does not automatically imply structural or permanent brain damage, nor does it imply a milder form of moderate to severe TBI. Concussion/mTBI is qualitatively different.

mTBI is most often sustained because of blast exposure. In their exploration of 4,623 explosive episodes encountered in Iraq between the years 2004 and 2007, Eskridge et al. (2012) found mTBI to be the most frequent single injury sustained, with nearly 11% of all documented International Classification of Diseases-9 codes identified as consistent with mTBI or concussion. In a sample of 2,074 US service members who had sustained TBIs of various severities during combat activities in Iraq, MacGregor et al. (2011) found that 89.3% were mild in severity, compared with far fewer moderate (4.3%) and severe (6.4%) TBIs. Blast resulting from IED exposure was far and away the most frequent injury mechanism across all severities of TBI (79.6%). Although IED was also a frequent source of injury in cases of moderate (65.6%) and severe (53.3%) TBI, it was a significantly more frequent cause of mTBI (82.1%) than injuries of greater severity. Moderate and severe TBIs were more frequently sustained as a result of gunshot wound to the head (13.3% and 31.8%, respectively) relative to mTBI (1.2%).

Still, the precise prevalence of combat-related mTBI (blast-related and otherwise) in OEF/OIF is unclear, with previous estimates ranging from 8–15% (Hoge et al., 2008; Kontos et al., 2013; Polusny et al., 2011; Schneiderman et al., 2008; Vanderploeg et al., 2012) to 19–23% (Polusny et al., 2011; Tanielian & Jaycox, 2008; Terrio et al., 2009). Prevalence estimates may vary according to several factors. Perhaps most basically, certain military cohorts participate in more regular combat activities than others, placing them at increased risk of sustaining blast-related mTBI. Variable prevalence may also reflect the level of scrutiny that researchers adopt when assigning a formal "positive" history of mTBI. Whereas some researchers assign mTBI status based upon screening instruments alone (e.g., Hoge et al., 2008; Schneiderman et al., 2008; Polusny et al., 2011), other researchers attempt to obtain a more refined and "clinician-confirmed" diagnosis of mTBI through detailed clinical interviews that follow an initial positive screen (e.g., Terrio et al., 2009; Terrio, Nelson, Betthauser, Harwood, & Brenner, 2011).

Rates of mTBI in OEF/OIF may also vary with the specific assessment tool that is implemented. The Departments of Defense (DoD) and Veterans Affairs (VA) have developed a variety of TBI screening instruments to promote identification of military personnel returning from OEF/OIF with mTBI histories (Belanger, Uomoto, & Vanderploeg, 2009b; General Accounting Office, 2008; Iverson, Langlois, McCrea, & Kelly, 2009; Schwab et al., 2007). As discussed later, available studies examining the psychometric properties and classification accuracies of these instruments have been quite mixed (Belanger, Vanderploeg, Soble, Richardson, & Groer, 2012; Donnelly et al., 2011; Terrio et al., 2011; Van Dyke, Axelrod, & Schutte, 2010), and it is plausible that prevalence variations are in part reflective of measurement error. Prevalence estimates are also affected by the time at which screening assessments are conducted; previous surveys have reported rates of mTBI at varying time points, from 1 month before return from deployment (Polusny et al., 2011), to a matter of days postdeployment (Terrio et al., 2009), to within a few months postdeployment (Hoge et al., 2008; Schneiderman et al., 2008), to a full year postdeployment (Polusny et al., 2011).

Regardless of the exact prevalence, blast-related mTBI has clearly evolved into an issue of major significance. Among clinicians, researchers, and others who work with OEF/OIF samples, few topics have received quite as much attention in the contemporary military and veteran literature. Combat-related mTBI has also resulted in substantially increased financial burden within the Veterans Health Administration. In their review of data associated with use of Veterans Health Administration services by 327,388 OEF/OIF veterans, Taylor et al. (2012) found that the median annual cost of care was approximately four times higher among veterans with diagnoses of TBI relative to those who had not been diagnosed with TBI. Costs increased even more with diagnostic complexity, with particularly high costs among those with comorbid TBI, pain, and posttraumatic stress disorder (PTSD).

Researchers have also examined the untoward effects of blast in civilian samples (Edwards et al., 2012; Patel, Dryden, Gupta, & Stewart, 2012). Edwards et al. describe the complex injury patterns that civilian children, adolescents, and adults sustained while receiving humanitarian care after blast exposure in Afghanistan and Iraq from 2002 to 2010. External burns represented the most frequent injury type (70%), although nonfatal blast-related injuries to the head and cervical spine (28%) and face (27%) were also common. Blast injuries to the head and cervical spine and face were among the most severe physical injuries sustained across ages. Hence, blast-related TBI represents a topic that is of potential significance not only to soldiers and veterans, but also to certain civilian samples.

Expanding upon the excellent review of blast-related injuries included in the preceding volume of this series (Vanderploeg et al., 2013), the current chapter provides an updated review of studies that have been published in the last couple of years, with occasional discussion of other important studies published before the year 2012 that may serve as important reference points. Although the circumstances surrounding the assessment and management of moderate and severe TBIs in OEF/OIF are in many ways unique (cf., DuBose et al., 2011; Tantawi, Armonda, Valerio, & Kumar, 2012; Weisbrod et al., 2012), the reality is that blast-related mTBI transpires with far greater regularity than TBIs of greater severity (MacGregor et al., 2011). As such, this chapter provides a specific review of blast-related mTBI. We conclude by offering suggestions for future research in the area of blast-related injury, particularly regarding the much-needed integration of acute-stage injury characteristics with late-stage self-report information pertaining to blast-related injuries in OEF/OIF samples.

BLAST IN HISTORICAL CONTEXT: BLAST PAST AND PRESENT

Blast from the Past

Blast as a potentially unique mechanism of concussive injury is not a new idea, and many of the same challenges and complexities that clinicians and researchers confront in their work with OEF/OIF soldiers and veterans today have been present at various times in history, particularly during war-time. In review of the historical literature, a recurrent problem stands out: researchers and treaters experience great difficulty conceptualizing and explaining the widespread nonspecific symptoms that so frequently follow exposure to explosive blast. This essential tension between disease (objective) and illness (the subjective experience of the patient) is long present throughout history, and the conflict drove competition between physiologic and psychological explanations for the symptomatic course of blast exposure.

Specific casualty statistics related to injuries sustained during 19th-century conflicts are scant (Jones & Wessely, 2001). Nevertheless, as early as Napoleonic times, writers proposed that brain injury might arise from the "wind" of cannon fire, leading to case descriptions of "windage" (Guthrie, 1842, as cited by Denny-Brown, 1945) or "wind contusion" (Jones, 2006). However, providers treated these cases with skepticism given that presenting symptoms were often reported in the absence of a readily identifiable physical cause. Interestingly, Jones (2006) notes that the label "windy," which was sometimes used to connote a lack of courage, may have arisen from the difficulties that providers had in explaining the causes of presenting symptoms in these blast-exposed soldiers.

Technologic advances in strategic warfare (e.g., development of mortars and mines) during the World War I resulted in a high rate of soldiers who were exposed to explosive blast. It was in this context that the label "shell shock" emerged to encompass the various nonspecific physical, cognitive, and emotional symptoms that a significant number of soldiers reported following their combat activities (refer to Jones & Wessely, 2005; Reid, 2010 for two excellent historical studies of shell shock). The frequency with which soldiers presented with debilitating symptoms, many of which were nonspecific, motivated experimental research to better understand potential causes. At the outset of World War I, some adopted the assumption that the various symptoms that accompanied shell shock were a direct result of central nervous system involvement itself. British neuropathologist Frederick Mott, for example, proposed that shell shock was the direct result of compressive and decompressive forces that followed explosive blast and that caused a cerebral lesion (Mott, 1917, as cited by Jones, Fear, & Wessely, 2007). However, the assumption of an underlying physiologic cause was not consistently embraced. In 1915, C. S. Myers, the consultant psychologist to the British war effort who has been credited with coinage of "shell shock," observed that many returning soldiers "had been nowhere near an explosion but had identical symptoms to those who had" (Jones et al., 2007, p. 1643). Myers therefore concluded that the symptoms of shell shock were better accounted for by psychological explanation.

The physiologic and psychological tension regarding etiology resurfaced during World War II. Once again, some researchers and clinicians (cf., Anderson, 1942; Cramer, Pastor, & Stephenson, 1947) adhered to the position that the various non-specific symptoms that some blast-exposed soldiers reported were the direct result of underlying, if ill-defined physiologic causes. Anderson (1942), for example, summarizes the presentations of a series of soldiers, each of whom presented with various psychiatric difficulties in the wake of blast exposure, to support the position of an "organic" cause. However, other researchers presented compelling data to support a psychological explanation (Fabing, 1947; Linn & Stein, 1945).

To illustrate, Linn and Stein (1945) described the divergent presentations of two groups of participants (Groups A and B) who presented for consultation in the context of an ear, nose, and throat evaluation. As depicted in Table 4.1, Group A included 40 participants with objective evidence of tympanic membrane (TM) rupture of either or both ears as a result of blast exposure that was accompanied by at least some period of alteration or loss of consciousness (LOC; ranging from momentary to up to 2 hours). None of the Group A participants exhibited sufficient symptoms of emotional distress to warrant psychiatric consultation. Group B consisted of 40 individuals who had also sustained some period of LOC as a result of blast exposure, but who did not evidence signs of TM rupture. Group B, unlike Group A, endorsed significant

Table 4.1 Historical Illustration of Presenting Features Following Blast-Related Concussion

Presenting Feature	Group A (n = 40)	Group B (n = 40)
Self-reported loss of consciousness	Momentary to 2 hours	Minutes to hours
Frequency of tympanic membrane perforation (one or both ears)	40 (100%)	0 (0%)*
Frequency of "neurotic symptoms" warranting psychiatric consultation	0 (0%)	40 (100%)
Disposition		
Full return to duty	27 (67%)	1 (2%)
Limited service	2 (5%)	37 (93%)
Hospital transfer	11 (28%)	2 (5%)

Source: Adapted from Linn and Stein (1945).

*Two participants presented with tympanic membrane perforation due to middle ear infections that predated combat activity.

psychiatric difficulties. The authors found that 27 (68%) of the Group A participants returned to full duty status (the remainder were transferred to general hospitals for further otologic management). By contrast, only one of the Group B participants (3%) resumed full duty status, and 37 (93%) were assigned "noncombatant status because of neurotic symptoms." The authors concluded that the LOC reported by Group B was likely to be "emotionally determined syncope, which should not be confused with the unconsciousness following concussion; it is this basic difference in the type of unconsciousness in these two groups which probably determines the subsequent difference in clinical course from a psychiatric standpoint" (p. 33). It is interesting to note the relevance of these findings to the more recent discussions of TM perforation as a potential objective indicator of blast-related concussion in OEF/OIF samples (cf., Howe, 2009; Xydakis, Bebarta, Harrison, Conner, & Grant, 2007), as well as the debate regarding TBI with LOC as potentially "protective" of chronic posttraumatic stress (cf., Bryant et al., 2009; Sbordone & Liter, 1995).

Researchers following both of the World Wars did not determine conclusively whether concussive injury might result from the primary (direct) result of explosive injury itself. The conclusions of Denny-Brown (1945) are particularly revealing in this regard. In his detailed review of the concussion research published at that time, he determined, "if such a condition as concussion from explosive force alone is to be established it is absolutely necessary to have full documentation of cases where all possibility of secondary injury is absent and amnesia both retrograde and immediate is verified. No such cases are on record" (p. 316). He concluded, "concussion, or indeed any similar physical damage to nervous tissue resulting from the force of an explosion transmitted by air or by water, therefore remains an unproven condition" (p. 320).

The study of blast-related concussion appears to have diminished in the decades that followed the times of the two World Wars. This is not to say that blast injuries were not relevant during the times of subsequent wars and conflicts. Indeed, data cited by Owens et al. (2008) suggests that injuries arising from blast exposure were very common in both the Korean (69%) and Vietnam (65%) conflicts. However, survival rates tend to be higher in OEF/OIF relative to previous conflicts; it has been suggested that advances in protective gear (e.g., Kevlar helmets) have contributed to blast-related concussions in OEF/OIF that would have resulted in loss of life as a result of blast exposure in previous conflicts. This may account for the greater level of attention that blast concussion has received in OEF/OIF relative to other recent conflicts. Furthermore, as noted by Vanderploeg et al. (2013), in recent years the difficulties that soldiers exhibited following combat activities have tended toward psychological conceptions. Hence, greater attention is being devoted to understanding the role of adjustment, anxiety, and posttraumatic stress. This may represent an additional reason why blast-related concussion remained understudied in the years leading up to OEF/OIF.

In summary, blast as a potential mechanism of TBI has been considered for many years, and this issue has received renewed attention with the onset of the wars in Iraq and Afghanistan. The need to understand the potential physiologic, psychological, and mixed physiologic/psychological factors that might underlie the symptoms and impairments that many OEF/OIF soldiers present with is greater now than ever to ensure that returning soldiers and veterans receive treatment and care that is appropriate to the causes of their difficulties.

Blast in the Present: Blast as a Unique Injury Mechanism

In view of the high reported frequency of blast-related concussion associated with OEF/OIF, and the unclear nature of causes of symptoms reported by blast-exposed solider samples, an extensive cross-disciplinary literature has emerged in recent years that attempts to isolate primary blast as a potentially distinct mechanism of TBI. Physicists, biologists, computer scientists, mechanical engineers, epidemiologists, neuroimaging experts, clinical psychologists, neuropsychologists, and researchers from other specialized disciplines have attempted to address this issue in their own distinctive ways.

The dynamic nature of explosive blast itself constitutes a unique injury mechanism that is qualitatively distinct relative to other potential causes of physical injury. As described by Taber, Warden, and Hurley (2006), explosive blast results in dramatic changes in atmospheric pressure, including an initial pressure increase (peak overpressure) that is followed by a relative vacuum that results in blast underpressure (negative blast phase). Physical injury may result as the "stress and shear waves" of the blast reaches the body. Blast-related injury may arise from four, nonmutually exclusive mechanisms (DePalma, Burris, Champion, & Hodgson, 2005; Mayorga, 1997; Taber et al., 2006), described as (1) primary, (2) secondary, (3) tertiary, and (4) quaternary effects. Primary blast injury is the direct effect of the blast wave itself. The TMs are highly susceptible to perforation following primary blast exposure, and some have suggested that TM perforation may represent a helpful proxy for TBI in OEF/OIF samples (Howe, 2009; Xydakis et al., 2007). Xydakis et al. reported a strong association between TM perforation and LOC. Air-filled organs (especially the lung and gastrointestinal tract) are also disproportionately vulnerable to the effects of primary blast, and individuals who are exposed to blast may be prone to expire as a result of injury to these organs (e.g., pulmonary hemorrhage, internal bleeding). Fluid-filled organs, including the eye and orbit, have also been shown to be vulnerable to blast (Rossi et al., 2012). Secondary blast effects include the displacement of debris or projectiles that are displaced as a result of blast, and secondary blast injury may result from penetrating trauma or fragmentation injuries (DePalma et al., 2005). Tertiary blast effects result from the collapse of structures or the displacement of the body by the blast wave itself, resulting in blunt trauma, or open or closed TBIs. Quaternary blast effects refer to burns, asphyxia, or toxic exposures that may arise from the explosion (DePalma et al., 2005; Taber et al., 2006).

As nicely described by Howe (2009), physical injury (including but not limited to TBI) may vary by a number of factors, such as the type of explosive, the level peak overpressure and duration, environmental hazards, and body orientation. Proximity to explosive blast is an important consideration with respect to the probability of sustaining injury. Howe (2009) notes that the blast wave dissipates by a cubed root of the distance from the source. For example, an individual who is 10 feet from a given blast source confronts nine times more overpressure than a person who is 20 feet from the blast source.

It should be noted that although OEF/OIF personnel frequently sustain TBIs as a result of secondary and tertiary blast effects as described previously, controversy surrounds the question as to whether mTBI is likely to result from primary blast exposure in humans (Saljo, Mayorga, Bolouri, Svensson, & Hamberger, 2011). Courtney and Courtney (2011) describe three theoretical means by which TBI may result from primary blast exposure: (1) thoracic, (2) head acceleration (translation or rotational) independent of blunt force, and (3) direct cranial entry of blast waves. Courtney and Courtney (2011, p. S60) conclude, "it is premature to greatly favor one likely mechanical mechanism of a blast wave leading to TBI to the exclusion of others. . . "

Just as researchers from previous conflicts developed animal models to better understand the potential effects of explosive blast on the central nervous system (Denny-Brown, 1945), contemporary researchers have attempted to understand primary blast by conducting blast experiments in various animal models with guinea pigs (Chen, Wang, Chen, Chen, & Chen, 2013); rabbits (Rafaels et al., 2011), ferrets (Rafaels et al., 2012), mice (Foley et al., 2013; Valiyaveettil et al., 2013), rats (Kamnaksh et al., 2012; Park, Eisen, Kinio, & Baker, 2013), and swine (Ahmed et al., 2012; Liu et al., 2012). Some of this research has been devoted to the identification of unique "biomarkers" that might herald a sign of previous blast exposure. Ahmed et al. (2012), for example, examined signs of the S100 protein at varying times after exposing animals to blast and found the protein to diminish in concentration within 2 weeks of blast exposure.

Other researchers have examined the potentially unique characteristics of blast exposure as a source of TBI by developing artificial surrogate head and brain models, which may consist of synthetic materials that allow researchers to simulate changes in brain structure following blast exposure (Alley, Schimizze, & Son, 2011; Ganpule et al., 2012; Roberts et al., 2012). The surrogate models are then exposed to explosive blast, and researchers examine the mechanics of blast wave and head interactions as the blast wave passes around and through the proxy brain.

A number of recent studies have implemented novel technologies to better understand possible brain changes associated with blast-related concussion. Through the implementation of functional magnetic resonance imaging (Graner, Oakes, French, & Ried, 2013; Jantzen, 2010; Matthews et al., 2011; McDonald, Saykin, & McAllister, 2012; Scheibel et al., 2012), cerebral blood flow (Foley et al., 2013), event-related brain potentials (Duncan, Summers, Perla, Coburn, & Mirsky, 2011), diffusion imaging (Matthews, Spadoni, Lohr, Strigo, & Simmons, 2012; Morey et al., 2012; Shenton et al., 2012), positron emission tomography (Peskind et al., 2011), and magnetoencephlography (Huang et al., 2012), researchers have attempted to elucidate underlying structural and/or functional signs of historical blast exposure that might not be as readily identified through the use of more conventional neuroimaging procedures (e.g., computed tomography, magnetic resonance imaging). As exciting as these technologies may be, however, it is essential to recognize that they remain *experimental* in nature. Diffusion imaging strategies, for example, "do not yet provide us with a gold-standard clinical diagnostic measure for TBI" (Silver, 2012, p. 1232), and "substantial work remains to be done to better characterize markers for mTBI as well as identify correlations between mTBI symptoms, test performance and diffusion measurements" (Fitzgerald & Crosson, 2011, p. 84).

As described in more detail later, neuropsychologists too have examined the potential psychological and cognitive impairments and symptoms that may be distinct to a history of blast-related concussion. Before turning to some of the latest neuropsychology outcomes and self-report findings in the area of blast concussion, we review other research related to the identification of blast- and other forms of combat-related concussion through contemporary screening instruments and more extended semistructured interviews.

CONTEMPORARY TBI SCREENING INSTRUMENTS

A variety of TBI screening instruments were developed in recent years. Their purpose is to assist the identification of individuals whose previous combat activities may have resulted in blast- and other combat-related TBIs (refer to Belanger et al., 2009b and Iverson et al., 2009 for excellent reviews of the potential benefits, risks, and challenges associated with TBI screening within the DoD and VA). The Brief Traumatic Brain Injury Screen (BTBIS; Schwab et al., 2007) was among the first screening instruments to be implemented, and the contents of the BTBIS are generally consistent with subsequent screening measures developed by independent researchers (e.g., Tanielian & Jaycox, 2008), the DoD Post-Deployment Health Assessment, and the VA TBI Screening Instrument (VATBISI; also known as the TBI Clinical Reminder; General Accounting Office, 2008). Although subtle differences exist across these screening tools, their formats and contents are in most ways consistent; each consists of an initial item that explores specific combat events (including blast exposure) that may have contributed to brain injury, followed by an exploration of potential acute-stage symptoms and signs, and a review of general symptoms to the present time.

The VATBISI (General Accounting Office, 2008) is reproduced in Table 4.2 to illustrate the general format and contents of one of the more commonly implemented TBI screening instruments among veterans. To provide a bit of context regarding the use and purpose of the instrument within VA, since April 2007, the administration of the VATBISI has been mandatory among veterans who (1) separated from military service after September 11, 2001; (2) served in either Iraq or Afghanistan; and/or (3) had not been diagnosed with TBI previously. Section one inquires about any specific events encountered in combat, including "blast or explosion." Veterans are asked to identify potential acute-stage disruptions (e.g., LOC) that may have resulted immediately after any of the specified events (section two), and whether any other general problems (e.g., memory problems) began or worsened over time (section three). Section four reviews any of the same symptoms from section three that may have persisted within the last week. A "positive" screen is obtained among

Table 4.2 Veterans Affairs Traumatic Brain Injury Clinical Reminder

Section 1: During any of your OEF/OIF deployment(s) did you experience any of the following events? (check all that apply)

☐ Blast or explosion
☐ Vehicular accident/crash (including aircraft)
☐ Fragment wound or bullet wound above shoulders
☐ Fall

Section 2: Did you have any of these symptoms IMMEDIATELY afterwards? (check all that apply)

☐ Losing consciousness/"knocked out"
☐ Being dazed, confused, or "seeing stars"
☐ Not remembering the event
☐ Concussion
☐ Head injury

Section 3: Did any of the following problems begin or get worse afterwards? (check all that apply)

☐ Memory problems or lapses
☐ Balance problems or dizziness
☐ Sensitivity to bright light
☐ Irritability
☐ Headaches
☐ Sleep problems

Section 4: In the past week, have you had any of the symptoms from section 3? (check all that apply)

☐ Memory problems or lapses
☐ Balance problems or dizziness
☐ Sensitivity to bright light
☐ Irritability
☐ Headaches
☐ Sleep problems

Source: Adapted from General Accounting Office (2008).

those who respond in the affirmative to events and symptoms across the four sections. Those who screen positive are provided suggestions for further assessment, and veterans who express interest in follow-up evaluation are referred for a more complete Comprehensive TBI Evaluation, typically with a physiatrist or other medical specialist (Belanger, Kretzmer, Yoash-Gantz, Pickett, & Tupler, 2009a). Providers who conduct the TBI secondary evaluation are tasked with either confirming or disconfirming the likelihood of combat-related TBI, identifying relevant comorbidities (physical, emotional, cognitive), conducting a complete physical examination, and administering a symptom checklist (Neurobehavioral Symptom Inventory; Cicerone & Kalmar, 1995). On the basis of information obtained following these procedures, examiners provide appropriate specialty service recommendations that often include neuropsychological evaluation. Thus, the VATBISI serves as an initial step in a sequence of service delivery that is meant to ensure that OEF/OIF and other veterans with possible histories of TBI receive the care and treatments appropriate to their combat histories.

Despite the good intentions behind the VATBISI and other screening instruments, evolving literature suggests significant limitations that may actually do more harm than good (Vanderploeg & Belanger, 2013). For example, DoD and VA TBI screening tools were initiated only after clinicians had identified concussion as a problem, suggesting that many OEF/OIF personnel have not been screened (Iverson et al., 2009). Postdeployment screening usually focuses on most recent deployments and single injuries, which limits understanding of events that may have transpired following multiple deployments and recurrent injuries, respectively. Perhaps of greatest importance, the psychometric utility of contemporary TBI screening instruments has been questioned in light of consistent false-positive rates of combat-related TBI.

False-positive identifications are likely to reflect the fundamental nature of all screening instruments: sensitivity is paramount. For example, the VA TBI Clinical Reminder was developed "to develop a highly sensitive screening tool that would err on the side of being overly-inclusive in identifying veterans who may be at risk for having a TBI" (General Accounting Office, 2008, p. 21). Nevertheless, researchers have raised concern regarding the psychometric utility of the VATBISI and other contemporary screening instruments, particularly with respect to equivocal reliabilities and stabilities (cf., Donnelly et al., 2011; Nelson et al., in review; Polusny et al., 2011; Van Dyke et al., 2010) and validities/classification accuracies (cf., Belanger et al., 2012; Donnelly et al., 2011; Terrio et al., 2011; Walker, McDonald, Ketchum, Nichols, & Cifu, 2012).

Van Dyke et al. (2010) examined the test-retest reliability of the VATBISI in a sample of 44 OEF/OIF veterans referred for neuropsychological evaluation following an initial positive screen. The average interval between the initial positive screen and readministration of the screening tool was approximately 6 months. The authors found frequent inconsistencies across each of the four VATBISI items. Although only 9% of the sample demonstrated inconsistent endorsement of previous blast exposure between assessment points, greater inconsistency was observed for other qualifying events, including previous motor vehicle accident (36% inconsistency), blunt trauma (43% inconsistency), and falls (48% inconsistency). Respondents also showed inconsistent endorsements of signs that followed immediately after previous injuries were sustained (section 2), including amnesia (32% inconsistency) and LOC (36%). Inconsistency was also noted with respect to postevent symptoms on section 3 (range, 24–39% inconsistency) and current symptoms (21–48% inconsistency). The authors described these results as "sobering" and called for further examination of the VATBISI reliability. They warned, "a measure that fails to obtain the same information about the same events is not a dependable tool for an accurate referral process" (p. 949).

Donnelly et al. (2011) reported more promising reliability findings on the VATBISI in a sample of 248 veterans referred for neuropsychological evaluation within a polytrauma setting. Internal consistency was fair (0.77) and test-retest reliability was also strong (0.80) compared with the findings of Van Dyke et al. (2010), although this may very well reflect the brief test-retest interval (approximately 2 weeks vs. approximately 6 months, respectively). Donnelly et al. also examined sensitivity and specificity of the VATBIST using a structured interview as a gold standard of TBI diagnosis. Results suggested high sensitivity (0.94), whereas specificity was more modest (0.59) overall. The diminished specificity was associated with an increased false-positive rate among veterans presenting with probable PTSD, with an especially high false-positive rate noted on section 1 (82%). In fact, endorsement of "blast or explosion" on section 1 was the most likely qualifying event to result in false-positive identification (76%).

Recently, Belanger et al. (2012) examined the sensitivity, specificity, and predictive values of the VATBIST using the Comprehensive TBI Evaluation as a gold standard of TBI status. In their review of a remarkable 48,175 veteran files, the authors found that although the VATBISI resulted in adequate sensitivity (0.87–0.90), it also showed relatively poor specificity (0.13–0.18). Furthermore, with an assumed TBI base rate of 15%, the VATBISI resulted in good negative predictive value (0.89) but poor positive predictive value (0.16). The authors concluded that the high false-positive rate was consistent with the underlying rationale of the VA TBI Clinical Reminder, which aimed to maximize identification of possible TBI even if this might result in increased false-positive error rates.

In their longitudinal investigation of health outcomes among National Guard soldiers deployed to Iraq, Polusny et al. (2011) surveyed 953 participants at two points in time, 1 month before leaving the combat zone (Time 1) and 1 year postdeployment (Time 2). Using an adaptation of the BTBIS (Schwab et al., 2007) as an indicator of possible TBI history, the authors found that approximately 9% of respondents endorsed a history of blast- or combat-related mTBI at Time 1. By contrast, approximately 22% of the same sample endorsed mTBI at Time 2. Although the authors provided hypothetical suggestions that might account for the more than twofold increase in self-reported mTBI over time (e.g., social influence, misattribution of symptoms, secondary gain issues), the authors did not explicitly examine variables predictive of inconsistent reports of mTBI over time.

Extending the results of Polusny et al. (2011), Nelson et al. (in press) aimed to document consistency of self-reported mTBI in the same group of 953 National Guard participants between Times 1 and 2, and identify factors that predict inconsistent report of mTBI over time (i.e., no mTBI at Time 1, positive mTBI at Time 2). As shown in Figure 4.1, most respondents (n = 739, 78%) denied any history of mTBI at either Time 1 or 2. However, a significant minority of respondents (n = 123; 13%) who denied mTBI at Time 1 went on to affirm a history of mTBI at Time 2. Relative to the reference group (No mTBI/No mTBI), the No mTBI/mTBI group showed significantly greater symptoms of PTSD and depression (Times 1 and 2), physical complaints (Time 2), active disability claims, and income distress relative to the No

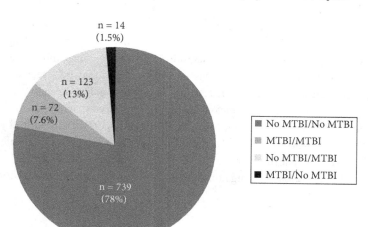

FIG 4.1 Frequencies of MTBI endorsement at 1 month prior to leaving Iraq (Time 1) and 1 year postdeployment (Time 2).

Source: Adapted from Nelson et al. (in press).

mTBI/No mTBI group. However, results of a final regression analysis revealed PTSD and physical symptoms (Time 2) to be the most optimal predictors of inconsistent report of mTBI. The authors offered that inconsistency in self-reported mTBI (i.e., No mTBI/mTBI) might represent a manifestation of augmented perceptions of combat events associated with chronic PTSD in the year following return from Iraq, postdeployment social stigmatization regarding mental health diagnoses, and/or interim iatrogenic influence.

The limitations of self-report of impaired consciousness should be obvious, especially if the injuring combat event is remote. For example, research suggests that soldiers and veterans often struggle to discriminate between blast-related LOC and/or posttraumatic amnesia (PTA). In a sample of 87 active duty OEF/OIF personnel and Veterans, Walker et al. (2012) examined respondents' consistency in responding to items specific to LOC and PTA following reported histories of blast exposure. Most of the sample endorsed items in a manner consistent with stated injuries. So, for example, of those participants who denied having experienced a "memory gap," 68 (78.2%) also endorsed having "continuous memory" following blast events. However, a meaningful proportion of the same sample endorsed these same items in a counterintuitive manner. For example, seven (8.0%) participants simultaneously endorsed having a "memory gap" and "continuous memory" following prior blast exposure, 11 (12.6%) simultaneously endorsed "continuous memory" and "LOC," and 11 (12.6%) endorsed "LOC" but denied having sustained a "memory gap." In light of these inconsistencies, the authors recommended that a more structured interview approach, as opposed to screening alone, "may improve specificity for making the diagnosis of mild TBI historically" (p. 75).

In light of screening instruments' limitations, some researchers have expressed concern about their continued use in OEF/OIF samples. In one especially compelling commentary, Vanderploeg and Belanger (2013) argued that the potential harms and costs of TBI screening (e.g., anxiety among those who screen positive, iatrogenesis, added expense, public misperception that mild TBI results in longstanding difficulty) outweigh the potential benefits (e.g., reassurance among those who screen negative). Noting that routine screening of mTBI violates basic medical screening assumptions (e.g., medical screening is meant for progressive disease, which mTBI is not), the authors concluded, "screening for mild TBI is unnecessary at best and potentially harmful at worst (p. 211)." To ensure that patients receive appropriate care, the authors argued that future screening could be conducted in a symptom-specific manner without necessarily tying nonspecific symptoms to a specific diagnostic condition (e.g., mTBI).

SEMISTRUCTURED TBI INTERVIEWS

Several semistructured TBI interview procedures have been developed in recent years to assist the assessment of blast- and combat-related TBI and improve upon the concerning classifications that have been reported on the basis of screening instruments alone (Brawn Fortier et al., 2014; Donnelly et al., 2011; Nelson et al., 2011a; Vanderploeg et al., 2012).

Structured Interview for TBI Diagnosis

Donnelly et al. (2011) developed the 22-item Structured Interview for TBI Diagnosis to define "the nature, probability, and severity of deployment-related TBI among OEF/OIF veterans and to provide the criterion for the sensitivity and specificity analyses" (p. 442). Following the suggested diagnostic criteria of Cifu et al. (2009), the Structured Interview includes a confirmed injury event that may have resulted in TBI, alteration of consciousness, and postconcussive symptoms (PCS). On the basis of the authors' clinical experience, they developed additional diagnostic items to allow for a detailed review of circumstances leading up to, during, and after the time of injury. As a result of information obtained, interviews resulted in various probability and severity ratings of reported TBI events, "based on the summary judgments of the interviewing psychologists in consideration of the totality of the responses" (p. 442). Injuries rated as "very likely" or "almost certainly" to have contributed to TBI were coded as positive for diagnosis. The Structured Interview was used as an independent indicator of TBI diagnosis in their investigation of the classification accuracy of the VATBISI. As with any semistructured interview, the authors acknowledge that the interview procedure represents an "imperfect" gold standard. However, specific reliability and validity of the Structured Interview were not reported.

Minnesota Blast Exposure Screening Tool

In light of the variable administration practices noted among providers who conducted the follow-up VA Comprehensive Evaluation following an initial positive screen on the VATBISI (Belanger et al., 2009b), Nelson et al. (2011) developed the Minnesota Blast Exposure Screening Tool (MN-BEST) as a strategy for maintaining a uniform approach to blast concussion assessment among OEF/OIF veterans. Based upon information obtained through a detailed blast concussion interview, the MN-BEST emphasizes three aspects of the concussion assessment process that are based upon acute-injury characteristics, identification of: (1) concussion *frequency*, (2) concussion *severity*, and (3) concussion *plausibility*.

A primary rationale in developing the MN-BEST was to generate a single, composite numerical rating of one or more blast concussions that represents a summary index of cumulative neurologic insult (information related to the three most significant non–blast-related concussions during respondents' lifetimes is also obtained). For each of the three blast events, as well as the three most significant non–blast-related events (typically prior to the time of military service), the research consensus team offers independent opinions as to whether it was more likely than not that reported blast events resulted in concussion as defined by an integration of the American Congress of Rehabilitation Medicine (Kay et al., 1993) criteria and those outlined by three concussion severity classifications outlined by Ruff and Richardson (1999). Preliminary interrater reliability for the MN-BEST was strong (Cohen alpha among the initial research team of .98; $p < .001$). However, the MN-BEST has not been independently validated and was developed as a research instrument that has not been implemented in routine clinical settings.

VA TBI Identification Clinical Interview

Vanderploeg et al. (2012) describe the sophisticated, multistep process that was implemented in the development of the VA TBI Identification Clinical Interview. The procedure was developed in consultation with a team of TBI subject matter experts, and is meant primarily for veteran populations. Aware of the limitations of previous interview approaches (e.g., lack of universal understanding of "loss of consciousness" and other injury terminology), the authors were interested in minimizing leading or close-ended questions that might influence the interviewee's description of previous injury events. As such, the interview begins with an open-ended set of questions that assist examinees to describe experiences "following a physically powerful event" (p. 554). It is only after this preliminary exploratory step that the interviewer inquires further with confirmatory questioning that assists the determination of whether criteria for TBI were met. Reliability and validity data were not reported. However, the authors obtained positive preliminary feedback from providers at three separate VA sites, and the procedure is typically completed in 15–20 minutes.

Boston Assessment of Traumatic Brain Injury

Brawn Fortier et al. (2014) developed the Boston Assessment of Traumatic Brain Injury—Lifetime (BAT-L). This semistructured interview evaluates blast exposures and other combat-related events that may have resulted in TBI and other physical injuries. The BAT-L explores two different aspects of previous blast exposure, including the number of blasts that were encountered within 100 m of the respondent, and the number of TBIs that resulted as a result of blast. Like the MN-BEST, the BAT-L summarizes histories of combat- and noncombat-related TBI, and rates the severity of these injuries on a graded scale. In a sample of 131 OEF/OIF veterans, the authors validated the BAT-L using the Ohio State University TBI Identification Method (Corrigan & Bogner, 2007) as the independent gold standard of TBI diagnosis. The BAT-L demonstrated impressive agreement with the Ohio State University TBI Identification Method procedure (Kappa >.80) and interrater reliability was also strong (Kappa >.80).

BLAST CONCUSSION AND NEUROPSYCHOLOGICAL OUTCOMES

The blast concussion literature in military and veteran samples is sparse by comparison to the sizeable civilian concussion literature that has emerged in recent decades (Lamberty, Nelson, & Yamada, 2013). Researchers have consistently documented the favorable course of recovery that is anticipated following conventional (i.e., non–blast-related) forms of concussive injury, with cognitive impairments typically resolving within days, weeks, to no more than a few months (Belanger & Vanderploeg, 2005; Binder, Rohling, & Larrabee, 1997; Frencham, Fox, & Maybery, 2005; Iverson, 2005; Schretlen & Shapiro, 2003).

Some of the highest quality concussion literature in neuropsychology has been conducted in sports concussion samples. As described by McCrea (2008), the various unique advantages associated with conducting neuropsychological outcomes research in athletes (e.g., limited comorbidities, readily available to conduct systematic longitudinal investigations) have facilitated researchers' ability to identify the "natural history" of favorable recovery that is anticipated following sports-related concussion. As a rule, blast concussion researchers do not enjoy these same advantages and have not been able to conduct neuropsychological outcomes research with the same level of methodologic rigor that has been true of sports concussion research. To illustrate the unique challenges that blast concussion researchers often confront in their work with OEF/OIF samples, Table 4.3 compares sports concussion and blast concussion research across the 11 "unique advantages" that McCrea (2008) has described of research with athletes. The distinct challenges that blast concussion researchers confront have in many ways restricted their ability to examine directly whether blast, as a potentially unique injury mechanism (Courtney & Courtney, 2011), might follow a similar or distinct trajectory of cognitive recovery relative to more conventional (i.e., non–blast-related) concussive injuries.

Nevertheless, amid these challenges and study weaknesses, several neuropsychological outcome studies have been conducted among OEF/OIF samples in recent

Table 4.3 Advantages of Sports Concussion Research Relative to Blast Concussion Research

Research Advantage*	Sports Concussion	Blast Concussion
1. Prospective identification of at-risk MTBI sample?	Yes (athletes high-risk population)	Yes (OEF/OIF high-risk population)
2. Defined period of MTBI risk exposure?	Yes (sports season)	Yes (deployment period)
3. Ability to obtain baseline testing?	Yes (preseason screening)	Yes (predeployment screening)
4. Witnessed; documented acute injury characteristics?	Yes (eyewitnesses abound)	Occasionally (e.g., MACE results)
5. Ability to conduct testing within minutes?	Yes	Occasionally (e.g., MACE results)
6. Systematic follow-up to track early outcomes?	Yes	Occasionally (e.g., MACE, ANAM)
7. Continuity of care?	Yes	Rarely (many postinjury providers)
8. Ready access to noninjured control subjects?	Yes	Variable (few deployment control)
9. Rare events (e.g., second impact syndrome)?	Yes	Rarely (undocumented recurrence)
10. "Clean sample"?	Yes	No (comorbidities highly prevalent)
11. Systematic longitudinal assessments?	Yes	No (limited to pre/post deployment)

Source: * Adapted from McCrea (2008).

MACE, Military Acute Concussion Evaluation.

years and these represent an important first step in clarifying potential cognitive effects that may be associated with blast-related concussion.

Acute-Stage Injury Outcomes

Some researchers have reported results of cognitive performances among OEF/ OIF personnel within the acute-stage (hours, days) of blast-related and other combat-related concussive injuries (Coldren et al., 2010, 2012; Kennedy et al., 2012; Luethcke, Bryan, Morrow, & Isler, 2011; Morrow, Bryan, & Isler, 2011). Coldren et al. (2012) examined cognitive performances on the Automated Neuropsychological Assessment Metrics (ANAM; 2007), a computerized, performance-based screening test of cognitive function, in a sample of 47 soldiers who sustained concussion during service in Iraq. Blast accounted for most concussions (45%), followed by impact (26%) and mixed (11%) concussive injuries. Performances in the concussion group were compared against 108 deployed control subjects at 72-hour, 5-day, and 10-day intervals postinjury. Although the concussion group demonstrated significantly lower ANAM performances at 72 hours, no significant group differences were observed on any of the six ANAM indices at 5- or 10-day assessments. A primary finding was "how rapidly all components of the ANAM normalize following a concussive injury in the combat setting, within 5 to 10 days" (p. 182). The authors regarded the findings as "highly consistent with the adult sports medicine literature" (p. 182) with respect to cognitive function, which typically resolve within the first 10 days postinjury.

Kennedy et al. (2012) describe results of acute concussion evaluations conducted in a group of 377 active duty military personnel who were evacuated from the battle zone in Afghanistan and who underwent assessments to inform return to duty status. Most concussions were deemed to be the direct result of primary blast following IED exposure. Participants were administered the Military Acute Concussion Evaluation (Defense and Veterans Brain Injury Center, 2007) as a component of the assessments. Although the Military Acute Concussion Evaluation performances were not associated with return to duty status or recovery within the acute-stage of injury, the authors perceived that it was of some benefit for use if administered on a serial basis if it was administered within 6 hours of injury.

Predeployment and Postdeployment Outcomes

Researchers have also compared postdeployment cognitive performances to those that were obtained at the time of baseline predeployment testing (Roebuck-Spencer et al., 2012; Vasterling et al., 2012). Roebuck-Spencer et al. compared predeployment and postdeployment ANAM performances of US Service personnel with self-reported mTBI who were either symptomatic (n = 197) or not symptomatic (n = 305) according to the BTBIS (Schwab et al., 2007); a symptomatic group with deployment-related injuries other than mTBI (n = 28); and a deployment control group (n = 400). Most deployment-related concussions were a result of blast (63%). Predeployment ANAM performances were not statistically different across groups. At postdeployment, the asymptomatic mTBI group did not demonstrate significantly different ANAM performances than the deployment control group. However, symptomatic mTBI participants demonstrated significantly lower ANAM performances than the control and asymptomatic mTBI groups, and also showed significantly lower performances relative to predeployment baseline. The authors emphasized that most of those with reported mTBI demonstrated no evidence of cognitive decline relative to predeployment assessment, with 70% showing no interim change in performance. They concluded that these results were "entirely consistent with the civilian literature" (p. 485) in which long-term cognitive impairments following mTBI is not anticipated. A substantial limitation of this study is that the interval of time between injury and postdeployment assessment was unavailable for review. In fact, the authors did not have access to any data regarding date of reported injuries. They also did not have access to comorbid diagnoses that may have impacted postdeployment performances.

Blast Versus Nonblast

Other researchers have examined neuropsychological performances of OEF/OIF personnel with reported histories of blast versus non–blast-related concussion (Belanger et al., 2009a; Cooper, Chau, Armistead-Jehle, Vanderploeg, & Bowles, 2012; Kontos et al., 2013; Lange et al., 2012; Luethcke et al., 2011). Cooper et al. compared Repeatable Battery for the Assessment of Neuropsychological Status (Randolph, 1998) performances of 32 service members with self-reported histories of blast-related concussion and 28 participants with self-reported histories of non–blast-related concussion. On average, the sample underwent the assessment approximately 6 months postinjury. The groups did not differ across any of the Repeatable Battery for the Assessment of Neuropsychological Status indices. Similar to previous investigations (Belanger et al., 2009a; Luethcke et al., 2011), results did not support the notion that blast contributed to a distinct pattern of cognitive limitation relative to concussions sustained by alternate nonblast mechanisms, "at least with respect to cognitive sequelae in the postacute timeframe" (p. 1159).

Lange et al. (2012) compared cognitive performances of US military service members with histories of reported blast-related mTBI (n = 35) and non–blast-related mTBI (n = 21) sustained as a result of activities in OEF/OIF. Both groups were assessed an average of 4 months after the time of injury. With exception of a minority of tasks (e.g., WAIS-III Similarities, Trail Making Test B), which were diminished in an unexpected direction (i.e., non–blast-related performed worse than blast-related mTBI group) and no longer significant after controlling for emotional distress, the authors did not identify any between-group differences on measures of cognitive performance. Findings were once again regarded as consistent with those obtained by previous researchers (Belanger et al., 2009a; Luethcke et al., 2011); the authors concluded, "these findings provide little evidence to suggest that blast exposure plus secondary blunt trauma results in worse cognitive or psychological recovery than blunt trauma alone" (p. 604).

More recently, Kontos et al. (2013) reported cognitive performances of a sizeable sample of US Army Special Operations Command personnel (n = 22,203), including 2,813 who had been diagnosed with at least one reported mTBI according to blast, blunt, or combination (blast-blunt) mechanisms. In addition to self-report measures of PCS and PTSD, participants completed a military adaptation of the Immediate Post-Concussion Assessment Cognitive Test as a measure of cognitive performance. Overall, participants with any history of mTBI performed significantly worse on select cognitive indices. For example, those with blast and combination injuries performed significantly worse on visual memory and reaction time indices than those with blunt mTBI and no mTBI history. Those with combined injuries also performed worse on verbal memory and processing speed indices than those with a history of blunt mTBI. The authors also conducted systematic analyses related to mTBI recurrence. Although there was evidence of a dose-response gradient with respect to PCS and PTSD (i.e., those with one, two, three or more concussions reported progressively more symptoms), there was not consistent evidence of dose-response with respect to cognitive performance, with exception of reaction time (which was significantly slower among those with three versus no diagnosis concussions).

Impact of Psychopathology on Cognitive Outcomes

Exploring the role of psychological factors in persistent symptoms has been a historical constant, based on the disease-illness conflict defined earlier. Drag, Spencer, Walker, Pangilinan, & Bieliauskas (2012) examined the relationships of self-reported mTBI injury characteristics (disorientation, LOC, PTA) and psychological symptoms (as assessed by measures of posttraumatic stress, depression, and anxiety) with self-reported cognitive symptoms (as assessed by cognitive items from the Neurobehavioral Symptom Inventory (NSI) and cognitive performances in a group of 167 OEF/OIF veterans with histories of combat-related mTBI referred for neuropsychological evaluation in a polytrauma clinic. Although participants who endorsed histories of LOC and PTA reported significantly higher psychological and cognitive symptoms than those who endorsed histories of disorientation, cognitive performances were not significantly different between these groups. Psychological symptoms significantly mediated the relationship between the injury parameters and report of cognitive symptoms. Subjective cognitive symptoms were no longer correlated with cognitive performances after controlling for the psychological symptoms. These findings suggested symptoms of psychological distress play an important role in both one's subjective experience of cognitive limitation and cognitive performance in the late stage of combat-related concussion.

Two recent studies (Nelson et al., 2012; Shandera-Ochsner et al., 2013) directly examined cognitive outcomes among OEF/OIF veterans as a function of remote, combat-related concussion status (present or absent) and ongoing psychiatric status (present or absent). Nelson et al. (2012) aimed to identify whether a remote history of blast-related concussion and/or current Axis I psychopathology (including, but not limited to PTSD) contributed to, either independently or in conjunction, significant long-term cognitive impairments in a sample of 104 OEF/OIF veterans with varied combat histories. Based on information obtained through independent blast concussion and psychopathology consensus meetings, participants were classified into the following four groups: (1) blast-concussion only, (2) Axis I psychopathology only, (3) comorbid blast-concussion/Axis I, and (4) deployment control. As hypothesized, veterans with self-reported histories of blast concussion and without Axis I pathology demonstrated comparable performances relative to the deployment control group. Furthermore, regardless of blast concussion history, those with Axis I psychopathology demonstrated significantly diminished performances relative to the deployment control group. No significant interaction was found between concussion history and Axis I.

In a follow-up study, Shandera-Ochsner et al. (2013) aimed to replicate and extend the findings of Nelson et al. (2012) in a sample of 81 OEF/OIF veterans with various histories of self-reported mTBI sustained during combat. The authors assigned participants to groups on the basis of concussion and psychopathology status, although the authors did not restrict concussions to those sustained as a result of blast alone and psychiatric status was restricted to PTSD alone. Cognitive performances were obtained among individuals with (1) mTBI histories only (blast or otherwise), (2) PTSD only, (3) comorbid mTBI/PTSD, and (4) deployment control. Similar to Nelson et al., the authors found that the PTSD-only and mTBI/PTSD groups performed significantly worse on select measures of verbal memory and executive function, whereas the mTBI-only group demonstrated performances that were not significantly different relative to the deployment control group.

Taking the findings of these two studies together (Nelson et al., 2012; Shandera-Ochsner et al., 2013), OEF/OIF veterans with remote histories of combat-related concussion (blast and nonblast) did not demonstrate cognitive performances that were significantly different than deployment control subjects. The combined findings suggest that regardless of self-reported concussion history, veterans with active psychiatric conditions (PTSD, depression) performed significantly worse than deployment control subjects. Stated differently, whereas the effect size difference in cognitive performance was small between mTBI-only and deployment control groups, OEF/OIF participants with PTSD and other Axis I conditions, regardless of mTBI status, demonstrated moderate effect size differences relative to deployment control subjects (see Figure 4.2 for effect size differences derived from both studies).

In their comprehensive review of mTBI outcomes in military and veteran samples, O'Neill et al. (2012) concluded, "although the overall strength of evidence evaluating outcomes following mTBI in Veteran or military populations is low, it is noteworthy that the findings are remarkably consistent with higher quality civilian literature. Both bodies of research suggest that many health consequences resolve within the

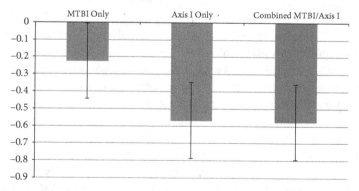

FIG 4.2 Cognitive effect size differences by MTBI and Axis I psychopathology status.
Note. Effect sizes, which are compared against OEF/OIF deployment control subjects (n = 49), are derived from a combination of 27 neuropsychological measures included in the Nelson et al. (2012) and Shandera-Ochsner et al. (2013) studies. N = 185 OEF/OIF participants, including "MTBI Only" (without Axis I psychopathology), n = 38; "Axis I Only" (without previous MTBI), n = 43; and "Combined MTBI/Axis I," n = 55. Error bars represent 95% confidence intervals.

first few months following injury, if not sooner" (p. 43). They noted that the strength of evidence was low because of limited or incomplete data and sampling procedures, failure to report time since injury, and the fact that most studies did not include an unblended approach and were single-center.

BLAST CONCUSSION AND SYMPTOM REPORT

In recent years, researchers have identified that OEF/OIF service members are not only at risk of sustaining blast-related mTBI, but are also at risk of developing a wide array of other physical and psychiatric comorbid/postmorbid difficulties. These include, but are not limited to, sleep disorder (Epstein, Babcock-Parziale, Haynes, & Herb, 2012), alcohol and substance use problems (Widome, Laska, Gulden, Fu, & Lust, 2011; Williams, McDevitt-Murphy, Murphy, & Crouse, 2012), depression (Hoge et al., 2008; Booth-Kewley et al., 2012), posttraumatic stress (Gates et al., 2012) and other anxiety disorder (Booth-Kewley, Highfill-McRoy, Larson, Garland, & Gaskin, 2012), sexual dysfunction (Nunnink, Fink, & Baker, 2012), relational difficulties (Erbes, Meis, & Polusny, 2011), and headache and chronic pain (Dobscha et al., 2009; Erickson, 2011; Theeler, Flynn, & Erickson, 2012). At least one recent study has also raised the possibility that premorbid psychological vulnerabilities predict the development of posttraumatic stress during the postdeployment phase (MacDonald, Proctor, Heeren, & Vasterling, 2013). Because these various conditions and difficulties are frequently accompanied by a variety of symptoms that influence symptom reports, OEF/OIF concussion researchers have appreciated the importance of considering the degree to which independent comorbidities underlie results of self-report measures of psychological and emotional functioning before inferring that they necessarily represent a manifestation of combat-related mTBI itself.

Stated differently, one should not retrospectively make a diagnosis of blast-related concussion on the basis of the various physical (e.g., headache, fatigue, dizziness), cognitive (e.g., inattention, memory difficulty), and emotional (e.g., irritability, anxiety) symptoms that many soldiers and veterans often endorse. Research conducted in civilian (cf., Iverson & Lange, 2003; Iverson, 2006; Iverson & McCracken, 1997; Lange, Iverson, & Rose, 2011) samples has demonstrated that various so-called PCS are not specific to concussion itself; these symptoms are frequently reported in psychiatric and healthy community samples without histories of mTBI. PCS have also been shown to be nonspecific to concussion in military and veteran samples (cf., Benge, Pastorek, & Thornton, 2009; Cooper et al., 2011; Donnell, Kim, Silva, & Vanderploeg, 2012; Fear et al., 2009). In veteran samples, PCS are not specific to brain injury severity after controlling for symptoms of emotional distress (Belanger et al., 2010) and typically lack an association with mTBI itself after controlling for psychiatric symptoms (Verfaellie, Lafleche, Spiro, Tun, & Bousquet, 2013). Additionally, aside from certain physical symptoms, such as blast-related tinnitus and hearing difficulty (Belanger et al., 2011; Luethcke et al., 2011), endorsements of PCS are generally quite comparable between those with self-reported histories of blast versus non–blast-related mTBI (Belanger et al., 2011; Lippa, Pastorek, Benge, & Thornton, 2010). In short, there is not consistent evidence that PCS are necessarily specific to blast exposure, although as described later, some researchers have implicated a possible dose-response relationship between blast exposure and PCS (Kontos et al., 2013).

To illustrate the nonspecific nature of PCS, consider the findings of Donnell et al. (2012), who recently conducted a retrospective review of symptoms endorsed by 4,462 Vietnam era veterans, including those with psychiatric difficulty, mTBI, and healthy control subjects. Whereas 32% of veterans with mTBI (and without other diagnosed conditions) met criteria for the Diagnostic and Statistical Manual-IV defined postconcussion syndrome, the latter criteria were fulfilled at even higher rates among those with psychiatric conditions, including PTSD (40%), generalized anxiety disorder (50%), and major depressive disorder (57%). Those fulfilling criteria for somatization disorder (91%) were especially prone to fulfill criteria for postconcussion syndrome.

Although research has not consistently supported the idea that blast is necessarily unique in its contribution to PCS, there is evidence that blast exposure represents a significant stressor that may increase risk of subsequent emotional difficulties, regardless of whether it contributed to mTBI or other physical injury. Lopes Cardozo et al. (2012), for example, conducted a mental health survey of Cambodian landmine survivors and found very high rates of depression (74%), anxiety (62%), and PTSD (34%) in this sample. That only a minority (8.4%) of the sample sustained head injuries illustrates that blast exposure itself, quite independent of whether it results in TBI, frequently results in significant symptoms of psychological and emotional distress that may persist long after the time of exposure.

Related, some of the latest self-report literature among OEF/OIF veterans suggests that those who sustain blast concussion are at increased risk of developing symptoms of posttraumatic stress and other emotional difficulties relative to those with non–blast-related mTBI or no history of mTBI (Kontos et al., 2013; Maguen, Madden, Lau, & Seal, 2012). In fact, the latter studies implicate a potential dose-response relationship between blast-related mTBI and psychological distress. In a sample of 1,082 OEF/OIF veterans who underwent TBI screening through the VA system of care, Maguen et al. (2012) examined the effect of injury mechanism (blast and other forms of mTBI) and injury recurrence (zero, one, two or more) on self-reported symptoms of PTSD and depression. Participants who reported multiple head injury mechanisms were at six times the risk of PTSD, four times the risk of depression, and two times the risk of screening positive for alcohol misuse relative to those without any history of head injury. Notably, those who endorsed a history of blast plus another type of head injury mechanism were at significantly increased risk of screening positive for all other psychiatric diagnoses.

Similarly, in the aforementioned Kontos et al. (2013) study, the authors not only examined cognitive performances in their sample of US Army personnel (n = 22,203; 2,813 with at least one mTBI), but also describe results of self-reported symptoms on the basis of injury mechanism (blunt, blast, or mixed) and recurrence (zero, one, two, three or more blasts). As a whole, respondents with reported histories of blast or blast-blunt mTBI histories endorsed significantly greater symptoms (both PCS and PTSD) than those with blunt mTBI histories or no history of mTBI. Notably, symptom endorsements increased significantly with each level of reported mTBI, consistent with an overall dose-response effect of blast and symptom report.

Most studies that recently examined self-reported symptoms in OEF/OIF mTBI samples relied upon brief, face valid self-report measures. Examples include the PTSD Checklist (PCL), Beck Depression Inventory—2nd Edition (Beck, Steer, & Brown, 1996), and Hamilton Depression and Anxiety Scales. Although these scales are expedient in identifying symptoms of emotional distress in a relatively timely fashion, they are not without limitations. The PCL, for example, is lacking in specificity and has been identified as an indicator of generalized emotional distress that is not specific to PTSD itself (Arbisi et al., 2011).

Relative to extended personality inventories (Minnesota Multiphasic Personality Inventory—2nd Edition [MMPI-2], Butcher, Dahlstrom, Graham, Tellegen, & Kaemmer et al., 1989; its Restructured Form [MMPI-2-RF], Ben-Porath & Tellegen, 2008; and the Personality Assessment Inventory [PAI], Morey, 1991), face valid self-report measures are limited in their ability to determine response validity, quality, and severity of symptoms. Relatively few recent researchers have implemented extended personality inventories to inform the validity, quality, and severity of psychological and emotional symptoms in OEF/OIF samples with histories of combat-related mTBI (Arbisi et al., 2011; Lange et al., 2012; Nelson et al., 2011).

Arbisi, Polusny, Erbes, Thuras, and Reddy (2011) examined MMPI-2-RF profiles in a sample of 251 National Guard soldiers who had recently returned from deployment to Iraq. Participants were classified according to results of mTBI screening (Schwab et al., 2007) and PTSD screening (PCL) to classify participants into four groups: (1) PTSD only, (2) mTBI only, (3) both PTSD and mTBI, and (4) neither condition. Scales associated with somatic complaints were significantly predictive of mTBI status, whereas a specific problem scale (Anxiety) effectively predicted PTSD status above and beyond the Restructured Clinical Scales. The sample included participants with histories of blast as well as other forms of mTBI, although the authors did not examine potential presentation differences according to injury mechanism. The authors concluded that a positive mTBI screen does not of itself predict significant emotional distress, and that the MMPI-2-RF had merit in assessing PTSD in non–treatment-seeking veterans.

In the aforementioned Lange et al. (2012) study, the authors describe PAI profiles in a group of 56 military service members classified by injury mechanism, either blast plus secondary injuries (n = 35) and non–blast-related injuries (n = 21). Although medium effect size differences were noted between those exposed to blast on the Depression (d = .49) and Stress (d = .47) scales, none of the differences were significantly different across 14 PAI clinical scales.

In their extensive review of the available literature relevant to combat-related concussion, O'Neill (2013) concluded, "though self-reported cognitive, physical, and mental health symptoms were common in the Veteran/military population, there was little evidence that symptoms were more common in those with mTBI than those without mTBI" (p. 2). However, similar to the conclusions that were offered on the basis of neurocognitive findings, the authors noted that the overall evidence base was weakened by inconsistent findings, significant methodologic weaknesses, and variations in outcomes and how they were measured.

COMPLICATING FACTORS

In addition to the various comorbid/postmorbid physical and psychiatric conditions described previously, other contextual factors may complicate the presentations of OEF/OIF soldiers and veterans who endorse a history of combat-related mTBI and contribute to persistent report of symptoms and/or cognitive impairments upon neuropsychological evaluation. Briefly reviewed in this section are secondary gain and response validity issues, and stigmatization and social influence issues.

Secondary Gain and Response Validity Issues

A growing literature suggests that issues of secondary gain, self-report bias, and performance validity are very important for clinicians and researchers to consider in their work with OEF/OIF soldiers and veterans. Much of postconcussion diagnosis is driven by self-reported histories of combat-related concussion and subsequent difficulties, and access to confirmatory medical and combat records is time consuming or impossible. Avoidance of combat duty in active personnel, and obtaining disability income in veterans, represent examples of external incentives that may motivate individuals to embellish their injury, and to appear more impaired than is actually the case. In light of the high rates at which symptom exaggeration and/or insufficiency transpire in civilian forensic contexts (Mittenberg, Patton, Canyock, & Condit, 2002), routine response validity assessment has become an essential component of any neuropsychological evaluation (Heilbronner et al., 2009). In OEF/OIF samples with histories of combat-related concussion, clinicians and researchers are encouraged to maintain awareness of "the potential pull for symptom embellishment due to multiple external incentives associated with establishment of injury" (Howe, 2009, p. 1329).

McNally and Frueh (2013) provide a compelling summary of the rates at which OEF/OIF veterans have applied for service-connected disability for PTSD and other conditions in recent years. Citing 2012 data published by the Associated Press and 2013 data from the Bureau of Labor Statistics, the authors reported that 45% of OEF/OIF veterans had applied for service-connected disability (including those without combat histories), compared with only 14% of other veterans. In spite of historically lower rates of fatality and injury in OEF/OIF relative to previous wars, far fewer disability compensation claims had been made at the times of previous wars, including World War II (11%), Vietnam War (16%), and the Gulf War (21%). Furthermore, the number of claimed disability conditions for OEF/OIF veterans ranged from 8 to 14, compared with an average of only two conditions for World War II veterans and four conditions for Vietnam veterans. The authors entertained multiple hypotheses that might account for these unprecedented rates of compensation-seeking, including questions of symptom validity and malingering.

In fact, several recent studies have directly examined issues of response validity assessment and malingering in OEF/OIF soldiers and veterans (Armistead-Jehle, 2010; Armistead-Jehle & Buican, 2012; Cooper et al., 2011b; Jones, 2013a,b; Jones & Ingram, 2011; Jones, Ingram, & Ben-Porath, 2012; Lange, Edmed, Sullivan, French, & Cooper, 2013; Nelson et al., 2010, 2011b; Whitney, Shepard, Williams, Davis, & Adams, 2009). Researchers have demonstrated relatively high rates of both symptom exaggeration and insufficient effort in OEF/OIF samples with reported histories of concussion. In active service members, rates of insufficient effort are significantly higher among those evaluated in context of pending disability evaluation (medical evaluation board) relative to those who are evaluated in clinical contexts (Armistead-Jehle & Buican, 2012). Similarly, relative to OEF/OIF veteran concussion samples that undergo neuropsychological evaluations in research settings, rates of both symptom exaggeration and insufficient effort are significantly higher in compensation/pension disability settings (Nelson et al., 2010, 2011b). OEF/OIF veterans who undergo concussion-related neuropsychological evaluations also show significantly higher rates of symptom exaggeration on the MMPI-2/RF validity scales if they have active disability claims relative to those without active claims (Nelson et al., 2011b).

These findings speak to the importance of developing reliable response validity indicators. These are divided into two types: symptom validity scales (self-report measures) and performance validity tests (skills assessment). With respect to the former, some researchers recently examined the potential use of the MMPI-2-RF validity scales in active duty and veteran samples with histories of concussion (Jones & Ingram, 2011; Jones et al., 2012). Regarding performance validity, recent efforts have been made to establish optimal cut-scores on effort measures that are commonly used in civilian postconcussion claimants. For example, researchers have attempted to develop optimal cut-scores for the Test of Memory Malingering (Jones, 2013a), and Victoria Symptom Validity Test (Jones, 2013b).

Other researchers have recently developed novel symptom validity tests explicitly for use in military and veteran samples. Cooper et al. (2011b) developed the Mild Brain Injury Atypical Symptoms Scale (a five-item scale consisting of content that was considered to be uncommonly endorsed in most individuals who sustain concussion. The Mild Brain Injury Atypical Symptoms Scale was designed to be administered simultaneous with the Neurobehavioral Symptom Inventory (NSI; Cicerone & Kalmar, 1995) and the PCL. A recent follow-up simulation study conducted in a sample of Australian undergraduate students provided preliminary support for use of the Mild Brain Injury Atypical Symptoms Scale in the detection of symptom exaggeration (Lange et al., 2013).

Stigmatization and Social Influence

Some research suggests that OEF/OIF soldiers and veterans express fear of stigmatization related to mental health diagnoses (Brenner, Vanderploeg, & Terrio, 2009; Hoge et al., 2004). Hoge et al. (2004) conducted a survey of OEF/OIF combat infantry personnel prior to deployment to Iraq (n = 2,530) or 3–4 months after deployment to Iraq or Afghanistan (3,671). Not surprisingly, the authors found a higher rate of major depression, PTSD, and alcohol use problems among those surveyed after deployment relative to those surveyed before deployment. However, only a small percentage of respondents indicated that they had received mental health services, and concerns regarding stigma were most significant among those who were most in need of such services. The authors found that participants who screened positive for some form of mental health disorder were approximately two times more likely to expressed concern regarding stigma. For example, 41% of those who met screening criteria for mental disorder endorsed that "it would be too embarrassing" to receive mental health services, compared with only 18% of those who did not meet screening criteria.

Relatively few studies have systematically assessed issues of stigmatization and social influence in the same manner as Hoge et al. (2004) in more recent years, although these have been topics of somewhat frequent discussion (Brenner et al., 2009; Howe, 2009; Jones et al., 2007; Nelson et al., 2012; Roth & Spencer, 2013; Spencer & Adams, 2012; Vanderploeg & Belanger, 2013). Spencer and Adams (2012) briefly summarize unpublished data derived from their survey of patients evaluated through a polytrauma clinic related to histories of TBI. The authors found that more than 90% of patients indicated that they had learned about TBI from at least one source prior to the time of their evaluation, more than 50% learned of TBI by word of mouth, and more than one-third used a pamphlet. Notably, only 32% reported getting information about TBI directly from medical providers.

It is conceivable that as a result of these fears, OEF/OIF soldiers and veterans with persistent mental health symptoms may identify mTBI as a more appealing or socially embraced diagnosis to explain the various difficulties. This was one hypothesis offered to account for inconsistent reports of mTBI during the postdeployment phase identified in significant proportion of OIF respondents who denied mTBI while in the combat zone who went on to affirm a history of mTBI 1 year later (Nelson et al., in review). Jones et al. (2007) too have offered that ascribing symptoms to mTBI, rather than mental health difficulties, may be associated with social influence issues in the same manner as it was during World War I:

> In states of uncertainty, it may be that contemporary service personnel prefer to be labeled as suffering from mild TBI than any psychological disorder, just as shell shock in its initial quasi-neurological formulation was very popular. It may be that such labels reduce stigma and encourage help seeking, a major issue for the present generation of service personnel. (p. 1644)

CONCLUSION

Although the notion that TBI might result from blast exposure (i.e., shock wave without blunt trauma) has been pondered for more than two centuries of warfare, the high rate of blasts reported among OEF/OIF soldiers and veterans has revived the need to understand whether this is a potentially unique injury mechanism and what distinct recovery pattern is associated with it. Recent research conducted in animals, artificial proxy models, and with novel neuroimaging technologies supports the idea that blast represents novel mechanism of TBI. However, the process by which concussive injury might result from primary (direct) blast effects is not well understood. As with more conventional (i.e., non–blast-related) forms of concussive injury, blast-related mTBI remains a clinical diagnosis.

The DoD and VA have conducted widespread screening of soldiers and veterans to identify those who may have sustained service-related mTBI. However, the psychometric properties and classification accuracies of contemporary TBI screening tools have come under critical scrutiny of late. Despite the good intentions for identifying at-risk soldiers and veterans, there are genuine concerns regarding their utility and benefits (Vanderploeg & Belanger, 2013). Blast-related concussion remains a clinical diagnosis that is offered on the basis of comprehensive interview, and several recent semistructured clinical interviews have been developed to improve clinicians' and researchers' ability to inform the likelihood that previous combat events resulted in mTBI.

In review of the latest neuropsychological outcome research, there is no consistent evidence that blast-related concussion (1) results in neuropsychological impairments beyond the acute-stage of injury, (2) contributes to cognitive limitations that are distinct from non–blast-related injuries, or (3) results in any long-term cognitive deficits. Although additional outcome studies are needed, available neuropsychology research suggests that behavioral outcome is injury-severity dependent. In other words, it matters only if the head trauma severity is mild versus moderate to severe. Whether it is blast versus nonblast seems to be irrelevant. Like civilian samples, soldiers and veterans who sustain blast-related concussion should anticipate favorable long-term recovery. However, methodologic weaknesses abound (O'Neill et al., 2012), and there is at least some indication of a potential cumulative effect of blast-related concussion (Kontos et al., 2013). The notion of a dose-response pattern between blast-related concussion and long-term outcomes is an area that will benefit from continued study. Blast exposure increases risk of developing psychological and emotional difficulties in both military/veteran and civilian samples, and various physical (e.g., chronic pain) and psychiatric (e.g., PTSD) comorbidities likely represent important contributors to any cognitive impairments and/or self-reported symptoms that may be present in the months and years that follow blast exposure.

Secondary gain, stigmatization, and social influence factors are also likely to represent important noninjury factors that reinforce and extend impairments and symptoms among a certain number of OEF/OIF soldiers and veterans. Similar to civilian concussion samples, particularly those evaluated in secondary gain contexts, OEF/OIF soldiers and veterans who undergo neuropsychological evaluations in relation to disabling blast- and other combat-related concussion show more frequent signs of response invalidity than those evaluated in other contexts. Response validity assessment is essential to neuropsychological evaluation of OEF/OIF soldiers and veterans. Although few recent studies have systematically examined prevalence of stigmatization and social influence, various researchers have suggested that these variables may account, at least in part, for the high rates of combat-related mTBI that have been reported in OEF/OIF soldiers and veterans. These represent important areas for future investigation.

FUTURE DIRECTIONS

The most noteworthy limitation of the contemporary OEF/OIF concussion literature is the heavy reliance on self-report information that researchers use to define and classify "mTBI" status. Despite the well-documented and concerning psychometric properties of TBI screening instruments (including poor stabilities and high false-positive rates), many mTBI outcome studies continue to rely upon the results of TBI screening instruments to define mTBI history (e.g., Kontos et al., 2013; Nelson et al., in review). Even among studies that include "clinician-confirmed" diagnoses of combat-related mTBI or make use of semistructured "comprehensive" interviews (e.g., Brawn Fortier et al., 2014; Nelson et al., 2012a), information related to mTBI is typically derived from self-report and is rarely corroborated by information obtained in the acute-stage of injury. Conversely, those studies that include acute-stage injury characteristics (e.g., Cooper et al., 2012; Kennedy et al., 2012) are rarely (if ever) followed longitudinally in subsequent months and years postinjury. In short, researchers have effectively documented pre-post outcomes, acute-stage impairments, and postdeployment outcomes; what is now needed is an integrated approach that combines these various forms of information, a task that will most likely be facilitated through large-scale DoD/VA collaboration. Until such a longitudinal approach is effectively implemented, as in sports concussion research, the true natural history of blast-related concussion will remain unclear.

Ongoing research devoted to the study of contemporary TBI screening instruments, and possible modifications that may improve reliabilities and classifications of mTBI, are well warranted. TBI screening instruments, including the VATBISI, were developed to err on the side of false-positive identification (General Accounting Office, 2008), and studies have shown that this is in fact how the instrument operates (Belanger et al., 2012). Future researchers might identify strategies by which the VATBISI and other screening instruments may be modified to simultaneously ensure that OEF/OIF soldiers and veterans who present with cognitive, physical, and emotional symptoms receive appropriate treatment, while minimizing the probability of reinforcing false expectations of cause. One might hypothesize, for example, that the current order of item administration, which begins with a specific precipitating event (item 1 pertains to blast exposure or other discrete event) that is followed by more general symptoms (item 4 pertains to current symptoms), results in a priming effect that accounts for the high false-positive rates that have been identified on the VATBISI.

The findings of Strack, Martin, and Schwarz (1988) are of potential relevance in this regard. The authors conducted a priming experiment among 180 undergraduates who were asked two questions: (1) "how happy are you with your life in general?" and (2) "how many dates did you have last month?" When the more general question (i.e., question 1) was asked before the more specific, event-related question (i.e., question 2), the correlation between the questions was minimal ($r = -.01$). By contrast, when the more specific question pertaining to dates in the last month preceded the more general question related to life satisfaction, the correlation between questions 1 and 2 was substantial ($r = .66$). The authors concluded that "answering a specific question makes specific information more accessible for use in answering a subsequent general question. As a consequence of the information priming, the answer to the general question becomes more similar to the answer to the previous specific question (i.e., assimilation" (p. 438). In this context, it is possible that the introduction of items related to specific events (e.g., previous blast exposure) primes respondents to endorse subsequent items related to generalized experience (e.g., symptoms within the last week). Whether the same link between the specific combat event and current symptoms would exist if the order of items was reversed (i.e., generalized symptoms followed by specific combat event) might warrant investigation.

Continued examination of contextual (political, monetary, personal) factors that influence long-term symptoms and outcomes is undeniably also warranted. This is a unique time in our history; the issue of concussion has received a remarkable amount of attention in the public media in recent years, and the frequent discussions of recurrent concussion among professional athletes and OEF/OIF soldiers as depicted in the media may partially reinforce false expectations regarding usual expectations of recovery following mTBI. Future researchers might examine more explicitly the possibility that public media exposure represents a significant source of "diagnosis threat" (Suhr & Gunstad, 2002, 2005) that has been identified as having a negative effect on cognitive performance in certain samples. Researchers might also explore further the various "malleable" factors (e.g., level of knowledge regarding TBI outcomes, self-efficacy, level of attribution) that accounted for a significant proportion of variance in report of PCS (Belanger et al., 2013). Extension of the previous study in blast concussion samples might be especially helpful in identifying appropriate treatment interventions among those with persisting symptoms.

Finally, most studies examining various outcomes following blast-related concussion have included samples with relatively few previous injuries, with many studies including samples with a median of a single blast-related event. Although a recent meta-analytic review did not find consistent evidence that recurrent concussion resulted in overall cognitive outcomes that were distinct relative to single uncomplicated concussions (Belanger et al., 2012), there is continued question as to whether recurrent blast concussion might be distinct in the way of long-term outcomes. In other words, continued exploration of a possible dose-response relationship between blast-related concussion and various outcomes should be considered (Kontos et al.,

2013; Maguen et al., 2012), although again it is important for researchers to establish a more detailed account of previous injury events as defined by acute-injury characteristics at discrete time points.

REFERENCES

Ahmed, F., Gyorgy, A., Kamnaksh, A., Ling, G., Tong, L., Parks, S., & Agoston, D. (2012). Time-dependent changes of protein biomarker levels in the cerebrospinal fluid after blast traumatic brain injury. *Electrophoresis, 33*, 3705–3711.

Alley, M. D., Schimizze, B. R., & Son, S. F. (2011). Experimental modeling of explosive blast-related traumatic brain injuries. *NeuroImage, 54*, S45–S54.

Anderson, E. W. (1942). Psychiatric syndromes following blast. *Journal of Mental Science, 88*, 328–340.

Arbisi, P. A., Polusny, M. A., Erbes, C. R., Thuras, P., & Reddy, M. K. (2011). The Minnesota Multiphasic Personality Inventory-2 Restructured Form in National Guard Soldiers screening positive for posttraumatic stress disorder and mild traumatic brain injury. *Psychological Assessment, 23*, 203–214.

Armistead-Jehle, P. (2010). Symptom validity test performance in US veterans referred for evaluation of mild TBI. *Applied Neuropsychology, 17*, 52–59.

Armistead-Jehle, P., & Buican, B. (2012). Evaluation context and symptom validity test performances in a U.S. military sample. *Archives of Clinical Neuropsychology, 27*, 828–839.

Automated Neuropsychological Assessment Metrics (Version 4) [Computer software]. (2007). Norman, OK: C-SHOP.

Beck, A. T., Steer, R. A., & Brown, G. K. (1996). *Beck Depression Inventory 2nd edition*. San Antonio, TX: The Psychological Corporation.

Belanger, H. G., Barwick, F. H., Kip, K. E., Kretzmer, T., & Vanderploeg, R. D. (2013). Postconcussive symptom complaints and potentially malleable positive predictors. *The Clinical Neuropsychologist, 27*, 343–355.

Belanger, H. G., Kretzmer, T., Vanderploeg, R. D., & French, L. M. (2010). Symptom complaints following combat-related traumatic brain injury: Relationship to traumatic brain injury symptoms and posttraumatic stress disorder. *Journal of the International Neuropsychological Society, 16*, 194–199.

Belanger, H. G., Kretzmer, T., Yoash-Gantz, R., Pickett, T., & Tupler, L. A. (2009a). Cognitive sequelae of blast-related versus other mechanisms of brain trauma. *Journal of the International Neuropsychological Society, 15*, 1–8.

Belanger, H. G., Proctor-Weber, Z., Kretzmer, T., Kim, M., French, L. M., & Vanderploeg, R. D. (2011). Symptom complaints following reports of blast versus non-blast mild TBI: Does mechanism of injury matter? *The Clinical Neuropsychologist, 25*, 702–715.

Belanger, H. G., Spiegel, E., & Vanderploeg, R. D. (2010). Neuropsychological performance following a history of multiple self-reported concussions: A meta-analysis. *Journal of the International Neuropsychological Society, 16*, 262–267.

Belanger, H. G., Uomoto, J. M., & Vanderploeg, R. D. (2009b). The Veterans Health Administration system of care for mild traumatic brain injury: Costs, benefits, and controversies. *Journal of Head Trauma Rehabilitation, 24*, 4–13.

Belanger, H. G., & Vanderploeg, R. D. (2005). The neuropsychological impact of sports-related concussion: A meta-analysis. *Journal of the International Neuropsychological Society, 11*, 345–357.

Belanger, H. G., Vanderploeg, R. D., Soble, J. R., Richardson, M., & Groer, S. (2012). Validity of the Veterans Health Administration's traumatic brain injury screen. *Archives of Physical Medicine Rehabilitation, 93*, 1234–1239.

Bell, R. S., Vo, A. H., Neal, C. J., Tigno, J., Roberts, R., Mossop, C., . . . Armonda, R. A. (2009). Military traumatic brain and spinal column injury: A study of the impact of blast and other military grade weaponry on the central nervous system. *The Journal of Trauma Injury, Infection, and Critical Care, 66*, S104–S111.

Benfield, R. J. Mamczak, C. N., Vo, K-C T., Smith, T., Osborne, L., Sheppard, F. R. & Elster, E. A. (2012). Initial predictors associated with outcome in injured multiple traumatic limb amputations: A Kandahar-based combat hospital experience. *Injury, 43*, 1753–1758.

Benge, J. F., Pastorek, N. J., & Thornton, G. M. (2009). Postconcussive symptoms in OEF-OIF veterans: Factor structure and impact of posttrauamtic stress. *Rehabilitation Psychology, 54*, 270–278.

Ben-Porath, Y. S., & Tellegen, A. (2008). MMPI-2-RF (Minnesota Multiphasic Personality Inventory-2 Restructured Form) Manual. Minneapolis: University of Minnesota Press.

Binder, L. M., Rohling, M. L., & Larrabee, G. J. (1997). A review of mild head trauma. Part I: Meta-analytic review of neuropsychological studies. *Journal of Clinical and Experimental Neuropsychology, 19*, 421–431.

Booth-Kewley, S., Highfill-McRoy, R. M., Larson, G. E., Garland, C. F., & Gaskin, T. A. (2012). Anxiety and depression in Marines sent to war in Iraq and Afghanistan. *Journal of Nervous and Mental Disorders, 200*, 749–757.

Brawn Fortier, C., Amick, M. M., Grande, L., McGlynn, S., Kenna, A., Morra, L., . . . McGlinchey, R. E. (2014). The Boston Assessment of Traumatic Brain Injury-Lifetime (BAT-L) Semistructured Interview: Evidence of research utility and validity. *Journal of Head Trauma Rehabilitation, 29*, 89–98.

Brenner, L. A., Vanderploeg, R. D., & Terrio, H. (2009). Assessment and diagnosis of mild traumatic rain injury, posttraumatic stress disorder, and other polytrauma conditions: Burden of adversity hypothesis. *Rehabilitation Psychology, 54*, 239–246.

Bryant, R. A., Creamer, M., O'Donnell, M., Silove, D., Clark, C. R., & McFarlane, A. C. (2009). Post-traumatic amnesia and the nature of post-traumatic stress disorder after mild traumatic brain injury. *Journal of the International Neuropsychological Society, 15*, 862–867.

Butcher, J. N., Dahlstrom, W. G., Graham, J. R., Tellegen, A. M., & Kaemmer, B. (1989). *MMPI-2, Minnesota Multiphasic Personality Inventory—2: Manual for administration and scoring.* Minneapolis, MN: University of Minnesota Press.

Chan, R. K., Siller-Jackson, A., Verrett, A. J., Wu, J., & Hale, R. G. (2012). Ten years of war: A characteristization of craniomaxillofacial injuries incurred during operations Enduring Freedom and Iraqi Freedom. *J Trauma Acute Care Surg, 73*, S453–S458.

Chen, W., Wang, J., Chen, J., Chen, J., & Chen, Z. (2013). Relationship between changes in the cochlear blood flow and disorder of hearing function induced by blast injury in guinea pigs. *International Journal of Clinical and Experimental Pathology, 6*, 375–384.

Cho, R. I., Bakken, H. E., Reynolds, M. E., Schlifka, B. A., & Powers, D. B. (2009). Concomitant cranial and ocular combat injuries during Operation Iraqi Freedom. *Journal of Trauma, 67*, 516–520.

Cicerone, K., & Kalmar, K. (1995). Persistent post-concussive syndrome: Structure of subjective complaints after mild traumatic brain injury. *Journal of Head Trauma Rehabilitation, 10*, 1–17.

Cifu, D., Bowles, A., Hurley, R., Cooper, D., Peterson, M., Drake, A., . . . Barth, J. (2009). Management of Concussion/mild Traumatic Brain Injury. *The Management of*

Concussion/mTBI Working Group. U.S. Department of Veterans Affairs and US Department of Defense. Washington, DC.

Cockerham, G. C., Lemke, S., Glynn-Milley, C., Zumhagen, L., & Cockerham, K. P. (2013). Visual performance and the ocular surface in traumatic brain injury. *The Ocular Surface, 11*, 25–34.

Coldren, R. L., Kelly, M. P., Parish, R. V., Dretsch, M., & Russell, M. L. (2010). Evaluation of the military acute concussion evaluation for use in combat operations more than 12 hours after injury. *Military Medicine, 175*, 477–481.

Coldren, R. L., Russell, M. L., Parish, R. V., Dretsch, M., & Kelly, M. P. (2012). The ANAM lacks utility as a diagnostic or screening tool for concussion more than 10 days following injury. *Military Medicine, 177*, 179–183.

Cooper, D. B., Chau, P. M., Armistead-Jehle, P., Vanderploeg, R. D., & Bowles, A. O. (2012). Relationship between mechanism of injury and neurocognitive functioning in OEF/OIF service members with mild traumatic brain injuries. *Military Medicine, 177*, 1157–1160.

Cooper, D. B., Kennedy, J. E., Cullen, M. A., Critchfield, E., Amador, R. R., & Bowles, A. O. (2011a). Association between combat stress and post-concussive symptom reporting in OEF/OIF service members with mild traumatic brain injuries. *Brain Injury, 25*, 1–7.

Cooper, D. B., Nelson, L., Armistead-Jehle, P., & Bowles, A. O. (2011b). Utility of the mild brain injury atypical symptoms scale as a screening measure for symptom over-reporting in Operation Enduring Freedom/Operation Iraqi Freedom service members with post-concussive complaints. *Archives of Clinical Neuropsychology, 26*, 718–727.

Corrigan, J. D., & Bogner, J. (2007). Initial reliability and validity of the Ohio State University TBI Identification Method. *Journal of Head Trauma Rehabilitation, 22*, 318–329.

Courtney, M. W., & Courtney, A. C. (2011). Working toward exposure thresholds for blast-induced thoracic and acceleration mechanisms. *NeuroImage, 54*, S55–S61.

Cramer, F., Pastor, S., & Stephenson, C. (1947). Cerebral injuries due to explosion waves: Blast concussion. *Journal of Nervous & Mental Disease, 106*, 602–605.

Defense and Veterans Brain Injury Center (2007). Military Acute Concussion Evaluation. Retrieved from www.dvbic.org

Denny-Brown, D. (1945). Cerebral concussion. *Physiological Reviews, 25*, 296–325.

DePalma, R. G., Burris, D. G., Champion, H. R., & Hodgson, M. J. (2005). Blast injuries. *The New England Journal of Medicine, 352*, 1335–1342.

Dobscha, S. K., Clark, M. E., Morasco, B. J., Freeman, M., Campbell, R., & Helfand, M. (2009). Systematic review of the literature on pain in patients with polytrauma including traumatic brain injury. *Pain Medicine, 10*, 1200–1217.

Donnell, A. J., Kim, M. S., Silva, M. A., & Vanderploeg, R. D. (2012). Incidence of postconcussion symptoms in psychiatric diagnostic groups, mild traumatic brain injury, and comorbid conditions. *The Clinical Neuropsychologist, 26*, 1092–1101.

Donnelly, K. T., Donnelly, J. P., Dunnam, M., Warner, G. C., Kittelson, C. J., Constance, J. E., . . . Alt, M. (2011). Reliability, sensitivity, and specificity of the VA traumatic brain injury screening tool. *Journal of Head Trauma Rehabilitation, 26*, 439–453.

Drag, L. L., Spencer, R. J., Walker, S. J., Pangilinan, P. H., & Bieliauskas, L. A. (2012). The contributions of self-reported injury characteristics and psychiatric symptoms to cognitive functioning in OEF/OIF veterans with mild traumatic brain injury. *Journal of the International Neuropsychological Society, 18*, 576–584.

DuBose, J. J., Barmparas, G., Inaba, K., Stein, D. M., Scalea, T., Cancio, L. C., . . . Blackbourne, L. (2011). Isolated severe traumatic brain injuries sustained during combat operations: Demographics, mortality outcomes, and lessons to be learned from contrasts to civilian counterparts. *The Journal of Trauma, 70*, 11–18.

Duncan, C. C., Summers, A. C., Perla, E. J., Coburn, K. L., & Mirsky, A. F. (2011). Evaluation of traumatic brain injury: Brain potentials in diagnosis, function, and prognosis. *International Journal of Psychopathology, 82*, 24–40.

Edwards, M. J., Lustik, M., Eichelberger, M. R., Elster, E., Azarow, K., & Coppola, C. (2012). Blast injury in children: An analysis from Afghanistan and Iraq, 2002-2010. *J Trauma Acute Care Surg, 73*, 1278–1283.

Epstein, D. R., Babcock-Parziale, J. L., Haynes, P. L., & Herb, C. A. (2012). Insomnia treatment acceptability and preferences of male Iraq and Afghanistan combat veterans and their healthcare providers. *Journal of Rehabilitation Research & Development, 49*, 867–878.

Erbes, C. R., Meis, L. A., & Polusny, M. A. (2011). Couple adjustment and posttraumatic stress disorder symptoms in National Guard veterans of the Iraq War. *Journal of Family Psychology, 25*, 479–487.

Erickson, J. C. (2011). Treatment outcomes of chronic post-traumatic headaches after mild head trauma in U.S. soldiers: An observational study. *Headache, 51*, 932–944.

Eskridge, S. L., Macera, C. A., Galarneau, M. R., Holbrook, T. L., Woodruff, S. I., MacGregor, A. J., . . . Shaffer, R. A. (2012). Injuries from combat explosions in Iraq: Injury type, location, and severity. *Injury, 43*, 1678–1682.

Fabing, H. D. (1947). Cerebral blast syndrome in combat soldiers. *Archives of Neurology and Psychiatry, 57*, 14–57.

Fear, N. T., Jones, E., Groom, M., Greenberg, N., Hull, L., Hodgetts, T. J., & Wessely, S. (2009). Symptoms of post-concussional syndrome are non-specifically related to mild traumatic brain injury in UK armed forces personnel on return from deployment in Iraq: An analysis of self-reported data. *Psychological Medicine, 39*, 1379–1387.

Fitzgerald, D. B., & Crosson, B. A. (2011). Diffusion weighted imaging and neuropsychological correlates in adults with mild traumatic brain injury. *International Journal of Psychopathology, 82*, 79–85.

Foley, L. M., O'Meara, A., Wisniewski, S. R., Hitchens, T. K., Melick, J. A., Ho, C., . . . Kochanek, P. M. (2013). MRI assessment of cerebral blood flow after experimental traumatic brain injury combined with hemorrhagic shock in mice. *Journal of Cerebral Blood Flow & Metabolism, 33*, 129–136.

Frencham, K. A., Fox, A. M., & Maybery, M. T. (2005). Neuropsychological studies of mild traumatic brain injury: A meta-analytic review of research since 1995. *Journal of Clinical and Experimental Neuropsychology, 27*, 334–351.

Ganpule, S., Alai, A., Plougonven, E., & Chandra, N. (2012). Mechanics of blast loading on the head models in the study of traumatic brain injury using experimental and computational approaches. *Biomech Model Mechanobiol.* Online Journal DOI 10.1007/s10237-012-0421-8.

Gates, M. A., Holowka, D. W., Vasterling, J. J., Keane, T. M., Marx, B. P., & Rosen, R. C. (2012). Posttraumatic stress disorder in veterans and military personnel: Epidemiology, screening and case recognition. *Psychological Services, 9*, 361–382.

General Accounting Office. (2008, February). VA Health Care. Mild traumatic brain injury screening and evaluation implemented for OEF/OIF veterans, but challenges remain. GAO-08-276. Washington, DC. Retrieved from www.gao.gov/new.items/d08276.pdf.

Graner, J., Oakes, T. R., French, L. M., & Ried, G. (2013). Functional MRI in the investigation of blast-related traumatic brain injury. *Frontiers in Neurology, 4*, 1–18.

Heilbronner, R. L., Sweet, J. J., Morgan, J. E., Larrabee, G. J. Millis, S. R., & Conference Participants (2009). American Academy of Clinical Neuropsychology consensus conference statement on the neuropsychological assessment of effort, response bias, and malingering. *The Clinical Neuropsychologist, 23*, 1093–1129.

Hoge, C. W., Castro, C. A., Messer, S. C., McGurk, D., Cotting, D. I., & Koffman, R. L. (2004). Combat duty in Iraq and Afghanistan, mental health problems, and barriers to care. *The New England Journal of Medicine, 351*, 13–22.

Hoge, C. W., McGurk, D., Thomas, J. L., Cox, A. L., Engel, C. C., & Castro, C. A. (2008). Mild traumatic brain injury in U.S. soldiers returning from Iraq. *New England Journal of Medicine, 358*, 453–463.

Howe, L. L. S. (2009). Giving context to post-deployment post-concussive-like symptoms: Blast-related potential mild traumatic brain injury and comorbidities. *The Clinical Neuropsychologist, 23*, 1315–1337.

Huang, M-X, Nichols, S., Robb, A., Angeles, A., Drake, A., Holland, M., . . . Lee, R. R. (2012). An automatic MEG low-frequency source imaging approach for detecting injuries in mild and moderate TBI patients with blast and non-blast causes. *NeuroImage, 61*, 1067–1082.

Ivanovic, A., Jovic, N., Vukelic-Markovic, S. (1996). Frontoethmoidal fractures as a result of war injuries. *Journal of Trauma, 40*, S177–S179.

Iverson, G. L. (2005). Outcome from mild traumatic brain injury. *Current Opinion in Psychiatry, 18*, 301–317.

Iverson, G. L. (2006). Misdiagnosis of the persistent postconcussion syndrome in patients with depression. *Archives of Clinical Neuropsychology, 21*, 303–310.

Iverson, G. L., & Lange, R. T. (2003). Examination of "postconcussion-like" symptoms in a healthy sample. *Applied Neuropsychology, 10*, 137–144.

Iverson, G. L., Langlois, J. A., McCrea, M. A., & Kelly, J. P. (2009). Challenges associated with post-deployment screening for mild traumatic brain injury in military personnel. *The Clinical Neuropsychologist, 23*, 1299–1314.

Iverson, G. L., & McCracken, L. M. (1997). "Postconcussive" symptoms in persons with chronic pain. *Brain Injury, 11*, 783–790.

Jantzen, K. J. (2010). Functional magnetic resonance imaging of mild traumatic brain injury. *Journal of Head Trauma Rehabilitation, 25*, 256–266.

Jones, A. (2013a). Test of memory malingering: Cutoff scores for psychometrically defined malingering groups in a military sample. *The Clinical Neuropsychologist, 27*, 1043–1059.

Jones, A. (2013b). Victoria symptom validity test: Cutoff scores for psychometrically defined malingering groups in a military sample. *The Clinical Neuropsychologist, 27*, 1373–1394.

Jones, A., & Ingram, M. V. (2011). A comparison of selected MMPI-2 and MMPI-2-RF validity scales in assessing effort on cognitive tests in a military sample. *The Clinical Neuropsychologist, 25*, 1207–1227.

Jones, A., Ingram, M. V., & Ben-Porath, Y. S. (2012). Scores on the MMPI-2-RF scales as a function of increasing levels of failure on cognitive symptom validity tests in a military sample. *The Clinical Neuropsychologist, 26*, 790–815.

Jones, E. (2006). Historical approaches to post-combat disorders. *Philosophical Transactions of the Royal Society, 361*, 533–542.

Jones, E., Fear, N. T., & Wessely, S. (2007). Shell shock and mild traumatic brain injury: A historical review. *American Journal of Psychiatry, 164*, 1641–1645.

Jones, E., & Wessely, S. (2001). Psychiatric battle casualties: An intra- and interwar comparison. *British Journal of Psychiatry, 178*, 242–247.

Jones, E., & Wessely, S. (2005). *Shell shock to PTSD: Military psychiatry from 1900 to the Gulf War*. Psychology Press: Hove.

Kamnaksh, A., Kwon, S-K, Kovesdki, E., Ahmed, F., Barry, E. S., Grunberg, N. E., . . . Agoston, D. (2012). Neurobehavioral, cellular, and molecular consequences of single and multiple mild blast exposure. *Electrophoresis, 33,* 3680–3692.

Kay, T., Harrington, D.E., Adams, R., Anderson, T., Berrol, S., Cicerone, K., . . . Malec, J. (1993). Definition of mild traumatic brain injury. *Journal of Head Trauma Rehabilitation, 8,* 86–87.

Kennedy, C. H., Evans, J. P., Chee, S., Moore, J. L., Barth, J. T., & Stuessi, K. A. (2012). Return to combat duty after concussive blast injury. *Archives of Clinical Neuropsychology, 27,* 817–827.

Kontos, A. P., Kotwal, R. S., Elbin, R. J., Lutz, R. H., Forsten, R. D., Benson, P. J., & Guskiewicz, K. M. (2013). Residual effects of combat-related mild traumatic brain injury. *Journal of Neurotrauma, 30,* 680–686.

Lamberty, G. J., Nelson, N. W., & Yamada, T. (2013). Effects and outcomes in civilian and military traumatic brain injury: Similarities, differences, and forensic implications. *Behavioral Sciences and the Law, 31,* 814–832.

Lange, R. T., Edmed, S. L., Sullivan, K. A., French, L. M., & Cooper, D. B. (2013). Utility of the mild brain injury atypical symptoms scale to detect symptom exaggeration: An analogue simulation study. *Journal of Clinical and Experimental Neuropsychology, 35,* 192–209.

Lange, R. T., Iverson, G. L., & Rose, A. (2011). Depression strongly influences postconcussion symptom reporting following mild traumatic brain injury. *Journal of Head Trauma and Rehabilitation, 26,* 127–137.

Lange, R. T., Pancholi, S., Brickell, T. A., Sakura, S., Bhagwat, A., Merritt, V., & French, L. M. (2012). Neuropsychological outcome from blast versus non-blast: Mild traumatic brain injury in U.S. military service members. *Journal of the Neuropsychological Society, 18,* 595–605.

Lesperance, K., Martin, M. J., Beekley, A. C., & Steele, S. R. (2008). The significance of penetrating gluteal injuries: An analysis of the Operation Iraqi Freedom experience. *Journal of Surgical Education, 65,* 61–66.

Lew, H. L., Jerger, J. F., Guillory, S. B., & Henry, J. A. (2007). Auditory dysfunction in traumatic brain injury. *Journal of Rehabilitation Research & Development, 44,* 921–928.

Linn, L., & Stein, M. H. (1945). Psychiatric studies of blast injuries of the ear. *War Medicine, 8,* 32–33.

Lippa, S. M., Pastorek, N. J., Benge, J. F., & Thornton, G. M. (2010). Postconcussive symptoms after blast and nonblast-related mild traumatic brain injuries in Afghanistan and Iraq War veterans. *Journal of the International Neuropsychological Society, 16,* 856–866.

Liu, H., Kang, J., Chen, J., Li, G., Li, X., & Wang, J. (2012). Intracranial pressure response to non-penetrating ballistic impact: An experimental study using a pig physical head model and live pigs. *International Journal of Medical Science, 9,* 655–664.

Lopes Cardozo, B., Blanton, C., Zalewski, T., Tor, S., McDonald, L., Lavelle, J., . . . Mollica, R. (2012). Mental health survey among landmine survivors in Siem Reap province, Cambodia. *Medicine, Conflict, and Survival, 28,* 161–181.

Luethcke, C. A., Bryan, C. J., Morrow, C. E., & Isler, W. C. (2011). Comparison of concussive symptoms, cognitive performance, and psychological symptoms between acute blast-versus nonblast-induced mild traumatic brain injury. *Journal of the International Neuropsychological Society, 17,* 36–45.

MacDonald, H. Z., Proctor, S. P., Heeren, T., & Vasterling, J. J. (2013). Associations of post-deployment PTSD symptoms with predepployment symptoms in Iraq-deployed Army soldiers. *Psychological Trauma: Theory, Research, and Policy, 5*, 470–476.

MacGregor, A. J., Dougherty, A. L., & Galarneau, M. R. (2011). Injury-specific correlates of combat-related traumatic brain injury in Operation Iraqi Freedom. *Journal of Head Trauma Rehabilitation, 26*, 312–318.

Maguen, S., Madden, E., Lau, K. M., & Seal, K. (2012). The impact of head injury mechanism on mental health symptoms in veterans: Do number and type of exposures matter? *Journal of Traumatic Stress, 25*, 3–9.

Matthews, S. C., Spadoni, A. D., Lohr, J. B., Strigo, I. A., & Simmons, A. N. (2012). Diffusion tensor imaging evidence of white matter disruption associated with loss versus alteration of consciousness in warfighters exposed to combat in Operations Enduring and Iraqi Freedom. *Psychiatry Research: Neuroimaging, 204*, 149–154.

Matthews, S. C., Strigo, I. A., Simmons, A. N., O'Connell, R. M., Reinhardt, L. E., & Moseley, S. A. (2011). Multimodal imaging study in U.S. veterans of Operations Iraqi and Enduring Freedom with and without major depression after blast-related concussion. *NeuroImage, 54*, S69–S75.

Mayorga, M. A. (1997). The pathology of primary blast overpressure injury. *Toxicology, 121*, 17–28.

McCrea, M. A. (2008). *Mild traumatic brain injury and postconcussion syndrome*. New York: Oxford University Press.

McCrea, M., Iverson, G. L., McAllister, T. W., Hammeke, T. A., Powell, M. R., Barr, W. B., & Kelly, J. (2009). An integrated review of recovery after mild traumatic brain injury (MTBI): Implications for clinical management. *The Clinical Neuropsychologist, 23*, 1368–1390.

McCrea, M., Pliskin, N., Barth, J., Cox, D, Fink, J., French, L., . . . Yoash-Gantz, R. (2008). Official Position of the Military TBI Task Force on the Role of Neuropsychology and Rehabilitation Psychology in the Evaluation, Management, and Research of Military Veterans with Traumatic Brain Injury. *The Clinical Neuropsychologist, 22*, 10–26.

McDonald, B. C., Saykin, A. J., & McAllister, T. W. (2012). Functional MRI of mild traumatic brain injury (mTBI): Progress and perspectives from the first decade of studies. *Brain Imaging and Behavior, 6*, 193–207.

McNally, R. J., & Frueh, B. C. (2013). Why are Iraq and Afghanistan War veterans seeking PTSD disability compensation at unprecedented rates? *Journal of Anxiety Disorders, 27*, 520–526.

Mittenberg, W., Patton, C., Canyock, E. M., & Condit, D. C. (2002). Base rates of malingering and symptom exaggeration. *Journal of Clinical and Experimental Neuropsychology, 24*, 1094–1102.

Mora, A. G., Ritenour, A. E., Wade, C. E., Holcomb, J. B., Blackbourne, L. H., & Gaylord, K. M. (2009). Posttraumatic stress disorder in combat casualties with burns sustaining primary blast and concussive injuries. *The Journal of Trauma, 66*, S178–S185.

Morey, L. C. (1991). *The Personality Assessment Inventory*. Odessa, FL: Psychological Assessment Inventory.

Morey, R. A., Haswell, C. C., Selgrade, E. S., Massoglia, D., Liu, C., Weiner, J., . . . McCarthy, G. (2012). Effects of chronic mild traumatic brain injury on white matter integrity in Iraq and Afghanistan War veterans. *Human Brain Mapping* (online journal). doi:10.1002/hbm.22117

Morrow, C. E., Bryan, C. J., & Isler, W. C. (2011). Concussive and psychological symptom predictors of aeromedical evacuation following possible brain injury among deployed military personnel. *Psychological Services, 8*, 224–235.

Murray, C. K., Reynolds, J. C., Schroeder, J. M., Harrison, M. B., Evans, O. M., & Hospenthal, D. R. (2005). Spectrum of care provided at an echelon II medical unit during Operation Iraqi Freedom. *Military Medicine, 170,* 516–520.

Nelson, N. W., Anderson, C. R., Thuras, P., Kehle-Forbes, S. M., Arbisi, P. A., Erbes, C. R., & Polusny, M.A. (in press). Factors associated with inconsistency in self-reported mild traumatic brain injury over time among U.S. National Guard Soldiers deployed to Iraq. *British Journal of Psychiatry.*

Nelson, N. W., Hoelzle, J. B., Doane, B. M., McGuire, K. A., Ferrier-Auerbach, A. G., Charlesworth, M. J., . . . Sponheim, S. R. (2012). Neuropsychological outcomes of U.S. veterans with report of remote blast concussion and current psychopathology. *Journal of the International Neuropsychological Society, 18,* 845–855.

Nelson, N. W., Hoelzle, J. B., McGuire, K. A., Ferrier-Auerbach, A. G., Charlesworth, M. J., & Sponheim, S. R. (2010). Evaluation context impacts neuropsychological performance of OEF/OIF veterans with reported combat-related concussion. *Archives of Clinical Neuropsychology, 25,* 713–723.

Nelson, N. W., Hoelzle, J. B., McGuire, K. A., Ferrier-Auerbach, A. G., Charlesworth, M. J., & Sponheim, S. R. (2011a). Neuropsychological evaluation of blast-related concussion: Illustrating the challenges and complexities through OEF/OIF case studies. *Brain Injury, 25,* 511–525.

Nelson, N. W., Hoelzle, J. B., McGuire, K. A., Sim, A. H., Goldman, D. J., Ferrier-Auerbach, A. G., . . . Sponheim, S. R. (2011b). Self-report of psychological function among OEF/OIF personnel who also report combat-related concussion. *The Clinical Neuropsychologist, 25,* 716–740.

Nunnink, S. E., Fink, D. S., & Baker, D. G. (2012). The impact of sexual functioning problems on mental well-being in U.S. veterans from the Operation Enduring Freedom and Operation Iraqi Freedom (OEF/OIF) conflicts. *International Journal of Sexual Health, 24,* 14–25.

O'Neil, M. E., Carlson, K. F., Storzbach, D., Brenner, L. A., Freeman, M., Quiñones, A., . . . Kansagara, D. (2013). *Complications of mild traumatic brain injury in veterans and military personnel: A systematic review.* VA-ESP Project #05-225; 2012

Owens, B. D., Kragh, J. F., Wenke, J. C., Macaitis, J., Wade, C. E., & Holcomb, J. B. (2008). Combat wounds in Operation Iraqi Freedom and Operation Enduring Freedom. *Journal of Trauma, 64,* 295–299.

Park, E., Eisen, R., Kinio, A., & Baker, A. J. (2013). Electrophysiological white matter dysfunction and association with deficits following low-level primary blast trauma. *Neurobiology of Disease, 52,* 150–159.

Patel, H. D. L., Dryden, S., Gupta, A., & Stewart, N. (2012). Human body projectiles implantation in victims of suicide bombings and implications for health and emergency care providers, the 7/7 experience. *Annals Royal College of Surgeons England, 94,* 313–317.

Peskind, E. R., Petrie, E. C., Cross, D. J., Pagulayan, K., McCraw, K., Hoff, D., . . . Minoshima, S. (2011). Cerebrocerebellar hypometabolism associated with repetitive blast exposure mild traumatic brain injury in 12 Iraq War veterans persistent postconcussive symptoms. *NeuroImage, 54,* S76–S82.

Petras, J. M., Bauman, R. A., & Elsayed, N. M. (1997). Visual system degeneration induced by blast overpressure. *Toxicology, 121,* 41–49.

Polusny, M. A., Kehle, S. M., Nelson, N. W., Erbes, C. R., Arbisi, P. A., & Thuras, P. (2011). Longitudinal effects of mild TBI and PTSD comorbidity on post-deployment outcomes in National Guard soldiers deployed to Iraq. *Archives of General Psychiatry, 68,* 79–89.

Rafaels, K. A., Bass, C. R. D., Panzer, M. B., Salzar, R. S., Woods, A., Feldman, S. H., . . . Derkunt, B. (2012). Brain injury risk from primary blast. *Journal of Trauma and Acute Care Surgery, 73*, 895–901.

Rafaels, K. A., Bass, C. R. D., Salzar, R. S., Panzer, M. B., Woods, A., Feldman, S. H., . . . Capehart, B. (2011). Survival risk assessment for primary blast exposures to the head. *Journal of Neurotrauma, 28*, 2319–2328.

Ramasamy, A., Harrisson, S. E., Clasper, J. C., Stewart, M. P. (2008). Injuries from road- side improvised explosive devices. *Journal of Trauma, 65*, 910–914.

Randolph, C. (1998). Repeatable Battery for the Assessment of Neuropsychological Status (RBANS) Manual. San Antonio, TX: The Psychological Corporation.

Reid, F. (2010). *Broken men: Shell shock, treatment and recovery in Britain 1914-30.* London: Continuum.

Roberts, J. C., Harrigan, T. P., Ward, E. E., Taylor, T. M., Annett, M. S., & Merkle, A. C. (2012). Human head-neck computational model for assessing blast injury. *Journal of Biomechanics, 45*, 2899–2906.

Roebuck-Spencer, T. M., Vincent, A. S., Twillie, D. A., Logan, B. W., Lopez, M., Friedl, K. E., . . . Gilliland, K. (2012). Cognitive change associated with self-reported mild traumatic brain injury sustained during the OEF/OIF conflicts. *The Clinical Neuropsychologist, 26*, 473–489.

Rossi, T., Boccassini, B., Esposito, L., Clemente, C., Iossa, M., Pacentino, L., & Bonora, N. (2012). Primary blast injury to the eye and orbit: Finite element modeling. *Investigative Ophthalmology & Visual Science, 53*, 8057–8066.

Roth, R. S., & Spencer, R. J. (2013). Iatrogenic risk in the management of mild traumatic brain injury among combat veterans: A case illustration and commentary. *J Palliative Care Med, 1*, 105.

Ruff, R., Richardson, A. M. Mild traumatic brain injury. In J. J. Sweet (Ed.), *Forensic neuropsychology: Fundamentals and practice* (pp. 315–338). Lisse: Swets & Zeitlinger.

Saljo, A., Mayorga, M., Bolouri, H., Svensson, B., & Hamberger, A. (2011). Mechanisms and pathophysiology of the low-level blast brain injury in animal models. *NeuroImage, 54*, S83–S88.

Sayer, N. A., Chiros, C. E., Sigford, B., Scott, S., Clothier, B., Pickett, T., & Lew, H. L. (2008). Characteristics and rehabilitation outcomes among patients with blast and other injuries sustained during the Global War on Terror. *Archives of Physical Medicine and Rehabilitation, 89*, 163–170.

Sbordone, R. J., & Liter, J. C. (1995). Mild traumatic brain injury does not produce post-traumatic stress disorder. *Brain Injury, 9*, 405–412.

Scheibel, R. S., Newsome, M. R., Troyanskaya, M., Lin, X., Steinberg, J. L., Radaideh, M., & Levin, H. S. (2012). Altered brain activation in military personnel with one or more traumatic brain injuries following blast. *Journal of the International Neuropsychological Society, 18*, 89–100.

Scherer, M. R., & Schubert, M. C. (2009). Traumatic brain injury and vestibular pathology as a comorbidity after blast exposure. *Physical Therapy, 89*, 980–992.

Schneiderman, A. I., Braver, E. R., & Kang, H. K. (2008). Understanding sequelae of injury mechanisms and mild traumatic brain injury incurred during the conflicts in Iraq and Afghanistan: Persistent postconcussive symptoms and post-traumatic stress disorder. *American Journal of Epidemiology, 167*, 1446–1452.

Schretlen, D.J., & Shapiro, A.M. (2003). A quantitative review of the effects of traumatic brain injury on cognitive functioning. *International Review of Psychiatry, 15*, 341–349.

Schwab, K. A., Ivins, B., Cramer, G., Johnson, W., Sluss-Tiller, M., Kiley, K., . . . Warden, D. (2007). Screening for traumatic brain injury in troops returning from deployment in Afghanistan and Iraq: Initial investigation of the usefulness of a short screening tool for traumatic brain injury. *Journal of Head Trauma Rehabilitation, 22*, 377–389.

Shandera-Ochsner, A. L., Berry, D. T. R., Harp, J. P., Edmundson, M., Graue, L. O., Roach, A., & Higher, W. M. (2013). Neuropsychological effects of self-reported deployment-related mild TBI and current PTSD in OIF/OEF veterans. *The Clinical Neuropsychologist, 27*, 881–907.

Shenton, M. E., Hamoda, H. M., Schneiderman, J. S., Bouix, S., Pasternak, O., Rathi, Y., . . . Zafonte, R. (2012). A review of magnetic resonance imaging and diffusion tensory imaging findings in mild traumatic brain injury. *Brain Imaging and Behavior, 6*, 137–192.

Silver, J. M. (2012). Diffusion tensor imaging and mild traumatic brain injury in soldiers: Abnormal findings, uncertain implications. *American Journal of Psychiatry, 169*, 1230–1232.

Spencer, R. J., & Adams, K. M. (2012). Neuropsychology and polytrauma services. In S. S. Bush (Ed.), *Neuropsychological practice for veterans* (pp. 77–98). New York, NY: Springer.

Strack, F., Martin, L. L., & Schwarz, N. (1988). Priming and communication: Social determinants of information use in judgments of life satisfaction. *European Journal of Social Psychology, 18*, 429–442.

Suhr, J. A., & Gunstad, J. (2002). "Diagnosis Threat": The effect of negative expectations on cognitive performance in head injury. *Journal of Clinical and Experimental Neuropsychology, 24*, 448–457.

Suhr, J. A., & Gunstad, J. (2005). Further exploration of the effect of "diagnosis threat" on cognitive performance in individuals with mild head injury. *Journal of the International Neuropsychological Society, 11*, 23–29.

Taber, K. H., Warden, D. L., & Hurley, R. A. (2006). Blast-related traumatic brain injury: What is known? *Journal of Neuropsychiatry and Clinical Neuroscience, 18*, 141–145.

Tanielian, T., & Jaycox, L. H. (2008). *Invisible wounds of war: Psychological and cognitive injuries, their consequences, and services to assist recovery.* Santa Monica, CA: Rand Corporation.

Tantawi, D., Armonda, R., Valerio, I., & Kumar, A. R. (2012). Management of decompressive craniectomy defects: Modern military treatment strategies. *The Journal of Craniofacial Surgery, 23*, 2042–2045.

Taylor, B. C., Hagel, E. M., Carlson, K. F., Cifu, D. X., Cutting, A., Bidelspach, D. E., & Sayer, N. A. (2012). Prevalence and costs of co-occuring traumatic brain injury with and without psychiatric disturbance among Afghanistan and Iraq War Veteran VA users. *Medical Care, 50*, 342–346.

Terrio, H., Brenner, L. A., Ivins, B. J., Cho, J. M., Schwab, K., Scally, K., . . . Warden, D. (2009). Traumatic brain injury screening: Preliminary findings in a U.S. Army Brigade combat team. *Journal of Head Trauma Rehabilitation, 24*, 14–23.

Terrio, H. P., Nelson, L. A., Betthauser, L. M., Harwood, J. E., & Brenner, L. A. (2011). Postdeployment traumatic brain injury screening questions: Sensitivity, specificity, and predictive values in returning soldiers. *Rehabilitation Psychology, 56*, 26–31.

Theeler, B. J., Flynn, F. G., & Erickson, J. C. (2012). Chronic daily headache in U.S. soldiers after concussion. *Headache, 52*, 732–738.

Valiyaveettil, M., Alamneh, Y., Wang, Y., Arun, P., Oguntayo, S., Wei, Y., . . . Nambiar, M. P. (2013). Contribution of systemic factors in the pathophysiology of repeated blast-induced neurotrauma. *Neuroscience Letters*, 1–6.

Van Dyke, S. A., Axelrod, B. N., & Schutte, C. (2010). Test-retest reliability of the traumatic brain injury screening instrument. *Military Medicine, 175*, 947–949.

Vanderploeg, R. D., & Belanger, H. G. (2013). Screening for a remote history of mild traumatic brain injury: When a good idea is bad. *Journal of Head Trauma Rehabilitation, 28*, 211–218.

Vanderploeg, R. D., Belanger, H. G., & Brenner, L. A. (2013). Blast injuries and PTSD: Lessons learned from the Iraqi and Afghanistan conflicts. In S. Koffler, J. Morgan, I. S. Baron, & M. F. Greiffenstein (Eds.), *Neuropsychology science & practice I* (pp. 114–148). Oxford: New York, NY.

Vanderploeg, R. D., Belanger, H. G., Horner, R. D., Spehar, A. M., Powell-Cope, G., Luther, S. L., & Scott, S. G. (2012). Health outcomes associated with military deployment: Mild traumatic brain injury, blast, trauma, and combat associations in the Florida National Guard. *Archives of Physical Medicine Rehabilitation, 93*, 1887–1895.

Vanderploeg, R.D., Groer, S., & Belanger, H.G. (2012). The Initial Developmental Process of a VA Semi-Structured Clinical Interview for TBI Identification. *Journal of Rehabilitation Research and Development, 49*, 545–556.

Vasterling, J. J., Brailey, K., Proctor, S. P., Kane, R., Heeren, T., & Franz, M. (2012). Neuropsychological outcomes of mild traumatic brain injury, post-traumatic stress disorder and depression in Iraq-deployed US Army soldiers. *British Journal of Psychiatry, 201*, 186–192.

Verfaellie, M., Lafleche, G., Spiro, A., Tun, C., and Bousquet, K. (2013). Chronic postconcussoin symptoms and functional outcomes in OEF/OIF veterans with self-report of blast exposure. *Journal of the International Neuropsychological Society, 19*, 1–10.

Walker, W., McDonald, S. D., Ketchum, J. M., Nichols, M., & Cifu, D. N. (2012). Identification of transient altered consciousness induced by military-related blast exposure and its relation to postconcussion symptoms. *Journal of Head Trauma Rehabilitation, 28*, 68–76.

Weichel, E. D., Colyer, M. H., Bautista, C., Bower, K. S., & French, L. M. (2009). Traumatic brain injury associated with combat ocular trauma. *Journal of Head Trauma Rehabilitation, 24*, 41–50.

Weisbrod, A. B., Rodriguez, C., Bell, R., Neal, C., Armonda, R., Dorlac, W., . . . Dunne, J. R. (2012). Long-term outcomes of combat causalities sustaining penetrating traumatic brain injury. *J Trauma Acute Care Surg, 73*, 1525–1530.

Whitney, K. A., Shepard, P. H., Williams, A. L., Davis, J. J., & Adams, K. M. (2009). The Medical Symptom Validity Test in the evaluation of Operation Iraqi Freedom/Operation Enduring Freedom soldiers: A preliminary study. *Archives of Clinical Neuropsychology, 24*, 145–152.

Widome, R., Laska, M. N., Gulden, A., Fu, S. S., & Lust, K. (2011). Health risk behaviors of Afghanistan and Iraq War veterans attending college. *American Journal of Health Promotion, 26*, 101–108.

Williams, J. L., McDevitt-Murphy, M. E., Murphy, J. G., & Crouse, E. M. (2012). Deployment risk factors and postdeployment health profiles associated with traumatic brain injury in heavy drinking veterans. *Military Medicine, 177*, 789–796.

Xydakis, M. S., Bebarta, V. S., Harrison, C. D., Conner, J. C., & Grant, G. A. (2007). Tympanic-membrane perforation as a marker of concussive brain injury in Iraq. *New England Journal of Medicine, 357*, 830–831.

5

NEUROPSYCHOLOGICAL EFFECTS OF SPORT-RELATED CONCUSSION

Michael McCrea, Peter D. Leo, and Lindsay D. Nelson

Sport-related concussion (SRC) is widely recognized as a major public health issue in the United States and worldwide.[1] SRC remains the focus of increasing concern from clinicians, researchers, sporting organizations, and athletes over the last 20 years (Barr & McCrea, 2001; DeKosky, Ikonomovic, & Gandy, 2010; Kelly, 1999; Langlois, Rutland-Brown, & Wald, 2006; McCrory et al., 2005, 2009). The annual incidence of nonfatal traumatic brain injuries (TBIs) from sports and recreation activities in persons aged 19 years or younger is estimated to be more than 2.6 million per year in the United States (Gilchrist, Thomas, Xu, McGuire, & Coronado, 2011). Concussion, commonly referred to as mild TBI (mTBI), is defined as a traumatically induced disturbance in brain function caused by a complex pathophysiologic process that is transient in nature (Gallagher et al., 2007).

Concussion is now among the most frequent injuries in contact and collision sports at all levels of participation, including youth sports (Guskiewicz, Weaver, Padua, & Garrett, 2000; Halstead & Walter, 2010; Powell & Barber-Foss, 1999). A recent study indicated that from 1997 to 2007 emergency department visits for 8- to 13-year-old children affected by concussion in organized sports doubled and increased by more than 200% in the 14- to 19-year-old group (Bakhos, Lockhart, Myers, & Linakis, 2010). The true incidence of SRC may even be higher than reported in conventional epidemiologic studies due to athletes' biases toward underreporting (McCrea, Hammeke, Olsen, Leo, & Guskiewicz, 2004).

Increases in the expected incidence of SRC over the last several years may be partially driven by increased awareness and identification of concussion among current-era athletes relative to earlier generations (Hootman, Dick, & Agel, 2007). Because of the high incidence of concussion and concern whether there exist long-term neurologic consequences (DeKosky et al., 2010; Gilchrist, Thomas, Wald, & Langlois, 2007; Kelly, 1999; Langlois et al., 2006; McCrory et al., 2005, 2009), nearly all states have recently enacted legislation. These laws require athletes, coaches, parents, and school organizations to be educated regarding the recognition, evaluation, and management of SRC. Based on current consensus guidelines and legislative law, any student athlete who is suspected of sustaining a concussion has to be removed from participation in the activity until they are evaluated and cleared to return to play by an appropriate healthcare professional.

Neuropsychologists are now leaders in the effort to develop evidenced-based guidelines for evaluation and management of SRC. Many neuropsychologists have made major contributions to advance scientific understanding of SRC, participated in the clinical treatment of athletes who have sustained a concussion, and disseminated information critical to injury prevention. Neuropsychologists benefit from a sophisticated understanding of the current literature in this field, which enables them to provide the highest level of care to patients and also educate the community regarding SRC. This chapter provides an overview of the science of SRC and an update on recent contributions to the literature over the past 18 months.

OVERVIEW OF THE SCIENCE OF SRC

Acute Clinical Effects and Recovery

Extensive research over the last decade has significantly advanced scientific understanding of the true natural history of SRC. In general, the clinical recovery is favorable. A 2003 report was the first to plot the continuous time course of acute recovery immediately and within several days after concussion, indicating that more than 90% of athletes reported symptom recovery within 1 week (McCrea et al., 2003, 2005). Figure 5.1 displays the recovery curves for symptoms, cognitive performance, and postural stability from this study (McCrea et al., 2003). Several other prospective studies have since demonstrated that most athletes achieve a complete recovery in symptoms, cognitive functioning, postural stability, and other functional impairments over a period of approximately 1 to 2 weeks following concussion (Belanger & Vanderploeg, 2005; Broglio & Puetz, 2008; Collins et al., 1999; Guskiewicz et al., 2003; Macciocchi, Barth, Alves, Rimel, & Jane, 1996).

Persistent postconcussion symptoms remain enigmatic. There are frequent anecdotal reports of athletes who remain symptomatic or impaired on functional testing well beyond the window of good recovery commonly reported in group studies. Based on the principle that the plural of anecdotes is not data, the challenge facing sports medicine clinicians and public health experts is how to understand, effectively manage, and reduce reinjury risk in the small subset of athletes who do not follow the "typical" course of recovery. The precise incidence of athletes who exhibit prolonged postconcussive symptoms or other functional impairments remains unclear but logically has to be in a range of less than 10%. To date, there is little empirical evidence as to which risk factors are most associated with prolonged recovery time or poor outcome, or how these risks can be reduced in a clinical setting prior to first concussion.

Limited research findings have suggested a lengthier recovery time in younger athletes (Field, Collins, Lovell, & Maroon, 2003), citing that roughly half of all

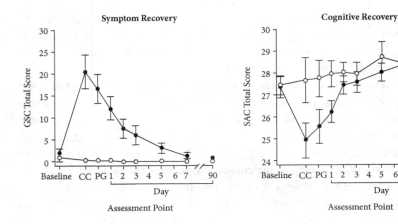

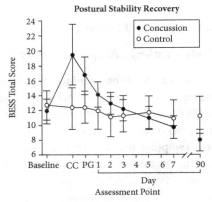

FIG 5.1 Symptom, cognitive, and postural stability recovery in concussion and control participants. Higher scores on the Graded Symptom Checklist (GSC) and Balance Error Scoring System (BESS) reflect increased symptoms and impairment in postural stability, respectively; lower scores on the Standardized Assessment of Concussion (SAC) indicate poorer cognitive performance. CC = time of injury; PG = postgame/postpractice. Error bars reflect 95% confidence intervals.

Adapted from McCrea et al., 2003.

high school athletes required more than 14 days to recover (Lau, Lovell, Collins, & Pardini, 2009; Lau, Collins, & Lovell, 2012). Unfortunately, these studies did not include control subjects and applied criteria for "recovery" that may have resulted in high false-positive rates due to criterion contamination that significantly complicated the interpretation of data from those studies. Other researchers have reported that women experience more symptoms (Colvin et al., 2009) and greater cognitive impairment than men (Dougan, Horswill, & Geffen, 2013) after SRC, although findings regarding gender differences in recovery are quite mixed (cf. Frommer et al., 2011; Zuckerman, Solomon, et al., 2012) and many studies that reported differences were hampered by small samples of female athletes, poorly matched male and female groups, or lack of preinjury baseline data.

A recent study of Australian Rules football players indicated that delayed return to sport after concussion was associated with acute symptom severity, but that study did not involve longitudinal tracking of concussed athletes beyond 7 days postinjury (Makdissi et al., 2010). Other studies (reviewed in subsequent sections) suggest that a subset of athletes experience symptoms and exhibit deficits on cognitive testing well beyond the typical 7–10 day window after SRC, and that prolonged recovery is associated with acute injury characteristics (loss of consciousness [LOC], posttraumatic amnesia [PTA]) and acute symptom severity. These findings raise speculation that a more severe biomechanical injury causes greater disruption of normal brain function, ultimately requiring a longer recovery time.

Physiologic Effects and Recovery

The time course of physiologic recovery after concussion is unclear. Earlier basic science studies using animal brain injury models have demonstrated that a complex cascade of ionic, metabolic, and physiologic events, culminating in axonal injury and neuronal dysfunction, follows concussion (Giza & Hovda, 2001; Hovda et al., 1995). Modern biomedical advances have enabled a powerful translation from earlier animal work to applied clinical research on the physiologic effects of concussion in humans. Studies using functional neuroimaging techniques and electrophysiologic testing have demonstrated that concussion is associated with metabolic and physiologic changes in the brain, which correlate with postconcussive symptoms and performance on neurocognitive testing during the acute postinjury phase.

Diffusion tensor imaging (DTI) and functional magnetic resonance imaging (fMRI) have shown particular promise in the study of concussion. Several studies have used DTI to investigate the physiologic effects of acute concussion (Chu et al., 2010; Mayer et al., 2010; Wilde et al., 2008). Lovell and colleagues (2007) and Jantzen, Anderson, Steinberg, and Kelso (2004) reported abnormal activation patterns on fMRI that correlated with clinical symptoms during the acute (7–10 days) postconcussion phase.

Several studies have correlated abnormalities on fMRI with persistent symptoms after SRC. Chen and colleagues found that atypical activation patterns on fMRI were highly related to persistent symptomatology during the subacute period months after SRC (Chen et al., 2004; Chen, Johnston, Petrides, & Ptito, 2008). Cubon Putukian, Boyer, and Dettwiler (2011) used DTI to evaluate 10 college athletes who experienced protracted symptoms for at least 1 month after SRC. Their findings indicated multiple areas of abnormality in concussed subjects, suggesting that DTI may be sensitive to structural changes after SRC that result in longer clinical recovery time.

Emerging data using translational technologies, such as DTI and fMRI, suggest that physiologic abnormalities may persist beyond the typical window of clinical recovery after concussion (Kraus et al., 2007; McGowan et al., 2000). A study by Mayer et al. (2010) evaluated 22 civilian (nonathlete) concussed patients an average of 12 days postinjury and revealed abnormalities on DTI that persisted beyond the point of clinical recovery in symptoms and on neurocognitive testing. Longitudinal follow-up 3–5 months postinjury in the same sample provided preliminary evidence of partial normalization of DTI values in several white matter tracts.

Unfortunately, extant research is insufficient to determine if similar physiologic abnormalities persist on neuroimaging in athletes beyond the point of clinical recovery. In addition, we know very little about the possible interaction between the time course of physiologic recovery and resumption of physical activity (e.g., return to play) after SRC.

Effects of Repetitive Concussion and Head Impact

With increased reporting of concussion, another concern has been the incidence of repeat concussion in athletes. Castile and colleagues (2011) used the National High School Sports-Related Injury Surveillance System database to look at epidemiologic data of new versus repeat concussions from 2005 to 2010. The results showed that there were 22.2 new concussions per 100,000 athletic exposures (AE) and 3.1 recurrent concussions per 100,000 AE. The authors used these data to estimate that nationally there were approximately 732,805 SRC during the 6-year study period, and they estimated that 86.6% of these injuries were new and 13.2% were recurrent. Based on the available epidemiologic data, concussion is a relatively common injury in contact and collision sports, but still is documented in only a small minority of participating athletes each season.

A review of the literature suggests that an athlete's risk of repeat concussion in the same sports season is essentially equivalent to the risk of a single concussion. In their study of 2,905 collegiate football players over three seasons (4,251 player seasons), Guskiewicz and colleagues (2003) found that 6.3% of players sustained a single concussion and 6.5% sustained a repeat concussion within the same season. Prior studies have illustrated that not only does clinical recovery typically occur over 7–10 days, but also that 75–90% of same-season repeat concussions occur within 7–10 days of an initial concussion (Guskiewicz et al., 2003; McCrea et al., 2009). It has long been held that a window of cerebral vulnerability may extend beyond the point of clinical recovery after SRC, during which the brain remains physiologically compromised and athletes are at heightened risk of repetitive injury or complications. The primary risk associated with repeat concussion is thought to be a slowed clinical recovery characterized by persistent symptoms or functional impairment. Historically, the greatest concern linked to repetitive concussion centered on the risk of catastrophic outcomes (i.e., death or permanent disability) associated with diffuse cerebral swelling or second-impact syndrome (Cantu, 1998; Kelly et al., 1991). Occurrences of catastrophic outcome are extremely rare and presumed to be caused by a second injury event encountered while the brain is still in a state of vulnerability from an initial concussion days earlier. However, the pathophysiology of delayed cerebral swelling remains the subject of great debate and it remains unclear whether closely spaced injuries are the true underlying mechanism (Cantu, 1998; McCrory, 2001; McCrory & Berkovic, 1998).

Basic science studies have used animal brain injury models to investigate the effects of a second concussion during the early window of vulnerability following initial injury (Vagnozzi et al., 2005). Using an experimental closed head injury model with rodents, Prins Hales, Reger, Giza, and Hovda (2010) reported that a second injury 24 hours after the first impact resulted in increased axonal injury, astrocytic reactivity, and more severe memory impairments. Vagnozzi investigated the existence of a temporal window of brain vulnerability in rats undergoing repeat concussion delivered at increasing time intervals (1, 2, 3, 4, 5 days after initial injury; Tavazzi et al., 2007; Vagnozzi et al., 2007). They discovered that a second concussive event within a period of days after initial injury resulted in profound derangement of mitochondrial function and severe disruption of brain metabolism.

Vagnozzi and colleagues have more recently studied the window of metabolic vulnerability and the effects of repeat concussion in human athletes by using proton magnetic resonance spectroscopy (H-MRS) to measure N-acetylaspartate (NAA; Vagnozzi et al., 2008). In a small sample of athletes who sustained a second concussion within 15 days of initial injury (n = 3), NAA normalization on H-MRS was prolonged by 15 days, rendering the first evidence in humans that repeat concussion during this window of cerebral vulnerability results in more severe, longer-lasting physiologic effects than a single concussion.

Scientific study of the effects of multiple concussions is difficult given the relatively low incidence of repeat injury. However, an emerging literature has begun to show that repeat concussions produce more severe symptoms, such as disorientation, LOC, and amnesia (Collins et al., 2002; Guskiewicz et al., 2003). Given the report of more severe symptoms, it is logical to expect longer periods of recovery postinjury following repeat concussions. Guskiewicz and colleagues (2003) showed that players with a self-reported history of multiple prior concussions take longer to recover (Guskiewicz et al., 2003), and there is also some evidence that the athlete's performance on balance testing (Bruce & Echemendia, 2004) and some cognitive measures (e.g., verbal memory and reaction time; Covassin, Stearne, & Elbin, 2008) may recover more slowly after repeat concussion. However, data capturing initial and repeated concussions prospectively have not revealed increased symptom duration between first and second concussions (McCrea et al., 2009).

There is evidence to suggest that sustaining concussions may increase an athlete's risk for subsequent injury. Studies have shown that individuals who report a prior history of concussion have 2.28–5.8 times the risk for sustaining subsequent concussions (Schulz et al., 2004; Zemper, 2003) in a given sports season and that there may be a dose-response type relationship, such that individuals reporting more concussions prior to study onset are at progressively increased risk for further injury (Guskiewicz, et al., 2003).

Chronic Effects

Historically, postconcussion syndrome has been the main concern of interest with respect to the chronic effects of concussion. Postconcussion syndrome is commonly referenced in clinical settings but is a poorly defined and often misunderstood term. Postconcussion syndrome or postconcussive disorder (PCD) has been proposed for diagnostic use when symptoms following concussion, such as neurologic, cognitive, behavioral, or somatic complaints, persist beyond the acute and subacute periods and become chronic (with chronic often operationalized as persisting beyond 3 months; Iverson, Zasler, & Lange, 2007). The cause of PCD is not entirely clear, as typically there is no identifiable neurologic cause for the persisting symptoms. PCD can also be difficult to diagnose and manage, as the symptoms commonly associated with PCD, such as chronic headache or decreased concentration, may be secondary to nonneurologic factors, such as musculoskeletal injury, chronic pain, or psychological factors. It has been reasonably well established that PCD, in lieu of other explanatory factors, is not a one-dimensional brain-based condition, but rather an outcome influenced by cognitive, emotional, medical, psychosocial, and motivational factors (Iverson et al., 2007; McCrea, 2007; Ruff, Camenzuli, & Mueller, 1996). Behavioral health interventions are often the most effective treatment for individuals with PCD, with therapeutic focus consisting of (1) symptom management (reduction), (2) cognitive restructuring, or (3) preventative education (Ferguson & Mittenberg, 1996; Mittenberg & Fischera, 1993; Mittenberg, Tremont, Zielinski, Fichera, & Rayls, 1996).

Beyond PCD, there is increasing concern whether long-term neurologic sequelae result from multiple concussions. There is, however, limited evidence that concussions sustained in athletic competition may increase the risk of late-life neurologic problems. Some epidemiologic research supports the idea that head injury is a risk factor for Alzheimer disease, with severity of injury (e.g., LOC) conferring particularly elevated risk (Guo et al., 2000; Mortimore et al., 1991). Not all studies have yielded significant results (Williams, Annegers, Kokmen, O'Brien, & Kurland, 1991), and few have evaluated how recurrent mild head injuries (e.g., SRCs) may impact risk for dementia and other neurodegenerative disorders.

In a large sample of retired professional football players, Guskiewicz and colleagues (2005) found that players with a history of three or more (vs. 0) prior concussions had a five-fold risk of being diagnosed with mild cognitive impairment, and although rates of Alzheimer disease were no different between the groups, those with multiple concussions and an Alzheimer diagnosis tended to be diagnosed earlier than those diagnosed with Alzheimer disease without a history of multiple concussions. Older rugby players who report histories of repeat concussion also report more subjective memory complaints than those without such a history (Thornton, Cox, Whitfield, & Fouladi, 2008).

Recent scholarship focused on the potential long-term risk of chronic traumatic encephalopathy (CTE), thought to be a unique pathologic syndrome and progressive neurodegenerative process found in individuals with a history of repetitive concussions or long-term exposure to "subconcussive" impacts (Stern et al., 2011). CTE typically develops years after the head injury history and is not considered a mere summation of acute or subacute brain damage or cognitive dysfunction. Understanding of CTE comes primarily from neuropathologically confirmed autopsy case studies or small cohorts of athletes with a history of head impacts (McKee et al., 2009).

CTE researchers assert that onset is insidious, with initial symptoms typically manifesting in midlife, often several years or even decades after exposure to concussive injury or subconcussive blows. Initial symptoms can be behavioral or emotional in nature and often involve irritability, impulsivity, depressed mood, apathy, substance abuse, and suicidality. Behavioral and emotional changes are often the primary concern of family and friends and prompt the initial evaluation by medical providers. Early cognitive symptoms are also reported to be common and typically involve a decline in memory and executive functioning. These symptoms gradually progress over the course of several years. Behavioral symptoms often evolve into frank outbursts, including physical aggression or marked apathy. Continued declines in memory and executive functioning, in addition to language problems (e.g., problems with speech output), are thought to be characteristic of relatively advanced disease (Stern et al., 2011; Welch, Nederberg, Bowden, Hilborn, & Stromme, 2007). Also of note, subsets of apparent CTE cases reportedly exhibit progressive motor neuron disease (e.g., weakness, atrophy, spasticity, and fasciculations) similar to amyotrophic lateral sclerosis (McKee et al., 2010).

Pathologically, CTE is reportedly characterized by generalized brain atrophy that is most evident in the frontal and temporal lobes, in keeping with the early deficits in memory and executive functioning. Other macroscopic abnormalities include dilation of the lateral and third ventricle; anterior cavum septum pellucidum and posterior fenestrations; atrophy of the olfactory bulbs, thalamus, mammillary bodies, basal ganglia, cerebellum, and brainstem; thinning of the hypothalamic floor; and pallor of the substantia nigra and locus coeruleus. Marked atrophy of the hippocampus, entorhinal cortex, and amygdala has also been found in more advanced cases (McKee et al., 2009).

Microscopically, CTE's signature is characterized as a diffuse tauopathy. In contrast to Alzheimer disease, the neurofibrillary pathology in CTE has a "patchy" distribution in the superficial layers of the frontal, temporal, and insular cortices. Pathologic tau aggregation has also been reported in subcortical structures (e.g., diencephalon, basal ganglia) and in subcortical white matter. Another differentiating feature is that β-amyloid plaques, a hallmark of Alzheimer disease, are found in only 40–45% of CTE cases (Stern et al., 2011; Wilson, Monaghan, Bowden, Parnell, & Cooper, 2007). In addition to neurofibrillary pathology, widespread TDP-43 proteinopathy was recently found in the brains of 10–12 athletes with neuropathologically confirmed CTE (McKee et al., 2009). Moreover, all three of the cases from that cohort that had progressive motor neuron disease showed TDP-43 in the anterior horns of the spinal cord and motor cortex, suggesting a link between sports-related head trauma and the development of motor neuron disease.

The scientific literature on CTE is in its infancy. There is general agreement that CTE represents a distinct tauopathy, but disagreement what the incidence is in former athletes. At the present time there are no epidemiologic, cohort, or prospective studies relating to CTE. Due to this lack of foundational scientific evidence, the assertion that CTE is caused by repeated concussive or subconcussive injury remains speculative and unproven. There are confounding factors to consider in future research, because it is unknown what role alcohol or drug use, psychiatric or mental health issues, age-related brain changes, or coexisting medical conditions play in the tauopathy process.

CONTRIBUTIONS TO THE LITERATURE, 2012–2013

Epidemiology

To date, most research investigating the incidence and risk factors associated with SRC in high school and collegiate athletes has focused on football, while other contact and collision sports (e.g., soccer, ice hockey, lacrosse) have received less attention. Marar, McIlvain, Fields, and Comstock (2012) recently used data from the National High School Sports-Related Injury Surveillance System to study the epidemiology of SRC in males and females across 20 sports. The National High School Sports-Related Injury Surveillance System is comprised of data submitted by certified athletic trainers associated with National Athletic Trainer's Association. The certified athletic trainers submit student athlete injury incidence and AE on a weekly basis during the academic year. For each injury the certified athletic trainers submitted data regarding athlete (age, height, weight, etc.), the injury (site, diagnosis, severity, etc.), and the injury event (activity, mechanism, etc.). The data were analyzed with respect to AE, which is defined as one athlete participating in one athletic practice or competition. Data were collected over two seasons from 2008 to 2010 with a total of 7,780,064 AE recorded. During this time 1,936 concussions were reported for an overall injury rate of 2.5 per 10,000 AE.

Previous studies had shown that athletes have a higher risk of concussion during competition (Powell & Barber-Foss, 1999; Schulz et al., 2004). This was replicated by Marar and colleagues, as athletes sustained 6.4 concussions per 10,000 AE during competition and 1.1 concussions per 10,000 AE during practice. As expected, football had the highest rate of concussion, with 6.4 concussions per 10,000 AE, followed by boy's hockey (5.4 per 10,000 AE), and boy's lacrosse (4.0 per 10,000 AE). In the same study, concussion represented 13.2% of total injuries, which is considerably higher than previous studies, where concussions accounted for 5.5–8.9% of reported injuries (Gessel, Fields, Collins, Dick, & Comstock, 2007; Powell & Barber-Foss, 1999; Schulz et al., 2004). Marar and colleagues found that girls had a higher rate of concussion than boys participating in parallel sports (e.g., soccer), which is consistent with previous literature (Upshaw, Gosserand, Williams, & Edwards, 2012) and more recent studies (Echlin et al., 2012).

The increase in SRC incidence over the past several years is not been limited to the United States. An Australian study of hospitalization due to SRC similarly showed a 61% increase from 2002–2003 to 2010–2011 (Finch, Clapperton, & McCrory, 2013). Although this figure could partially be explained by increased sports during the reporting period, there remained a 39% increase over this time after adjusting for rate of participation. Finch and colleagues attributed some of these increases to enhanced awareness and better identification of concussion symptoms but not necessarily due to increased incidence of concussion.

Previous work showed that large number of concussions were unreported or underreported. McCrea and colleagues (2004) found that less than half of high school football players that sustained symptoms related to concussion reported their symptoms. A study of collegiate athletes showed that only 17% reported sustaining a concussion, even though 48% reported sustaining a head injury that was followed by signs and symptoms of a concussion (LaBotz, Martin, Kimura, Hetzler, & Nichols, 2005). Given national efforts to increase awareness of the signs and symptoms of concussion, one would expect a corresponding decrease in recent years in unreported concussion. Meehan, Mannix, O'Brien, and Collins (2013) asked whether student athletes clinically evaluated for SRC had a history of unreported concussion. Results from 486 patients showed that approximately one-third reported a previously undiagnosed concussion. They also found that a history of previous unreported concussion was associated with higher scores on the Post Concussion Symptoms Scale and also more severe injury characteristics (i.e., LOC) compared to patients who had not had a previous concussion. Results should be interpreted cautiously, however, as this was a cross sectional study that relied upon retrospective data of past injuries provided by the patients. In addition, some of the patients included in the sample did not sustain a SRC, but rather a concussion that was determined by the authors to be "mechanistically similar" to a SRC.

Acute Injury Diagnosis, Assessment, and Recovery

Although understanding of the natural course of mTBI and SRC advanced considerably over the past two decades, there remain challenges in diagnosis and evaluation. Because most cases are not accompanied by LOC, abnormal neuroimaging studies (e.g., computed tomography, MRI), or obvious neurologic symptoms, SRC diagnosis remains clinically based on the real-time observation of the actual injury, and the signs and symptoms reported by the athlete.

Several standardized performance-based assessment measures have been developed and have been shown to be useful in the evaluation of concussion, but they appear to supplement rather than replace traditional assessment of self-reported symptoms. McCrea, Iverson, Echemendia, Makdissi, and Raftery (2013) recently performed an extensive review of the literature from 1982 to 2012 to classify the measures typically used on the day of injury in SRC assessment. Results indicated that symptom assessment, in spite of concerns regarding underreporting, remains a critical component in the diagnosis of concussion and that the effect size of symptoms reported on the day of the injury is typically larger than on performance-based measures. However, given that SRC produces a complex combination of effects and presents differently among athletes, a multimodal approach that takes into account injury characteristics, acute symptoms, cognitive functioning, and balance should be included in the assessment at the time of injury and over the course of postinjury recovery.

Several tools reported in the literature have been developed to aid in the assessment of concussion. The Sport Concussion Assessment Tool 3 (SCAT3) is a multimodal assessment tool that shows promise in the acute (i.e., sideline) assessment of SRC. The SCAT3 (McCrory, Meeuwisse, Aubry, et al., 2013), a recent revision of the original SCAT and earlier SCAT2, allows examiners to document acute injury characteristics and physical examination findings and to aggregate scores from several other measures, including a postconcussive symptom scale, a coordination rating scale, and several well-known assessment measures including the Glasgow Coma Scale, Maddock Orientation Score, Standardized Assessment of Concussion (SAC), and modified Balance Error Scoring System (BESS). There have been several studies that have investigated the reliability, sensitivity, and clinical use of components of the original SCAT and SCAT2 in the assessment of SRC, including the symptoms scale, BESS, and SAC (Barr & McCrea, 2001; McCrea et al., 2005), and given that these components of the SCAT3 examination remain identical to those of the SCAT2, these findings can be extended to the new form.

Furman and colleagues (2013) investigated whether an intermediate technology, an accelerometer worn by the athlete during balance testing, may be more sensitive and reliable than the person-rated method used by the BESS. The Balance Accelerometer Measure, a dual-axis accelerometer attached anteriorly at the midline on the pelvis using a gait belt, was used in the study of concussed high school athletes. Although the Balance Accelerometer Measure was not sensitive to concussion and was deemed not a useful tool for such assessment, their findings replicated earlier findings that the BESS was able to discriminate concussed from healthy individuals. Additional findings regarding the BESS showed that the tandem stance trial (one of three positions athletes maintain during the task) was best at discriminating concussed from healthy individuals. The authors also explored the conditions of the modified BESS (only firm surface conditions) that are used on the SCAT2 and found that this did not discriminate between groups. It should be noted that the BESS was scored via videotape in this study and the raters were allowed to rewind the tape to ensure the most accurate rating. This is not the standard of clinical practice so the results should be viewed cautiously.

Concerns about the BESS and other clinical measures used acutely (at or shortly after SRC) is that testing conditions differ widely from conditions present at baseline measurement. Typically, athletes undergo baseline BESS testing prior to the season in an athletic training room wearing sneakers. However, postinjury evaluation primarily takes place on a playing surface that may not be firm or completely level, with an athlete in cleats who may also have ankles taped or braced, and in a distracted state (Harmon et al., 2013). These factors likely impact the quality of the data when comparing to baseline.

Recent studies showed that level of exertion has an impact on measures of balance. Normal healthy volunteers perform more poorly on balance tests after heavy physical exertion (Schneiders, Sullivan, Handcock, Gray, & McCrory, 2012). Weber and colleagues (2013) were interested in how the effects of dehydration and weight-cutting techniques in wrestling may impact outcomes on concussion measures. In this study, 32 Division I healthy collegiate male wrestlers completed preseason baseline concussion testing in September and then underwent prewrestling and postwrestling practice follow-up testing in October after starting weight-cutting tactics the day before. Data from the SCAT2, BESS, Graded Symptom Checklist (GSC), and Simple Reaction Time scores from the Automated Neuropsychological Assessment Metrics were acquired at each time point. Results indicated that BESS error scores were higher postpractice when compared to baseline. In addition, athletes performed worse on the SCAT2 and endorsed more symptoms on the GSC at both prepractice and postpractice when compared to baseline. The authors concluded that wrestlers who are using weight-cutting tactics should be evaluated in a rehydrated state to ensure that dehydration is not influencing clinical measures. Although this finding is specific to wrestling and may not generalize to other sports, it reasserts the point that clinical baseline testing should be done under conditions that are as similar as possible with those of the sporting environment that exists at the time of a SRC.

Even though high technology forceplate measurements of balance are not available to most clinicians, these technologies have value in the management of SRC. In a more severe TBI population, the use of forceplate technologies has shown promise in detecting static and dynamic control of posture deficits in patients who do not otherwise show deficits on routine neurological exam. In addition, these deficits can be observed as far out as two years post injury in some patients (Geurts, Ribbers, Knoop, & van Limbeek, 1996). Powers, Kalmar, and Cinelli (2013) investigated whether this technology could be used to identify balance deficits in concussed athletes who had been cleared to return to play. Results of the study indicated that balance control of athletes who had sustained a concussion did not completely return to baseline at the time of return to play on all measures of balance. The authors advocate for the development of more objective balance assessment tools to ensure that athletes do not return to play with persistent or subtle sensorimotor deficits. This study had a number of limitations, including a small sample size of concussed athletes (n = 9), lack of baseline testing, and follow-up intervals that varied greatly between testing time points. Given these limitations, the results of this study should be interpreted cautiously, but it does provide support for the use of more sophisticated balance measurements in prospective studies of SRC and TBI.

Another consideration receiving insufficient attention is the appropriateness of postexertion cognitive testing. The most recent Zurich Consensus Statement on Concussion in Sport recommends the protocol of a graduated return to play; the athlete slowly returns to full participation in a stepwise fashion. After a defined symptom-free period of rest, athletes return to light exercise and then slowly increase activity until full sport-specific participation occurs without relapse of postconcussive symptoms (McCrory, Meeuwisse, Aubry, et al., 2013). Although "asymptomatic" is typically interpreted to mean lack of self-reported problems, some assert that athletes may continue to experience cognitive difficulties provoked by exertional testing that are reported or obvious in behavior to the observer supervising these activities. McGrath and colleagues (2013) explored postexertion cognitive performance among student athletes who sustained a SRC and had recovered to baseline cognitive functioning at rest following injury. After each athlete was symptom-free at rest and cognitive testing results had normalized, they participated in moderate cardiovascular exercise (e.g., stationary cycling) and/or noncontact sport-specific activity (e.g., skating) for 15–25 minutes. Following a brief rest period (~5–10 minutes) they completed the ImPACT test. Results showed that 27.7% of those athletes who had returned to cognitive baseline and were symptom-free at rest still showed signs of continued cognitive dysfunction following moderate exertion exercises. Based on their results, the authors advocated that postexertion cognitive testing should be a component of the return to play protocol.

It has been well established in the scientific literature that the natural course of recovery from mTBI/SRC occurs over a relatively brief period of time following injury, typically 7–10 days, and that most individuals make a complete recovery within 2–4 weeks postinjury. There is a minority of individuals, however, whose symptoms persist past this typical window of recovery. McCrea, Guskiewicz, and colleagues (2013) used data from a multicenter prospective study from 1999 through 2008 investigating acute effects and recovery after SRC. In total, 18,531 player seasons (i.e., total sport seasons of participation by all athletes) were under study. All athletes enrolled in the study had baseline data collected on the GSC, BESS, SAC, and a brief battery of neuropsychological tests. During the study period, 570 athletes sustained a SRC. Of those, 57 (10%) were classified as having a prolonged recovery, based on the study definition of postconcussive symptoms lasting more than 7 days. In addition to having longer-lasting symptoms, the prolonged recovery group performed more poorly on several objective measures of cognition during the acute period compared to the typical recovery group (see Figure 5.2 for a depiction of symptom, cognitive, and postural stability recovery for the prolonged recovery, typical recovery, and control groups). The recovery curve of the prolonged group did not differ from the typical group on the measure of postural stability, indicating similar recovery of balance functions. Nearly a quarter (25%, or 2.5% of total injured sample) of the prolonged recovery group's symptoms persisted until the long-term follow-up date of the study (either Day 45 or 90 postinjury) without evidence of differences on objective measures of cognitive functioning or balance. Factors found to be associated with prolonged recovery included the occurrence of unconsciousness, PTA, and higher symptom severity within 24 hours of injury. Athletes who suffered LOC had 4.15 times higher odds of prolonged recovery than those who did not lose consciousness. Although some prior work has found that lower age is associated with prolonged recovery from SRC (Zuckerman, Lee, et al., 2012), this was not found in the current study, which included high school and collegiate athletes (McCrea, Guskiewicz, et al., 2013). Future research in this area should focus on clarifying the extent to which individual factors (e.g., age, gender, psychological factors) other than acute injury characteristics may be related to prolonged recovery in athletes after SRC.

There is evidence that neurocognitive deficits may persist past the point at which athletes report being symptom-free (Broglio, Macciocchi, & Ferrara, 2007). This observation has, in part, fueled the movement toward more sophisticated neurocognitive testing in hopes of maximizing the sensitivity to detect subtle cognitive deficits in athletes who are otherwise reporting complete symptom recovery and could be cleared for return to competition before clinical recovery is complete. In line with this idea, Howell et al. (2013) recently used two laboratory-based tests of executive function and attention, the Attentional Network Task (Fan, McCandliss, Sommer, Raz, & Posner, 2002) and a modified Task Switching Test (Mayr, 2006), to evaluate cognitive recovery following SRC in high school athletes. The athletes were evaluated within

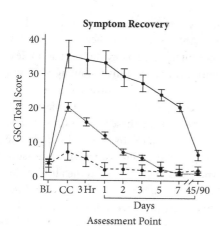

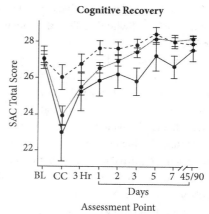

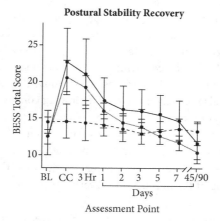

FIG 5.2 Symptom, cognitive, and postural stability recovery in two groups of concussed participants (prolonged recovery vs. typical recovery; defined by persistence of symptoms) and control participants. Higher scores on the Graded Symptom Checklist (GSC) and Balance Error Scoring System (BESS) indicate more severe symptoms and balance problems, respectively; lower scores on the Standardized Assessment of Concussion (SAC) indicate poorer cognitive performance. Error bars reflect 95% confidence intervals. BL = baseline; CC = time of concussion; 3HR = 3 hours postinjury. Predictors of prolonged recovery included loss of consciousness, posttraumatic amnesia, retrograde amnesia, and postinjury symptom severity. Adapted from McCrea, Guskiewicz, et al., 2013.

72 hours of injury, as well as 1 week, 2 weeks, 1 month, and 2 months postinjury. There was also a control group matched by gender, height, weight, age, and sport. The Attentional Network Task is designed to measure three types of distinct attention responses: (1) alerting (alerting effect), (2) spatial orientation (orienting effect), and (3) executive control (cognitive conflict). The Task Switching Test measures a person's ability to switch between competing tasks or stimulus-response rules (switch cost). There were no differences between the injured and control groups on either the alerting or spatial orientation component of the Attentional Network Task test. However,

on the more complex executive control component of the Attentional Network Task and on the Task Switching Test, the concussed athletes showed deficits that persisted for 2 months postinjury. These findings were interpreted as evidence that adolescences have more difficulty recovering executive function skills following SRC and that they may require an extended time period for complete cognitive recovery. The authors also advocate for postinjury cognitive testing to include several measures of executive function and complex attention, as they believe these to be most sensitive to the effects of concussion. This study was limited by a relatively small sample size of concussed athletes (n = 20) and a lack of baseline data against which to measure changes in cognitive test performance and track recovery. Although the authors did attempt to match control subjects on several variables, it is possible that matching control subjects on factors related to premorbid cognitive functioning would have led to a better match between injured and control players.

Another cognitive measure shown to be sensitive to acute concussion is the King-Devick test (KDT). The KDT can be performed in less than 1 minute. The respondent reads a series of numbers whose placement on three cards requires saccadic (fast alternating) eye movements to fixed targets. The KDT combined with a modified SCAT2 (without balance testing) was given to a sample of 27 professional hockey players during preseason baseline testing. Of those 27 athletes who were baseline tested, two were also tested on the KDT following concussion. In the baseline sample there was a significant relationship between performance on the KDT and SAC scores, but the KDT appeared more sensitive to the acute effects of concussion in the small injured sample. Specifically, the 2 injured athletes showed increases of 4.2 and 6.4 seconds on the KDT despite no apparent change in SAC scores. Both players also showed worsening of the number and severity of symptoms on the SCAT2 following SRC (Galetta et al., 2013).

The KDT was also used in a sample of 37 rugby players participating in the premier amateur division in New Zealand. All players had baseline testing on the KDT and SCAT2 and completed concussion history questionnaires prior to the start of the season. The team participated in 24 games over the course of the season and there were five reported concussions. In addition, postmatch testing on the KDT identified impairments in 17 players who had sustained meaningful head injuries but did not show or report symptoms of concussion. The authors classified these athletes as having unrecognized concussions. There were no statistically significant differences between the recognized and unrecognized concussions on the SCAT2 following the match. It should be noted that there were differences between the groups on some variables (e.g., immediate and delayed memory scores), so the lack of statistical significance may stem from the insufficient statistical power in the study. The athletes that had recognized concussions performed more poorly on the KDT than the unrecognized group when compared to baseline. It was also found that players with unrecognized concussion returned to baseline levels on the SCAT2 faster than those with recognized concussions (King, Brughelli, Hume, & Gissane, 2013).

King and colleagues also replicated earlier findings that exercise alone does not lead to a worsening of the KDT (Galetta, Brandes, et al., 2011). Consistent with other standardized assessments of concussion that have been advocated recently for the assessment of SRC (e.g., the SCAT2, SAC, BESS, etc.), there is growing evidence that the KDT is sensitive to the effects of SRC (Galetta, Barrett, et al., 2011; Galetta, Brandes, et al., 2011; King, Clark, & Gissane, 2012). This joins a growing body of studies indicating that reported symptoms or observation of behavior may not be as sensitive as standardized measures in detecting subtle deficits resulting from concussion (Macciocchi, Barth, Littlefield, & Cantu, 2001).

Physiologic Studies

SRC and mTBI can cause changes in brain structure and function. The changes cannot be directly observed, only inferred by scores on surrogate measures of behavior, symptoms, cognition, balance, and other functional abilities. Given the diagnostic difficulties associated with SRC, several lines of research are exploring the viability of using advanced imaging techniques, such as DTI, fMRI, electroencephalography (EEG), and magnetoencephalography, to better understand the physiologic effects of SRC. The clinical diagnosis of a concussion is primarily based on description of the acute injury characteristics, reported symptoms following the injury, and clinical measures of cognition or other functional activities. More recently, there is stronger pursuit in the scientific community toward finding a definitive "biomarker" that could enable a more objective diagnosis of concussion and indicate when an athlete has achieved a complete physiologic recovery and, therefore, is fit to safely return to play. To date, no such biomarker exists for clinical use.

In addition to the direct effects of concussive injury, there is also concern whether repetitive sub-concussive head impacts lead to physiological brain changes. Koerte, Ertl-Wagner, Reiser, Zafonte, and Shenton (2012) used DTI to compare male soccer players without a history of concussion to age, sex, and handedness matched competitive swimmers. DTI reportedly detected widespread differences in white matter integrity in the brains of soccer players despite there being no history of concussion. A similar finding was also described in a sample of college-aged football players, which showed DTI changes from baseline even in the absence of an observed concussion (Marchi et al., 2013). The changes on DTI correlated with an autoantibody marker (SB100B), suggesting that blood-brain barrier disruption resulted from repeated "subconcussive" head impacts. Another study investigating DTI changes in 25 hockey players over the course of the season reported changes in white matter diffusivity over the course of the season (Koerte, Kaufmann, et al., 2012). Bazarian, Zhu, Blyth, Borrino, and Zhong (2012) also found DTI changes in a sample of high school boys' football and hockey players who did not sustain a concussion, but had many subconcussive head impacts during routine participation.

Recent DTI studies appear more consistent when investigating recovery beyond the subacute phase. In a sample of adolescents who were evaluated 2–8 weeks after concussive injuries, DTI showed differences compared to control subjects, even though there were no statistically significant differences observed on the SCAT2 (Virji-Babul et al., 2013). Similarly, mean diffusivity differences were found over

7 months postinjury in a sample of female athletes who had concussion compared to normal control subjects (Chamard et al., 2013) indicating the possible presence of microstructural changes. These results indicate that DTI may have promise in studying the underlying pathophysiology of SRC, but further study is required for the method to be appropriate for clinical use.

Functional MRI may be more sensitive to mTBI in symptomatic patients, in the absence of deficits on objective cognitive testing, as suggested by (McAllister et al., 1999). However, fMRI results have varied widely, sometimes in opposite directions. Some studies have reported decreased activation following the subacute phase of recovery in injured athletes (Gosselin et al., 2011) and still others have not shown any difference in brain activation patterns as measured by fMRI following the subacute recovery period (Elbin et al., 2012; Terry et al., 2012). Hammeke and colleagues (2013) used an event-related fMRI design with a working memory task to investigate brain activation patterns in high school football players who had sustained two or three concussions, according to the American Academy of Neurology grading system (Quality Standards Subcomittee of the American Academy of Neurology, 1997). Injured athletes and control teammates (matched on age, preseason Glasgow Coma Scale, and SAC score) were initially tested approximately 13 hours postinjury and then again during the subacute phase of the injury approximately 7 weeks later. During the acute phase, the injured group showed the expected postconcussive symptoms and cognitive decline when compared to the healthy control subjects. Brain activation patterns showed decreases in the injured group compared to the control subjects in attention networks during this acute phase. During the subacute phase, the injured athletes showed the expected improvement in symptoms and cognitive performance. Brain activation patterns showed the reverse of the acute-phase activation patterns, in that the attention network of the concussed athletes was greater than the activation in the healthy control subjects. These results suggest that there is less activation during the acute symptomatic phase, which is indicative of underlying brain dysfunction. Conversely, after a period of recovery, the increase in brain activation is likely due to compensatory increases in brain activity to support normal behavioral performance.

The fMRI studies mentioned previously used a task-state fMRI design. The participant actively engages in a cognitive task, which is correlated with brain activity. Resting state fMRI (R-fMRI) is another method to investigate brain function. R-fMRI involves data collection while the participant is at rest, rather than while the participant is performing a cognitive activation task. Work that began in the early 1990s showed that an individual's brain at rest demonstrates important information about functional organization (for a review, see Biswal, 2012). In that respect, there is a specific network of brain regions referred to as the default network, which is consistently active during rest and has shown to be sensitive to a number of neurologic and psychiatric disorders (Buckner, 2012; Raichle et al., 2001). Johnson, Zhang, and colleagues (2012) used R-fMRI to assess brain activation patterns in athletes who were asymptomatic following a SRC. Athletes reporting at least a 24-hour symptom-free period (approximately 10 ± 2 days) postinjury, were recruited to participate in a R-fMRI task. These asymptomatic patients showed a reduced number of connections in the default network when compared to healthy control subjects. Furthermore, a regression analysis indicated that the magnitude of the connections between the left dorsal lateral prefrontal cortex and the left lateral parietal cortex decreased with an increase in the number of concussions. Other studies have shown that resting state differences between concussed and healthy control subjects first become apparent after light physical activity (Zhang et al., 2012).

There are a number of studies suggesting that quantitative EEG (QEEG) is sensitive to brain dysfunction following concussion (Nuwer, Hovda, Schrader, & Vespa, 2005). QEEG's use as a clinical tool to measure possible physiological vulnerability following a concussion is of interest, but there are limited data on QEEG during the course of recovery following SRC. Barr, Prichep, Chabot, Powell, and McCrea (2012) recently used a number of clinical measures (Concussion Symptom Inventory, SAC, BESS, and Automated Neuropsychological Assessment Metrics and QEEG at the time of injury, at recovery Day 8 and recovery Day 45. As expected, the injured subjects demonstrated impairments on clinical measures at the time of injury, but these impairments resolved by Day 8 postinjury. The QEEG measure, however, showed abnormal findings in the concussed group when compared to control subjects on the day of injury that persisted through Day 8 (and resolved by Day 45). These data support the notion that a period of physiologic recovery persists beyond the point of full recovery on clinical measures. During this period of ongoing physiologic recovery, athletes may continue to be vulnerable to the effects of repeat concussion even after being asymptomatic.

Although functional imaging has received the greatest attention in recent years, advanced imaging techniques that explore metabolic changes in the brain (MRS), blood biomarkers, and cerebral spinal fluid studies following mTBI have also been areas of interest among researchers (Gasparovic et al., 2009; Zetterberg, Smith, & Blennow, 2013). They asserted that MRS is sensitive to brain changes following head injury and brain recovery may be different depending on concussion history. For their study, 28 student-athletes who sustained a SRC were compared to 20 healthy control subjects. The SRC athletes were scanned within 24 hours of meeting criteria consistent with the return to play guidelines set forth by the Zurich consensus statement (i.e., self-reported symptom resolution, return to baseline on clinical measures, and clearance from a medical professional for the first stage of aerobic activity; McCrory et al., 2009). Results showed that a concussive episode leads to a reduction in the NAA/Cho and NAA/Cr ratios in the genu of the corpus callosum relative to healthy control subjects. However, when individuals in the SRC group were stratified according to concussion history (i.e., 1, 2, or 3+), results showed less decrease in those individuals that had a prior concussion history. Interpretation of this result is complicated due to variability in the time postinjury that the athletes were evaluated (athletes with multiple concussions took longer to recover so were further removed from the injury), but it could be argued that these findings indicate there may be an adaptive process in the neurons following multiple concussions (Johnson, Gay, et al., 2012).

Other reports investigating long-term consequences of concussion show that brain changes can be identified in middle-aged individuals years after the last concussive event. Tremblay and colleagues (2013) recruited 30 male former college hockey and American football players aged 51–75. Fifteen of the individuals had a history of concussion limited to the years that they were in college and 15 had no history of concussions. Exclusion criteria were any history of drug or alcohol abuse, psychiatric illness, medical condition that required daily medication or treatment, learning disability, or neurologic history and, therefore, all were considered to be healthy. Results showed neurometabolic abnormalities in the left medial temporal lobe and the right prefrontal cortex in concussion group when compared to healthy control subjects. Others have suggested that biomarkers extracted from blood tests may be beneficial to diagnosing concussion or identifying mild blows to the head that do not lead to a clinically recognized concussion (Neselius et al., 2013).

Chronic Effects

Interest has grown recent years regarding the possible long-term effects of repeat head injuries and subconcussive head impacts, although there is a dearth of high-quality, methodologically sound research in this area. In particular, there is a growing concern about potential risk of CTE resulting from repetitive head trauma or impacts over the course of a person's lifetime (for a review, see Yi, Padalino, Chin, Montenegro, & Cantu, 2013). This literature has suffered from a lack of well-designed epidemiologic and prospective studies; heavy reliance on individual autopsy studies; small cohorts of patients that are identified retrospectively; reliance on self-report of injuries, which can be inaccurate; and poor control conditions in many studies (Jenkins et al., 2007; McCrory, Meeuwisse, Kutcher, Jordan, & Gardner, 2013). Earlier studies have reported that there is a higher incidence of mild cognitive impairment and depression in former National Football League players who sustained concussions when compared to players that did not have a concussion history (Guskiewicz et al., 2005). Kerr and colleagues recently showed the 9-year risk of depression increases with self-report of a greater history of concussion in a cohort of retired National Football League players (Kerr, Marshall, Harding, & Guskiewicz, 2012). More recent findings showed that retired National Football League players showed greater cognitive deficits and higher levels of depression when compared to healthy age-matched control subjects. In addition, these deficits were correlated with white matter abnormalities and changes in cerebral blood flow according to Arterial Spin Labeling analysis (Hart et al., 2013). However, not all individuals that have a history of repeat head injury and develop neurocognitive decline show neuropathologic signs consistent with CTE. In a consecutive case series brain autopsy study of six players from the Canadian Football league with histories of multiple concussions and cognitive decline, only three showed evidence of CTE on autopsy. The other three showed evidence of Alzheimer disease, amyotrophic lateral sclerosis, and Parkinson disease (Hazrati et al., 2013).

Studies have shown a possibility of increased cognitive difficulty following one season of contact sports versus a season of playing noncontact sports (McAllister et al., 2012). The extent to which these athletes may be susceptible to long term deficits or future declines is not known. In a recent study, a cohort of male students who played high school football from 1946 to 1956 was compared to a group of male students at the same school who participated in glee club, band, and choir to investigate whether there was a relationship between playing football (sustaining head injuries) and the development of neurodegenerative disease later in life. The football players and control group were identified from the high school yearbooks from those years and a subsequent review of medical records was conducted. Results of the study showed that high school football players did not have a higher risk of developing neurodegenerative diseases, such as dementia, Parkinson's disease, or amyotrophic lateral sclerosis, when compared to other classmates that did not participate in contact sports (Savica, Parisi, Wold, Josephs, & Ahlskog, 2012). This study was limited by poor documentation of concussion frequency or severity and the completeness and accuracy of medical records was unclear.

Injury Management

As stated earlier, the most recent Zurich Consensus statement on Concussion in Sport recommends a graduated return to play protocol in which the athlete returns to full participation in a stepwise fashion. According to these guidelines (depicted in Table 5.1), the athletes progress to the next rehabilitative stage when they have

Table 5.1 Zurich Consensus Conference Graduated Return to Play Protocol

Rehabilitation Stage	Functional Exercise at Each Stage of Rehabilitation	Objective of Each Stage
1. No activity	Symptom-limited physical and cognitive rest	Recovery
2. Light aerobic exercise	Walking, swimming, or stationary cycling keeping intensity <70% maximum permitted heart rate. No resistance training	Increase heart rate
3. Sport-specific exercise	Skating drills in ice hockey, running drills in soccer. No head impact activities	Add movement
4. Noncontact training drills	Progression to more complex training drills (e.g., passing drills in football and ice hockey) May start progressive resistance training	Exercise, coordination, and cognitive load
5. Full-contact practice	Following medical clearance participate in normal training activities	Restore confidence and assess functional skills by coaching staff
6. Return to play	Normal game play	

Source: Adapted from McCrory, Meeuwisse, Aubry, et al. (2013)

been asymptomatic for at least 24 hours. There are a total of six stages with the first stage being symptom-limited physical and cognitive rest. The second stage is light aerobic activity, then sport-specific exercise (e.g., skating drills in hockey, running drills in soccer), noncontact training drills (e.g., passing drills in football), full contact practice, and then finally return to play. If at any time the athlete becomes symptomatic, they are to return to the previous stage until asymptomatic for a 24-hour period. As each step in this process should take approximately 1 day, the whole process is expected to take approximately 1 week (McCrory, Meeuwisse, Aubry, et al., 2013).

Previous consensus guidelines recommended cognitive and physical rest following a SRC, as activity was thought to exacerbate symptoms and possibly delay recovery. Although the evidence that rest is therapeutic following a concussion is limited, this recommendation has led many clinicians to keep student athletes out of school for extended periods of time. A recent study looking at 184 patients evaluated in a SRC clinic did not find a relationship between cognitive rest and duration of symptoms following concussion (Gibson, Nigrovic, O'Brien, & Meehan, 2013). The authors concluded that a few days off of school during the acute phase following a concussion is likely beneficial but that caution should be exerted regarding extended absences from school due to concussion. In fact, a greater proportion of individuals in the cognitive rest group experienced prolonged concussion-related symptoms (>30 days). Schneider and colleagues (2013) performed a review of the literature and concluded that cognitive rest immediately following concussion is warranted but that there is not convincing evidence that extended rest periods improve outcomes. This review did find a benefit for light exercise in athletes who are slow to recover from SRC. However, the authors did not provide guidelines for when to transition from acute periods of rest to activity (Schneider et al., 2013). Benefit for complete rest soon after or several weeks following a SRC was found in one study of high school and college-aged student athletes who presented to a SRC clinic (Moser, Glatts, & Schatz, 2012). This study was limited by a selection bias in the clinic sample, great variability in time postinjury that the athletes were evaluated (range, 2–234 days), and lack of use of a standardized rest intervention.

Future research is required to ultimately determine the effects of rest on recovery after SRC, and the parameters of rest that provide the greatest benefit.

SUMMARY AND CONCLUSION

Major advances in the basic and clinical science of concussion have been made over the past 20 years. New contributions to the literature in the past 2 years have further accelerated this scientific movement. Neuropsychologists, in particular, made major contributions to science and practice. This includes advancing through research an understanding of the nature of SRC, developing guidelines for best practices in the clinical evaluation and management of SRC, and guiding educational campaigns geared at SRC prevention. Recent scientific discoveries have incrementally advanced understanding of the defining characteristics of concussion, the true natural history of clinical recovery following SRC, the issues involved in measuring various domains of functioning postinjury, and the potential long-term or persistent consequences of repetitive injury. In the basic science arena, major scientific breakthroughs have shed light on the underlying pathophysiology of concussion, which in turn has implications for understanding of the time course and nature of the effects and recovery of injury. These research advances directly influenced the development of evidence-based, best practice guidelines for the diagnosis, assessment, and management of SRC, including protocols that drive the decision-making process on an athlete's fitness to return to participation after concussion.

Ongoing and future research on SRC continues to address pressing questions on the risks, recovery, and outcome associated with one of the most common injuries encountered by athletes participating in contact sports. The continued accumulation of large-scale prospective studies of SRC and the incorporation of technological advances including accelerometer technology and neuroimaging methods are a key to the advancement of knowledge about the complex, multifaceted injury that is concussion. Ongoing and planned scientific work will continue to drive injury management strategies that protect the health and safety of athletes, preserve the integrity of sports, and minimize the societal impact of concussion in sports.

NOTE

1. The authors thank Adam Pfaller for his contribution to the literature search.

REFERENCES

Bakhos, L. L., Lockhart, G. R., Myers, R., & Linakis, J. G. (2010). Emergency department visits for concussion in young child athletes. *Pediatrics, 126*(3), e550–556.

Barr, W. B., & McCrea, M. (2001). Sensitivity and specificity of standardized neurocognitive testing immediately following sports concussion. *Journal of the International Neuropsychological Society, 7*(6), 693–702.

Barr, W. B., Prichep, L. S., Chabot, R., Powell, M. R., & McCrea, M. (2012). Measuring brain electrical activity to track recovery from sport-related concussion. *Brain Injury, 26*(1), 58–66. doi:10.3109/02699052.2011.608216

Bazarian, J. J., Zhu, T., Blyth, B., Borrino, A., & Zhong, J. (2012). Subject-specific changes in brain white matter on diffusion tensor imaging after sports-related concussion. *Magnetic Resonance Imagng, 30*(2), 171–180. doi:10.1016/j.mri.2011.10.001

Belanger, H. G., & Vanderploeg, R. D. (2005). The neuropsychological impact of sports-related concussion: A meta-analysis. *Journal of the International Neuropsychological Society, 11*(4), 345–357.

Biswal, B. B. (2012). Resting state fMRI: A personal history. *NeuroImage, 62*(2), 938-944. doi:10.1016/j.neuroimage.2012.01.090

Broglio, S. P., Macciocchi, S. N., & Ferrara, M. S. (2007). Neurocognitive performance of concussed athletes when symptom free. *Journal of Athletic Training, 42*(4), 504–508.

Broglio, S. P., & Puetz, T. W. (2008). The effect of sport concussion on neurocognitive function, self-report symptoms and postural control: a meta-analysis. *Sports Med, 38*(1), 53–67.

Bruce, J. M., & Echemendia, R. J. (2004). Concussion history predicts self-reported symptoms before and following a concussive event. *Neurology, 63*(8), 1516–1518.

Buckner, R. L. (2012). The serendipitous discovery of the brain's default network. *NeuroImage, 62*(2), 1137–1145. doi:10.1016/j.neuroimage.2011.10.035

Cantu, R. C. (1998). Second-impact syndrome. *Clinics in Sports Medicine, 17*(1), 37–44.

Castile, L., Collins, C. L., McIlvain, N. M., & Comstock, R. D. (2011). The epidemiology of new versus recurrent sports concussions among high school athletes, 2005–2010. *British Journal of Sports Medicine, 46*(8), 603–610.

Chamard, E., Lassonde, M., Henry, L., Tremblay, J., Boulanger, Y., De Beaumont, L., & Theoret, H. (2013). Neurometabolic and microstructural alterations following a sports-related concussion in female athletes. *Brain Injury, 27*(9), 1038–1046. doi:10.3109/02699052.2013.794968

Chen, J. K., Johnston, K. M., Frey, S., Petrides, M., Worsley, K., & Ptito, A. (2004). Functional abnormalities in symptomatic concussed athletes: An fMRI study. *Neuroimage, 22*(1), 68–82.

Chen, J. K., Johnston, K. M., Petrides, M., & Ptito, A. (2008). Recovery from mild head injury in sports: Evidence from serial functional magnetic resonance imaging studies in male athletes. *Clin J Sport Med, 18*(3), 241–247.

Chu, Z., Wilde, E. A., Hunter, J. V., McCauley, S. R., Bigler, E. D., Troyanskaya, M., . . . Levin, H. S. (2010). Voxel-based analysis of diffusion tensor imaging in mild traumatic brain injury in adolescents. *AJNR Am J Neuroradiol, 31*(2), 340–346.

Collins, M. W., Grindel, S. H., Lovell, M. R., Dede, D. E., Moser, D. J., Phalin, B. R., . . . McKeag, D. B. (1999). Relationship between concussion and neuropsychological performance in college football players. *Journal of the American Medical Association, 282*(10), 964–970.

Collins, M. W., Lovell, M. R., Iverson, G. L., Cantu, R. C., Maroon, J. C., & Field, M. (2002). Cumulative effects of concussion in high school athletes. *Neurosurgery, 51*(5), 1175–1179; discussion 1180–1171.

Colvin, A. C., Mullen, J., Lovell, M. R., West, R. V., Collins, M. W., & Groh, M. (2009). The role of concussion history and gender in recovery from soccer-related concussion. *American Journal of Sports Medicine, 37*(9), 1699–1704. doi:10.1177/0363546509332497

Covassin, T., Stearne, D., & Elbin, R. (2008). Concussion history and postconcussion neurocognitive performance and symptoms in collegiate athletes. *Journal of Athletic Training, 43*(2), 119–124. doi:10.4085/1062-6050-43.2.119

Cubon, V. A., Putukian, M., Boyer, C., & Dettwiler, A. (2011). A diffusion tensor imaging study on the white matter skeleton in individuals with sports-related concussion. *J Neurotrauma, 28*(2), 189–201.

DeKosky, S. T., Ikonomovic, M. D., & Gandy, S. (2010). Traumatic brain injury—football, warfare, and long-term effects. *New England Journal of Medicine, 363*(14), 1293–1296.

Dougan, B. K., Horswill, M. S., & Geffen, G. M. (2013). Athletes' age, sex, and years of education moderate the acute neuropsychological impact of sports-related concussion: A meta-analysis. *Journal of the International Neuropsychological Society*, 1–17. doi:10.1017/S1355617712001464

Echlin, P. S., Skopelja, E. N., Worsley, R., Dadachanji, S. B., Lloyd-Smith, D. R., Taunton, J. A., . . . Johnson, A. M. (2012). A prospective study of physician-observed concussion during a varsity university ice hockey season: Incidence and neuropsychological changes. Part 2 of 4. *Neurosurgical Focus, 33*(6), E2: 1–11. doi:10.3171/2012.10.FOCUS12286

Elbin, R. J., Covassin, T., Hakun, J., Kontos, A. P., Berger, K., Pfeiffer, K., & Ravizza, S. (2012). Do brain activation changes persist in athletes with a history of multiple concussions who are asymptomatic? *Brain Injury, 26*(10), 1217–1225. doi:10.3109/02699052.2012.672788

Fan, J., McCandliss, B. D., Sommer, T., Raz, A., & Posner, M. I. (2002). Testing the efficiency and independence of attentional networks. *Journal of Cognitive Neuroscience, 14*(3), 340–347. doi:10.1162/089892902317361886

Ferguson, R. J., & Mittenberg, W. (1996). Cognitive-behavioral treatment of postconcussion syndrome. In V. B. Van Hasselt & M. Hersen (Eds.), *Sourcebook of psychological treatment manuals for adult disorders* (pp. 615–655). New York: Plenum Press.

Field, M., Collins, M. W., Lovell, M. R., & Maroon, J. (2003). Does age play a role in recovery from sports-related concussion? A comparison of high school and collegiate athletes. *J Pediatr, 142*(5), 546–553.

Finch, C. F., Clapperton, A. J., & McCrory, P. (2013). Increasing incidence of hospitalisation for sport-related concussion in Victoria, Australia. *The Medical Journal of Australia, 198*(8), 427–430.

Frommer, L. J., Gurka, K. K., Cross, K. M., Ingersoll, C. D., Comstock, R. D., & Saliba, S. A. (2011). Sex differences in concussion symptoms of high school athletes. *Journal of Athletic Training, 46*(1), 76–84. doi:10.4085/1062-6050-46.1.76

Furman, G. R., Lin, C. C., Bellanca, J. L., Marchetti, G. F., Collins, M. W., & Whitney, S. L. (2013). Comparison of the balance accelerometer measure and balance error scoring system in adolescent concussions in sports. *American Journal of Sports Medicine, 41*(6), 1404–1410. doi:10.1177/0363546513484446

Galetta, K. M., Barrett, J., Allen, M., Madda, F., Delicata, D., Tennant, A. T., . . . Balcer, L. J. (2011). The King-Devick test as a determinant of head trauma and concussion in boxers and MMA fighters. *Neurology, 76*(17), 1456–1462. doi:10.1212/WNL.0b013e31821184c9

Galetta, K. M., Brandes, L. E., Maki, K., Dziemianowicz, M. S., Laudano, E., Allen, M., . . . Balcer, L. J. (2011). The King-Devick test and sports-related concussion: Study of a rapid visual screening tool in a collegiate cohort. *Journal of the Neurological Sciences, 309*(1-2), 34–39. doi:10.1016/j.jns.2011.07.039

Galetta, M. S., Galetta, K. M., McCrossin, J., Wilson, J. A., Moster, S., Galetta, S. L., . . . Master, C. L. (2013). Saccades and memory: Baseline associations of the King-Devick and SCAT2 SAC tests in professional ice hockey players. *Journal of the Neurological Sciences, 328*(1-2), 28–31. doi:10.1016/j.jns.2013.02.008

Gallagher, C. J., Keene, K. L., Mychaleckyj, J. C., Langefeld, C. D., Hirschhorn, J. N., Henderson, B. E., . . . Sale, M. M. (2007). Investigation of the estrogen receptor-alpha gene with type 2 diabetes and/or nephropathy in African-American and European-American populations. *Diabetes, 56*(3), 675–684. doi:10.2337/db06-0303

Gasparovic, C., Yeo, R., Mannell, M., Ling, J., Elgie, R., Phillips, J., . . . Mayer, A. R. (2009). Neurometabolite concentrations in gray and white matter in mild traumatic brain injury: An 1H-magnetic resonance spectroscopy study. *Journal of Neurotrauma, 26*(10), 1635–1643. doi:10.1089/neu.2009-0896

Gessel, L. M., Fields, S. K., Collins, C. L., Dick, R. W., & Comstock, R. D. (2007). Concussions among United States high school and collegiate athletes. *Journal of Athletic Training, 42*(4), 495–503.

Geurts, A. C., Ribbers, G. M., Knoop, J. A., & van Limbeek, J. (1996). Identification of static and dynamic postural instability following traumatic brain injury. *Archives of Physical Medicine and Rehabilitation, 77*(7), 639–644.

Gibson, S., Nigrovic, L. E., O'Brien, M., & Meehan, W. P., 3rd. (2013). The effect of recommending cognitive rest on recovery from sport-related concussion. *Brain Injury, 27*(7-8), 839–842. doi:10.3109/02699052.2013.775494

Gilchrist, J., Thomas, K.E., Wald, M. M., & Langlois, J. (2007). Nonfatal traumatic brain injuries from sports and recreation activities—United States. *Morbidity and Mortality Weekly Report, 56*(29), 733–737.

Gilchrist, J., Thomas, K.E., Xu, L., McGuire, L.C., & Coronado, V. (2011). Nonfatal traumatic brain injuries related to sports and recreation activities among persons aged </= 19 years—United States, 2001-2009. *Morbidity and Mortality Weekly Report, 60*(39), 1337–1342.

Giza, C. C., & Hovda, D. A. (2001). The neurometabolic cascade of concussion. *Journal of Athletic Training, 36*(3), 228–235.

Gosselin, N., Bottari, C., Chen, J. K., Petrides, M., Tinawi, S., de Guise, E., & Ptito, A. (2011). Electrophysiology and functional MRI in post-acute mild traumatic brain injury. *Journal of Neurotrauma, 28*(3), 329–341. doi:10.1089/neu.2010.1493

Guo, Z., Cupples, L. A., Kurz, A., Auerbach, S. H., Volicer, L., Chui, H., . . . Farrer, L. A. (2000). Head injury and the risk of AD in the MIRAGE study. *Neurology, 54*(6), 1316–1323.

Guskiewicz, K. M., Marshall, S. W., Bailes, J., McCrea, M., Cantu, R. C., Randolph, C., & Jordan, B. D. (2005). Association between recurrent concussion and late-life cognitive impairment in retired professional football players. *Neurosurgery, 57*(4), 719–726.

Guskiewicz, K. M., McCrea, M., Marshall, S. W., Cantu, R. C., Randolph, C., Barr, W., . . . Kelly, J. P. (2003). Cumulative effects associated with recurrent concussion in collegiate football players: The NCAA Concussion Study. *Journal of the American Medical Association, 290*(19), 2549–2555.

Guskiewicz, K. M., Weaver, N. L., Padua, D. A., & Garrett, W. E., Jr. (2000). Epidemiology of concussion in collegiate and high school football players. *American Journal of Sports Medicine, 28*(5), 643–650.

Halstead, M. E., & Walter, K. D. (2010). Sport-related concussion in children and adolescents. *Pediatrics, 126*(3), 597–615.

Hammeke, T. A., McCrea, M., Coats, S. M., Verber, M. D., Durgerian, S., Flora, K., . . . Rao, S. M. (2013). Acute and subacute changes in neural activation during the recovery from sport-related concussion. *Journal of the International Neuropsychological Society, 19*(8), 863–872. doi:10.1017/S1355617713000702

Harmon, K. G., Drezner, J., Gammons, M., Guskiewicz, K., Halstead, M., Herrin, S., et al. (2013). American Medical society for sports medicine position statement: Concussion in sport. *Clinical Journal of Sports Medicine, 23*, 1–18.

Hart, J., Jr., Kraut, M. A., Womack, K. B., Strain, J., Didehbani, N., Bartz, E., . . . Cullum, C. M. (2013). Neuroimaging of cognitive dysfunction and depression in aging retired National Football League players: A cross-sectional study. *Journal of the American Medical Association—Neurology, 70*(3), 326–335. doi:10.1001/2013.jamaneurol.340

Hazrati, L., Tartaglia, M., Diamandis, P., David, K., Green, R. E., Wennberg, R., et al. (2013). Absence of chronic traumatic encephalopathy in retired football players with multiple concussions and neuroplogical symptomatology. *Frontiers in Human Neuroscience, 7*(222), 1–9.

Hootman, J. M., Dick, R., & Agel, J. (2007). Epidemiology of collegiate injuries for 15 sports: Summary and recommendations for injury prevention initiatives. *Journal of Athletic Training, 42*(2), 311–319.

Hovda, D. A., Lee, S. M., Smith, M. L., Von Stuck, S., Bergsneider, M., Kelly, D., . . . et al. (1995). The neurochemical and metabolic cascade following brain injury: moving from animal models to man. *J Neurotrauma, 12*(5), 903–906.

Howell, D., Osternig, L., van Donkelaar, P., Mayr, U., & Chou, L. (2013). Effects of concussion on attention and executive function in adolescents. *Medicine & Science in sports and Exercise, 45*(6), 1030–1037.

Iverson, G. L., Zasler, N. D., & Lange, R. T. (2007). Post-concussive disorder. In N. D. Zasler, D. I. Katz & R. D. Zafonte (Eds.), *Brain injury medicine: Principles and practice* (pp. 373–405). New York: Demos Medical Publishing.

Jantzen, K. J., Anderson, B., Steinberg, F. L., & Kelso, J. A. (2004). A prospective functional MR imaging study of mild traumatic brain injury in college football players. *AJNR Am J Neuroradiol, 25*(5), 738–745.

Jenkins, G. J., Mikhail, J., Alhamdani, A., Brown, T. H., Caplin, S., Manson, J. M., ... Baxter, J. N. (2007). Immunohistochemical study of nuclear factor-kappaB activity and interleukin-8 abundance in oesophageal adenocarcinoma: A useful strategy for monitoring these biomarkers. *Journal of Clinical Pathology, 60*(11), 1232–1237. doi:10.1136/jcp.2006.043976

Johnson, B., Gay, M., Zhang, K., Neuberger, T., Horovitz, S. G., Hallett, M., ... Slobounov, S. (2012). The use of magnetic resonance spectroscopy in the subacute evaluation of athletes recovering from single and multiple mild traumatic brain injury. *Journal of Neurotrauma, 29*(13), 2297–2304. doi:10.1089/neu.2011.2294

Johnson, B., Zhang, K., Gay, M., Horovitz, S., Hallett, M., Sebastianelli, W., & Slobounov, S. (2012). Alteration of brain default network in subacute phase of injury in concussed individuals: Resting-state fMRI study. *NeuroImage, 59*(1), 511–518. doi:10.1016/j.neuroimage.2011.07.081

Kelly, J. P. (1999). Traumatic brain injury and concussion in sports. *Journal of the American Medical Association, 282*(10), 989–991.

Kelly, J. P., Nichols, J. S., Filley, C. M., Lillehei, K. O., Rubinstein, D., & Kleinschmidt-DeMasters, B. K. (1991). Concussion in sports. Guidelines for the prevention of catastrophic outcome. *Journal of the American Medical Association, 266*(20), 2867–2869.

Kerr, Z. Y., Marshall, S. W., Harding, H. P., Jr., & Guskiewicz, K. M. (2012). Nine-year risk of depression diagnosis increases with increasing self-reported concussions in retired professional football players. *American Journal of Sports Medicine, 40*(10), 2206–2212. doi:10.1177/0363546512456193

King, D., Brughelli, M., Hume, P., & Gissane, C. (2013). Concussions in amateur rugby union identified with the use of a rapid visual screening tool. *Journal of the Neurological Sciences, 326*(1-2), 59–63. doi:10.1016/j.jns.2013.01.012

King, D., Clark, T., & Gissane, C. (2012). Use of a rapid visual screening tool for the assessment of concussion in amateur rugby league: A pilot study. *Journal of the Neurological Sciences, 320*(1-2), 16–21. doi:10.1016/j.jns.2012.05.049

Koerte, I. K., Ertl-Wagner, B., Reiser, M., Zafonte, R., & Shenton, M. E. (2012). White matter integrity in the brains of professional soccer players without a symptomatic concussion. *Journal of the American Medical Association, 308*(18), 1859–1861. doi:10.1001/jama.2012.13735

Koerte, I. K., Kaufmann, D., Hartl, E., Bouix, S., Pasternak, O., Kubicki, M., ... Shenton, M. E. (2012). A prospective study of physician-observed concussion during a varsity university hockey season: White matter integrity in ice hockey players. Part 3 of 4. *Neurosurgical Focus, 33*(6), E3: 1–7. doi:10.3171/2012.10.FOCUS12303

Kraus, M. F., Susmaras, T., Caughlin, B. P., Walker, C. J., Sweeney, J. A., & Little, D. M. (2007). White matter integrity and cognition in chronic traumatic brain injury: A diffusion tensor imaging study. *Brain, 130*(Pt 10), 2508–2519.

LaBotz, M., Martin, M. R., Kimura, I. F., Hetzler, R. K., & Nichols, A. W. (2005). A comparison of a preparticipation evaluation history form and a symptom-based concussion survey in the identification of previous head injury in collegiate athletes. *Clin J Sport Med, 15*(2), 73–78.

Langlois, J. A., Rutland-Brown, W., & Wald, M. M. (2006). The epidemiology and impact of traumatic brain injury: A brief overview. *Journal of Head Trauma Rehabilitation, 21*(5), 375–378.

Lau, B., Lovell, M., Collins, M. W., & Pardini, J. (2009). Neurocognitive and symptom predictors of recovery in high school athletes. *Clin J Sport Med, 19*(3), 216–221.

Lau, B. C., Collins, M. W., & Lovell, M. R. (2012). Cutoff scores in neurocognitive testing and symptom clusters that predict protracted recovery from concussions in high school athletes. *Neurosurgery, 70*(2), 371–379.

Lovell, M. R., Pardini, J. E., Welling, J., Collins, M. W., Bakal, J., Lazar, N., . . . Becker, J. T. (2007). Functional brain abnormalities are related to clinical recovery and time to return-to-play in athletes. *Neurosurgery, 61*(2), 352–359; discussion 359-360.

Macciocchi, S. N., Barth, J. T., Alves, W., Rimel, R. W., & Jane, J. A. (1996). Neuropsychological functioning and recovery after mild head injury in collegiate athletes. *Neurosurgery, 39*(3), 510–514.

Macciocchi, S. N., Barth, J. T., Littlefield, L., & Cantu, R. C. (2001). Multiple concussions and neuropsychological functioning in collegiate football players. *Journal of Athletic Training, 36*(3), 303–306.

Makdissi, M., Darby, D., Maruff, P., Ugoni, A., Brukner, P., & McCrory, P. R. (2010). Natural history of concussion in sport: markers of severity and implications for management. *Am J Sports Med, 38*(3), 464–471.

Marar, M., McIlvain, N. M., Fields, S. K., & Comstock, R. D. (2012). Epidemiology of concussions among United States high school athletes in 20 sports. *American Journal of Sports Medicine, 40*(4), 747–755. doi:10.1177/0363546511435626

Marchi, N., Bazarian, J. J., Puvenna, V., Janigro, M., Ghosh, C., Zhong, J., . . . Janigro, D. (2013). Consequences of repeated blood-brain barrier disruption in football players. *PloS One, 8*(3), e56805. doi:10.1371/journal.pone.0056805

Mayer, A. R., Ling, J., Mannell, M. V., Gasparovic, C., Phillips, J. P., Doezema, D., . . . Yeo, R. A. (2010). A prospective diffusion tensor imaging study in mild traumatic brain injury. *Neurology, 74*(8), 643–650. doi:10.1212/WNL.0b013e3181d0ccdd

Mayr, U. (2006). What matters in the cued task-switching paradigm: Tasks or cues? *Psychonomic Bulletin & Review, 13*(5), 794–799.

McAllister, T. W., Flashman, L. A., Maerlender, A., Greenwald, R. M., Beckwith, J. G., Tosteson, T. D., . . . Turco, J. H. (2012). Cognitive effects of one season of head impacts in a cohort of collegiate contact sport athletes. *Neurology, 78*(22), 1777–1784. doi:10.1212/WNL.0b013e3182582fe7

McAllister, T. W., Saykin, A. J., Flashman, L. A., Sparling, M. B., Johnson, S. C., Guerin, S. J., . . . Yanofsky, N. (1999). Brain activation during working memory 1 month after mild traumatic brain injury: A functional MRI study. *Neurology, 53*(6), 1300–1308.

McCrea, M. (2007). *Mild traumatic brain injury and post-concussion syndrome: The New evidence base for diagnosis and treatment.* New York: Oxford Press.

McCrea, M., Barr, W. B., Guskiewicz, K., Randolph, C., Marshall, S. W., Cantu, R., . . . Kelly, J. P. (2005). Standard regression-based methods for measuring recovery after sport-related concussion. *Journal of the International Neuropsychological Society, 11*(1), 58–69.

McCrea, M., Guskiewicz, K. M., Marshall, S. W., Barr, W., Randolph, C., Cantu, R. C., . . . Kelly, J. P. (2003). Acute effects and recovery time following concussion in collegiate football players: The NCAA Concussion Study. *Journal of the American Medical Association, 290*(19), 2556–2563.

McCrea, M., Guskiewicz, K., Randolph, C., Barr, W. B., Hammeke, T. A., Marshall, S. W., & Kelly, J. P. (2009). Effects of a symptom-free waiting period on clinical outcome and risk of reinjury after sport-related concussion. *Neurosurgery, 65*(5), 876–882.

McCrea, M., Guskiewicz, K., Randolph, C., Barr, W. B., Hammeke, T. A., Marshall, S. W., . . . Kelly, J. P. (2013). Incidence, clinical course, and predictors of prolonged recovery time following sport-related concussion in high school and college athletes. *Journal of the International Neuropsychological Society, 19*(1), 22–33. doi:10.1017/S1355617712000872

McCrea, M., Hammeke, T., Olsen, G., Leo, P., & Guskiewicz, K. (2004). Unreported concussion in high school football players: Implications for prevention. *Clinical Journal of Sport Medicine, 14*(1), 13–17.

McCrea, M., Iverson, G. L., Echemendia, R. J., Makdissi, M., & Raftery, M. (2013). Day of injury assessment of sport-related concussion. *British Journal of Sports Medicine, 47*(5), 272–284. doi:10.1136/bjsports-2013-092145

McCrory, P. (2001). Does second impact syndrome exist? *Clinical Journal of Sport Medicine, 11*(3), 144–149.

McCrory, P., & Berkovic, S. F. (1998). Second impact syndrome. *Neurology, 50*(3), 677–683.

McCrory, P., Johnston, K., Meeuwisse, W., Aubry, M., Cantu, R., Dvorak, J., . . . Schamasch, P. (2005). Summary and agreement statement of the 2nd International Conference on Concussion in Sport, Prague 2004. *British Journal of Sports Medicine, 39*(4), 196–204.

McCrory, P., Meeuwisse, W. H., Aubry, M., Cantu, B., Dvorak, J., Echemendia, R. J., . . . Turner, M. (2013). Consensus statement on concussion in sport: The 4th International Conference on Concussion in Sport held in Zurich, November 2012. *Journal of the American College of Surgeons, 216*(5), e55–71. doi:10.1016/j.jamcollsurg.2013.02.020

McCrory, P., Meeuwisse, W. H., Kutcher, J. S., Jordan, B. D., & Gardner, A. (2013). What is the evidence for chronic concussion-related changes in retired athletes: Behavioural, pathological and clinical outcomes? *British Journal of Sports Medicine, 47*(5), 327–330. doi:10.1136/bjsports-2013-092248

McCrory, P., Meeuwisse, W., Johnston, K., Dvorak, J., Aubry, M., Molloy, M., & Cantu, R. (2009). Consensus statement on concussion in sport: The 3rd International Conference on Concussion in Sport held in Zurich, November 2008. *British Journal of Sports Medicine, 43 (Suppl 1)*, i76–90.

McGowan, J. C., Yang, J. H., Plotkin, R. C., Grossman, R. I., Umile, E. M., Cecil, K. M., & Bagley, L. J. (2000). Magnetization transfer imaging in the detection of injury associated with mild head trauma. *AJNR Am J Neuroradiol, 21*(5), 875–880.

McGrath, N., Dinn, W. M., Collins, M. W., Lovell, M. R., Elbin, R. J., & Kontos, A. P. (2013). Post-exertion neurocognitive test failure among student-athletes following concussion. *Brain Injury, 27*(1), 103–113. doi:10.3109/02699052.2012.729282

McKee, A. C., Cantu, R. C., Nowinski, C. J., Hedley-Whyte, E. T., Gavett, B. E., Budson, A. E., . . . Stern, R. A. (2009). Chronic traumatic encephalopathy in athletes: Progressive tauopathy after repetitive head injury. *J Neuropathol Exp Neurol, 68*(7), 709–735.

McKee, A. C., Gavett, B. E., Stern, R. A., Nowinski, C. J., Cantu, R. C., Kowall, N. W. et al. (2010). TDP-43 proteinopathy and motor neuron disease in chronic traumatic encephalopathy. *Journal of Neuropathology & Experimental neurology, 69*(9), 918–929.

Meehan, W. P., 3rd, Mannix, R. C., O'Brien M, J., & Collins, M. W. (2013). The prevalence of undiagnosed concussions in athletes. *Clinical Journal of Sport Medicine, 23*, 339–342. doi:10.1097/JSM.0b013e318291d3b3

Mittenberg, W., & Fischera, S. (1993). Recovery from mild head injury: A treatment manual for patients. *Psychotherapy in Private Practice, 12*, 37–52.

Mittenberg, W., Tremont, G., Zielinski, R. E., Fichera, S., & Rayls, K. R. (1996). Cognitive-behavioral prevention of postconcussion syndrome. *Arch Clin Neuropsychol, 11*(2), 139–145.

Mortimore, J. A., van Duijn, C. M., Chandra, V., Fratiglioni, L., Graves, A. B., Heyman, A., . . . Hofman, A. (1991). Head truama as a risk factor for Alzheimer's disease: A collaborative re-analysis of case-control studies. *International Journal of Epidemiology, 20*(2 Suppl. 2), S28–S35.

Moser, R. S., Glatts, C., & Schatz, P. (2012). Efficacy of immediate and delayed cognitive and physical rest for treatment of sports-related concussion. *Journal of Pediatrics, 161*(5), 922–926. doi:10.1016/j.jpeds.2012.04.012

Neselius, S., Zetterberg, H., Blennow, K., Randall, J., Wilson, D., Marcusson, J., & Brisby, H. (2013). Olympic boxing is associated with elevated levels of the neuronal protein tau in plasma. *Brain Injury, 27*(4), 425–433. doi:10.3109/02699052.2012.750752

Nuwer, M. R., Hovda, D. A., Schrader, L. M., & Vespa, P. M. (2005). Routine and quantitative EEG in mild traumatic brain injury. *Clinical Neurophysiology, 116*(9), 2001–2025. doi:10.1016/j.clinph.2005.05.008

Powell, J. W., & Barber-Foss, K. D. (1999). Traumatic brain injury in high school athletes. *Journal of the American Medical Association, 282*(10), 958–963.

Powers, K. C., Kalmar, J. M., & Cinelli, M. E. (2013). Recovery of static stability following a concussion. *Gait & Posture.* doi:10.1016/j.gaitpost.2013.05.026

Prins, M. L., Hales, A., Reger, M., Giza, C. C., & Hovda, D. A. (2010). Repeat traumatic brain injury in the juvenile rat is associated with increased axonal injury and cognitive impairments. *Dev Neurosci, 32*(5–6), 510–518.

Quality Standards Subcommittee of the American Academy of Neurology. (1997). Practice parameter: The management of concussion in sports (summary statement). Report of the Quality Standards Subcommittee. *Neurology, 48*(3), 581–585.

Raichle, M. E., MacLeod, A. M., Snyder, A. Z., Powers, W. J., Gusnard, D. A., & Shulman, G. L. (2001). A default mode of brain function. *Proceedings of the National Academy of Sciences of the United States of America, 98*(2), 676–682. doi:10.1073/pnas.98.2.676

Ruff, R. M., Camenzuli, L., & Mueller, J. (1996). Miserable minority: Emotional risk factors that influence the outcome of a mild traumatic brain injury. *Brain Injury, 10*(8), 551–565.

Savica, R., Parisi, J. E., Wold, L. E., Josephs, K. A., & Ahlskog, J. E. (2012). High school football and risk of neurodegeneration: A community-based study. *Mayo Clinic Proceedings, 87*(4), 335–340. doi:10.1016/j.mayocp.2011.12.016

Schneider, K. J., Iverson, G. L., Emery, C. A., McCrory, P., Herring, S. A., & Meeuwisse, W. H. (2013). The effects of rest and treatment following sport-related concussion: A systematic review of the literature. *British Journal of Sports Medicine, 47*(5), 304–307. doi:10.1136/bjsports-2013-092190

Schneiders, A. G., Sullivan, S. J., Handcock, P., Gray, A., & McCrory, P. R. (2012). Sports concussion assessment: The effect of exercise on dynamic and static balance. *Scandinavian Journal of Medicine & Science in Sports, 22*(1), 85–90. doi:10.1111/j.1600-0838.2010.01141.x

Schulz, M. R., Marshall, S. W., Mueller, F. O., Yang, J., Weaver, N. L., Kalsbeek, W. D., & Bowling, J. M. (2004). Incidence and risk factors for concussion in high school athletes, North Carolina, 1996-1999. *American Journal of Epidemiology, 160*(10), 937–944.

Stern, R. A., Riley, D. O., Daneshvar, D. H., Nowinski, C. J., Cantu, R. C., & McKee, A. C. (2011). Long-term consequences of repetitive brain trauma: Chronic traumatic encephalopathy. *PM&R, 3*(10 Suppl 2), S460–467. doi:10.1016/j.pmrj.2011.08.008

Tavazzi, B., Vagnozzi, R., Signoretti, S., Amorini, A. M., Belli, A., Cimatti, M., . . . Lazzarino, G. (2007). Temporal window of metabolic brain vulnerability to concussions: Oxidative and nitrosative stresses—part II. *Neurosurgery, 61*(2), 390–395; discussion 395–396.

Terry, D. P., Faraco, C. C., Smith, D., Diddams, M. J., Puente, A. N., & Miller, L. S. (2012). Lack of long-term fMRI differences after multiple sports-related concussions. *Brain Injury, 26*(13-14), 1684–1696. doi:10.3109/02699052.2012.722259

Thornton, A. E., Cox, D. N., Whitfield, K., & Fouladi, R. T. (2008). Cumulative concussion exposure in rugby players: Neurocognitive and symptomatic outcomes. *Journal of Clinical & Experimental Neuropsychology, 30*(4), 398–409. doi:10.1080/13803390701443662

Tremblay, S., De Beaumont, L., Henry, L. C., Boulanger, Y., Evans, A. C., Bourgouin, P., . . . Lassonde, M. (2013). Sports concussions and aging: A neuroimaging investigation. *Cerebral Cortex, 23*(5), 1159–1166. doi:10.1093/cercor/bhs102

Upshaw, J. E., Gosserand, J. K., Williams, N., & Edwards, J. C. (2012). Sports-related concussions. *Pediatric Emergency Care, 28*(9), 926–932. doi:10.1097/PEC.0b013e318267f674

Vagnozzi, R., Signoretti, S., Tavazzi, B., Cimatti, M., Amorini, A. M., Donzelli, S., . . . Lazzarino, G. (2005). Hypothesis of the postconcussive vulnerable brain: Experimental evidence of its metabolic occurrence. *Neurosurgery, 57*(1), 164–171; discussion 164–171.

Vagnozzi, R., Signoretti, S., Tavazzi, B., Floris, R., Ludovici, A., Marziali, S., . . . Lazzarino, G. (2008). Temporal window of metabolic brain vulnerability to concussion: a pilot 1H-magnetic resonance spectroscopic study in concussed athletes—part III. *Neurosurgery, 62*(6), 1286–1295; discussion 1295–1286.

Vagnozzi, R., Tavazzi, B., Signoretti, S., Amorini, A. M., Belli, A., Cimatti, M., . . . Lazzarino, G. (2007). Temporal window of metabolic brain vulnerability to concussions: mitochondrial-related impairment—part I. *Neurosurgery, 61*(2), 379–388; discussion 388–379.

Virji-Babul, N., Borich, M. R., Makan, N., Moore, T., Frew, K., Emery, C. A., & Boyd, L. A. (2013). Diffusion tensor imaging of sports-related concussion in adolescents. *Pediatric Neurology, 48*(1), 24–29. doi:10.1016/j.pediatrneurol.2012.09.005

Weber, A. F., Mihalik, J. P., Register-Mihalik, J. K., Mays, S., Prentice, W. E., & Guskiewicz, K. M. (2013). Dehydration and performance on clinical concussion measures in collegiate wrestlers. *Journal of Athletic Training, 48*(2), 153–160. doi:10.4085/1062-6050-48.1.07

Welch, K., Nederberg, F., Bowden, T., Hilborn, J., & Stromme, M. (2007). Molecular dynamics of a biodegradable biomimetic ionomer studied by broadband dielectric spectroscopy. *Langmuir, 23*(20), 10209–10215. doi:10.1021/la7009012

Wilde, E. A., McCauley, S. R., Hunter, J. V., Bigler, E. D., Chu, Z., Wang, Z. J., . . . Levin, H. S. (2008). Diffusion tensor imaging of acute mild traumatic brain injury in adolescents. *Neurology, 70*(12), 948–955.

Williams, D. B., Annegers, J. F., Kokmen, E., O'Brien, P. C., & Kurland, L. T. (1991). Brain injury and neurologic sequelae: A cohort study of dementia, parkinsonism, and amyotrophic lateral sclerosis. *Neurology, 41*(10), 1554–1557.

Wilson, R., Monaghan, P., Bowden, S. A., Parnell, J., & Cooper, J. M. (2007). Surface-enhanced Raman signatures of pigmentation of cyanobacteria from within geological samples in a spectroscopic-microfluidic flow cell. *Analytical Chemistry, 79*(18), 7036–7041. doi:10.1021/ac070994c

Yi, J., Padalino, D. J., Chin, L. S., Montenegro, P., & Cantu, R. C. (2013). Chronic traumatic encephalopathy. *Current Sports Medicine Reports, 12*(1), 28–32. doi:10.1249/JSR.0b013e31827ec9e3

Zemper, E. D. (2003). Two-year prospective study of relative risk of a second cerebral concussion. *American Journal of Physical Medicine & Rehabilitation, 82*(9), 653–659.

Zetterberg, H., Smith, D. H., & Blennow, K. (2013). Biomarkers of mild traumatic brain injury in cerebrospinal fluid and blood. *Nature Reviews Neurology, 9*(4), 201–210. doi:10.1038/nrneurol.2013.9

Zhang, K., Johnson, B., Gay, M., Horovitz, S. G., Hallett, M., Sebastianelli, W., & Slobounov, S. (2012). Default mode network in concussed individuals in response to the YMCA physical stress test. *Journal of Neurotrauma, 29*(5), 756–765. doi:10.1089/neu.2011.2125

Zuckerman, S. L., Lee, Y. M., Odom, M. J., Solomon, G. S., Forbes, J. A., & Sills, A. K. (2012). Recovery from sports-related concussion: Days to return to neurocognitive baseline in adolescents versus young adults. *Surgical Neurology International, 3*, 130. doi:10.4103/2152-7806.102945

Zuckerman, S. L., Solomon, G. S., Forbes, J. A., Haase, R. F., Sills, A. K., & Lovell, M. R. (2012). Response to acute concussive injury in soccer players: Is gender a modifying factor? *Journal of Neurosurgery: Pediatrics, 10*(6), 504–510. doi:10.3171/2012.8.PEDS12139

6

EXECUTIVE FUNCTIONING IN CHILDREN WITH ATTENTION-DEFICIT/HYPERACTIVITY DISORDER

Jeffrey M. Halperin, Sarah O'Neill, Ashley N. Simone,
and Elizaveta Bourchtein

INTRODUCTION

The notion that attention-deficit/hyperactivity disorder (ADHD) is due to primary deficits in executive functions mediated via neural circuits involving the prefrontal cortex dates back more than three decades. This association was initially inferred from observations that deficits and impairments in children with ADHD appear strikingly similar to those of monkeys and human adults with known frontal lobe lesions (Fuster, 1997; Mattes, 1980; Pontius, 1973) and was further supported by early data indicating impaired performance on neuropsychological tests measuring these functions (Benson, 1991; Chelune, Ferguson, Koon, & Disckey, 1986; Shue & Douglas, 1992).

These initial observations and findings led to a very substantial literature examining the performance of children with ADHD on neuropsychological measures of executive functions and, within the past decade, several comprehensive meta-analyses that leave little doubt that as a group, children with ADHD perform more poorly than their typically developing peers on a wide array of tests and measures of executive function (Frazier, Demaree, & Youngstrom, 2004; Willcutt, Doyle, Nigg, Faraone, & Pennington, 2005). Most prominently, deficits have been reported in working memory (Martinussen, Hayden, Hogg-Johnson, & Tannock, 2005; Willcutt et al., 2005), inhibitory control (Barkley, 1997; Barkley, Grodzinsky, & DuPaul, 1992; Casey et al., 1997), planning (Willcutt et al., 2005), and vigilance (Willcutt et al., 2005). However, these reviews and meta-analyses also indicated that the magnitude of the effect size for executive function deficits is moderate (Willcutt et al., 2005) and that a substantial portion of children with ADHD do not perform poorly on neuropsychological tests of executive functions (Nigg, Willcutt, Doyle, & Sonuga-Barke, 2005). The well-known heterogeneity characteristic of children with ADHD has further complicated the picture as it seems likely that different children with the disorder have distinct patterns of deficits, raising the possibility of separable neuropsychological subtypes of ADHD (Nigg et al., 2005; Sonuga-Barke, 2003). Additionally, some data raise questions regarding the extent to which poor performance on executive function tests by children with ADHD are due to primary "top-down" executive deficits as opposed to their being secondary to deficits in more basic information processing systems (e.g., Rommelse et al., 2007; Marks et al., 2005). Together, these findings have raised key theoretical issues regarding the role of executive functions in ADHD and the extent to which neuropsychological tests of executive functions should play a role in the diagnostic process. Throughout the past 2 years, research has begun to grapple with these and other issues related to the neuropsychology of ADHD, including, but not limited to, whether distinct subtypes (Diagnostic and Statistical Manual [DSM]-IV) or presentations (DSM-V) of the disorder differ in neuropsychological functioning, the impact of comorbidity, and the extent to which executive function measures not only differentiate children with ADHD from their typically developing peers, but also from children with other disorders.

This chapter systematically examines peer-reviewed research on executive functions and ADHD in children published between January 1, 2012 and May 1, 2013. To maximally capture the research published within this time-frame, we searched PubMed, PsycINFO, and Medline databases using variations on "ADHD" (e.g., attention-deficit/hyperactivity disorder, attention deficit disorder, and so forth) in combination with "executive functions" and an array of search terms related to specific types of executive functions (e.g., inhibitory control, working memory, planning, fluency, attention, and so forth). Finally, we examined the tables of contents from several journals in the fields of neuropsychology (i.e., *Neuropsychology, Journal of the International Neuropsychological Society, Developmental Neuropsychology, Child Neuropsychology, Journal of Clinical and Experimental Neuropsychology*), psychiatry (i.e., *American Journal of Psychiatry, Archives of General Psychiatry, Biological Psychiatry, Journal of Abnormal Psychology, Journal of Attention Disorders*), and child psychopathology (i.e., *Journal of Child Psychology and Psychiatry, Journal of Abnormal Child Psychology, Journal of the American Academy of Child and Adolescent Psychiatry*) to capture additional papers that we might have missed. To define the parameters of this review, we limited it to studies of children with a diagnosis of ADHD, largely excluding studies focusing on the symptom dimensions of inattention and hyperactivity/impulsivity. Furthermore, our primary focus is on neuropsychological *tests* of executive functions rather than ratings of these characteristics. We did not include behavioral/neuropsychological data derived while children were in a functional neuroimaging (i.e., magnetic resonance imaging, electroencephalogram) environment due to the facts that such an environment is likely to affect performance and, for the most part, nonstandardized variations of neuropsychological tests are used in such research. Finally, we limit this review to papers written in English with human participants younger than age 18 years.

The chapter is divided into five partially overlapping sections that focus on (1) executive function differences between children with ADHD and their typically developing peers, (2) differences in executive functioning among ADHD subtypes, (3) parsing the heterogeneity of ADHD, (4) whether poor performance on executive function tests could be accounted for by more basic nonexecutive processing problems, and (5) the extent to which measures of executive function distinguish between ADHD and other psychiatric disorders. Not surprisingly, several of the reviewed papers are broad in scope and address multiple issues. To avoid redundancy and improve readability of the chapter, we chose to not review such papers in multiple sections. Rather, we placed the discussion of such papers in the section that we believed best captured the primary emphasis of the research.

ADHD YOUTH VERSUS TYPICALLY DEVELOPING PEERS

Recent research has continued to find that children and adolescents with ADHD exhibit poorer performance on a wide array of measures assessing executive functions compared to their typically developing peers. Although the comparison of ADHD versus non-ADHD groups on neuropsychological measures of executive functioning appears in many recently published studies, more often than not, this contrast is a small part of research that tackles more complex issues related to the heterogeneity of ADHD, the extent to which executive function deficits are better accounted for by impairments in more basic nonexecutive processes, or the degree to which such measures distinguish youth with ADHD from other clinical groups. This section is limited to studies in which the primary focus was either (1) the simple comparison of children with and without ADHD, (2) the comparison of children with and without ADHD with the aim of more precisely narrowing-down the nature of the executive deficit associated with ADHD, or (3) the elucidation of the functional consequences of executive function deficits in children with ADHD. In later sections targeting specific theoretical or clinical issues such contrasts are indicated, but framed within the broader questions addressed by the research.

Two recent meta-analyses examined the published research literature to determine the magnitude of differences between children with and without ADHD on specific aspects of executive functions.

Hasson and Fine (2012) conducted a meta-analysis to examine gender differences in continuous performance test (CPT) errors of omission and commission in 6- to 18-year-old children and adolescents with and without ADHD. Articles published between 1980 and 2009 that allowed for gender differentiation were included. Participants from all included studies were medication-free at the time of testing and any studies in which children/adolescents had a primary diagnosis of learning disability, conduct disorder (CD), oppositional-defiant disorder (ODD), anxiety, or depression were excluded. The included sample comprised 772 boys and 325 girls with ADHD from eight studies in which several different types of CPTs were used, including AX-CPT, Conners' CPT-II (respond to all stimuli except X), and an auditory CPT. Boys with ADHD were found to make more errors of commission than girls ($d = .31$), but no gender differences in omission errors was observed ($d = -.09$). Normative gender differences in commission errors was examined by comparing control males to control females, with boys emerging as significantly more likely to commit errors of commission in that group as well. Within-gender comparisons (i.e., ADHD boys vs. control boys; ADHD girls vs. control girls) revealed that children with ADHD were more likely to commit errors of commission, and that the magnitude of the difference was significantly greater for boys than for girls. The authors conclude that inhibitory control may be moderated by gender.

Given the marked interest in working memory functioning of children with ADHD over the past 10 years, Kasper, Alderson, and Hudec (2012) aimed to update previous meta-analytic reviews in this area. As well as looking at group differences in working memory functioning, they also examined potential moderating effects of gender, age, and task parameters. To achieve this they analyzed 45 studies published from 1989 to 2011 that measured phonological or visual-spatial working memory in children aged 8 to 16 years old. All studies allowed for between-group comparisons of children with and without ADHD. Children with ADHD showed deficits in both phonological and visual-spatial working memory compared with typically developing children, with large effect sizes obtained (.74 for visual-spatial and .69 for phonological). However, significant heterogeneity among effect sizes was observed for both the phonological and visual-spatial domains. Exploration of possible moderating variables using weighted multiple regression revealed a model able to explain a significant proportion of effect size variability. Studies that included fewer females, a larger number of trials, recall tasks, and tasks that placed high demands on the central executive were associated with larger between-group differences for both systems. Thus, these findings provide further evidence that children with ADHD perform more poorly on tests of phonological and visual-spatial working memory when compared to their typically developing peers. Notably, effect sizes found in this meta-analysis, particularly for phonological working memory, were larger than those previously reported (Martinussen et al., 2005; Willcutt et al., 2005).

Together, these reviews support previous data indicating verbal and spatial working memory as well as inhibitory control deficits in ADHD. They also identify possible moderators of these well-established effects. Notably, the data did not support the notion that attention, at least as measured by CPTs, is impaired in youth with ADHD.

Several recent studies have compared children with and without ADHD to determine the diagnostic and clinical utility of new or existing measures for distinguishing between these groups. To determine the utility of the computerized Cambridge Neuropsychological Test Automated Battery (CANTAB; Robbins, James, Owen, Sahakian, & Rabbitt, 1994) for evaluating executive functioning deficits in children with ADHD, Fried, Hirshfeld-Becker, Petty, Batchelder, and Biederman (2012) administered it to 6- to 16-year-old unmedicated children with (n = 107) and without (n = 45) ADHD. The test battery included the following subtests: Stockings of Cambridge, Intra-Extra Dimensional Set Shift, Spatial Working Memory, Rapid Visual Information Processing, Reaction Time, Affective Go/No-go, and the California Verbal Learning Test. ADHD participants performed significantly worse than those without ADHD on all outcome measures except Affective Go/No-go total omission errors, with effect sizes generally falling in the medium range. The authors concluded that the results are consistent with data reported in studies using traditional neuropsychological tests and thus support the utility of the CANTAB to assess neuropsychological deficits in children with ADHD.

In a sample of 8- to 11-year-old Israeli boys with (n = 25) and without (n = 25) ADHD, Shimoni, Engel-Yeger, and Tirosh (2012) aimed to examine the relation between executive functioning as measured by standardized neuropsychological tests and as observed in everyday life by the children's parents. Children completed the Behavioral Assessment of Dysexecutive Functions for Children (BADS-C; Emslie, Wilson, Burden, Nimmo-Smith, & Wilson, 2003) and their parents completed the Behavior Rating Inventory of Executive Functions (BRIEF; Gioia, Isquick, Guy, & Kenworthy, 2000). Compared to children without ADHD, boys with ADHD achieved lower scores on most, but not all, subtests of the BADS-C. Similarly, parents of children with ADHD rated them as showing deficits on most, but not all, subscales of the BRIEF when compared to children without ADHD. Significant correlations were obtained between BADS-C and BRIEF total scores, and between BADS-C total score and BRIEF metacognition scale and emotion control, working memory, planning, monitoring, and inhibition subscales, but not organization of materials, initiation, and attention shift. The authors concluded that boys with ADHD showed executive function deficits on both objective measures and parent reports of everyday functioning. Integrating information from both types of assessment may provide a more ecologically valid profile of children's strengths and weaknesses.

Similarly, Rauch, Gold, and Schmitt (2012) noted that impulsivity is commonly measured in clinical settings using personality questionnaires, whereas more objective laboratory or neuropsychological tests are typically used in research. Yet, the degree of convergence between these two measurement approaches is unclear. To evaluate the relative value of each method, Rauch et al. recruited a sample of 9- to 12-year-old children with (n = 18) and without (n = 17) ADHD. Children completed a German adaptation of Eysenck, Easting, and Pearson's (1984) impulsivity questionnaire and a computerized Go/No-go task. In addition, a combined measure of impulsiveness, based on both approaches, was generated. The associations between these measures of impulsivity as well as with group status and parent-reported ADHD symptoms were investigated. Children with ADHD differed significantly from non-ADHD control children on both measures, but there was also significant distributional overlap. Scores on the two measures correlated weakly with one another, yet both correlated robustly with parent ratings of ADHD severity, with each measure explaining unique variance of parent ratings. As such, the combination of scores from the two impulsivity measures outperformed the individual measures in diagnostic accuracy. The authors concluded that on their own, these measures are not good at classifying children as having ADHD, because many children score in the "normal" range. However, by combining the measures, classification accuracy can be improved, particularly with regards to sensitivity. These findings provided further support for the heterogeneity observed among children with ADHD.

Bioulac et al. (2012) used a virtual reality task to examine performance decrements over time in 20 7- to 10-year-old children with ADHD as compared to 16 age-matched non-ADHD children. In addition, children were administered the CPT-II (Conners & Staff, 2000) to assess comparability of the virtual reality task and a more traditional measure of vigilance. For the virtual reality task, children wore a head monitor through which they saw a classroom that included distractions outside the classroom door and window as well as inside the classroom. Within the virtual classroom, letters were presented on the blackboard and the task, like a more traditional CPT, was to press a button when they saw a specified sequence of letters (i.e., K preceded by A). Children with ADHD had significantly fewer hits and a greater number of commissions relative to control participants on the virtual reality task, but the groups did not differ on reaction time measures. On the CPT-II, the ADHD group had fewer hits, and longer and more variable reaction times, but the groups did not differ with regard to the number of commission errors. Notably, the virtual reality test was more sensitive to time-on-task deficits in the children with ADHD. The authors suggest that the virtual reality classroom task offers several advantages compared to classical tools in that it is more realistic and lifelike, and that classroom distractions can be added in a standardized manner. They concluded that the virtual classroom is a good clinical tool for evaluation of attention in children with ADHD, especially to explore time-on-task effects.

Ferrin and Vance (2012) examined the utility of assessing nonexecutive neurological subtle signs as a clinical tool for diagnosing ADHD. They also explored the relations between these signs and spatial working memory in 1,055 children and adolescents with ADHD and 130 age-matched typically developing youth. Neurological subtle signs were measured using the Scored Developmental Neurological Examination (Taylor, Schachar, Thorley, & Wieselberg, 1986) and spatial working memory was assessed using the CANTAB. As expected, youth with ADHD had significantly higher levels of all forms of neurological subtle signs (i.e., choreiform/athetoid movements, smoothness/accuracy of movements, mirror movements, conjugate eye gaze, and cerebellar signs). Receiver operating curve analyses indicated that smoothness/accuracy, cerebellar signs, and choreoathetoid movement scores, as well as total subtle sign score, were associated with good indicators of ADHD. Furthermore, several measures of subtle signs distinguished between individuals with good (>75th percentile) and poor (<25th percentile) working memory, most prominently spatial span. These data suggest that neurological subtle signs, which are more closely linked to subcortical as opposed to executive processes, may be good indicators of ADHD and working memory deficits in children and adolescents. Nevertheless, the authors acknowledge that future studies are needed to clarify whether neurological subtle signs can aid in routine clinical diagnosis of ADHD.

Several investigators have suggested that children with ADHD have impairments with time perception (e.g., Barkley, Koplowitz, Anderson, & McMurray, 1997; Toplak, Rucklidge, Hetherington, John, & Tannock, 2003), which in particular, could account for their characteristically impulsive behavior. Although not necessarily considering diagnostic utility, Walg, Oepen, and Prior (2012) used a forced choice paradigm to study judgments of time duration in 10- to 14-year-old children with (n = 31) and without (n = 29) ADHD. Due to data suggesting distinct neural systems associated with short- and long-duration timing, children participated in two test sessions separated by 5 days. On one day the task focused on "long"-duration time judgments, with stimuli lasting up to 8.1 seconds in duration; on the other day the focus was on short-duration judgments with stimuli lasting up to 500 ms. Furthermore, within sessions, context varied using ascending and descending duration probes to enable the assessment of temporal set shifts. The primary dependent measure for this study was the point of subjective equality, which is the value of a time duration that is judged with a 50% probability as long and a 50% probability as short. During the long-duration conditions, children with ADHD showed significantly lower point of subjective equality values, indicating more long judgments than control particpants; point of subjective equality values did not differ in the short/millisecond condition. However, unlike controls, the ADHD group's judgments during millisecond trials varied as a function of ascending versus descending contexts. For durations on the seconds scale, children with ADHD seemed to perceive time intervals as longer than control participants did, suggesting that they have a faster internal clock. On the milliseconds scale, those with ADHD were less efficient in shifting, suggesting an alteration in temporal set-shifting in ADHD. Overall, the authors suggested that timing ability might represent a core deficit in a subset of children with ADHD.

Finally, based on the idea that phonological working memory is comprised of two separate subsystems, Bolden, Rapport, Raiker, Sarver, and Kofler (2012) compared 8- to 12-year-old boys with (n = 18) and without (n = 15) ADHD on measures of phonological short-term storage (<3 seconds) and longer-term rehearsal mechanisms (12 and 21 seconds). The children were initially administered short word lists (two, four, and six one-syllable words) and were then required to recall the list within 3 seconds. There were no group differences with two-word lists, but boys with ADHD performed worse on the four- and six-word lists, suggesting difficulties with phonological short-term storage. Subsequently, based on performance during the short-term storage part of the study (length at which they got at least 50% correct), the children received 21 trials each with 3-, 12-, and 21-second delays. A significant interaction emerged such that boys with ADHD had a steeper drop in performance across delay intervals. The authors interpreted the findings to indicate that children with ADHD have weaknesses in both short-term storage and longer-term rehearsal mechanisms, although the latter are of greater magnitude and may be a target for intervention. Future research could investigate how well this measure classifies children as having ADHD, and whether positive response to intervention improves symptom severity.

Studies that investigate the clinical and diagnostic utility of assessment tools for ADHD, particularly objective measures, are critical. Decreasing sole reliance of informants' descriptions of children's behavior and developing multimethod approaches to assessment should help to improve the reliability and validity of diagnostic decisions. Empirical studies that address the prognostic usefulness of these measures over time would be an even greater addition to the field.

Given the protracted and nonlinear developmental trajectory of executive functions, it is quite possible that relations between ADHD and executive functions vary as a function of age. This has been the focus of two recent studies.

Gau and Chiang (2013), using a developmental approach, examined the association between symptoms of ADHD in early childhood and working memory in later childhood and adolescence as assessed using Digit Span Backwards from the WISC-III and the Spatial Working Memory task of the CANTAB. The participants consisted of 401 youth with ADHD, 213 of their siblings, and 176 unaffected comparison children ranging in age from 8 to 17 years. Parents were interviewed twice by separate examiners to retrospectively assess the presence of ADHD symptoms when their child was aged 6–8 years; and to assess current ADHD symptoms and diagnosis. Based on these interviews, the sample was divided into those with ADHD (full diagnosis at both time-points), subthreshold ADHD, and non-ADHD. Both the ADHD and subthreshold ADHD groups performed significantly worse on both measures of working memory compared to those without ADHD. The ADHD and subthreshold groups did not differ from each other. Most notably, after controlling for a number of covariates, greater severity of childhood inattention symptoms, as retrospectively assessed, was significantly associated with poorer verbal and spatial working memory at the current assessment. The authors suggest that earlier inattention symptoms are associated with impaired verbal and visuospatial working memory later in development, and that perhaps impaired working memory in adolescence can be detected earlier by screening for the severity of inattention in childhood. However, prospective longitudinal data are required to more adequately test this hypothesis because retrospective reports of ADHD symptoms and diagnosis are highly suspect (Miller, Newcorn, & Halperin, 2010).

Another cross-sectional study employed a large sample of Han Chinese children. Qian, Shuai, Chan, Qian, and Wang (2013) examined the trajectory of executive function development for children with (n = 515) and without (n = 249) ADHD. Specifically, the authors were interested in investigating whether children with ADHD show a lag versus complete deviation in executive function development. Several different executive functions were examined, including inhibition, working memory, shifting, and planning. Children were grouped into four age bands: 7–8, 9–10, 11–12, and 13–15 years. The impact of age and diagnostic status on executive function, controlling for intelligence quotient (IQ), was examined using multiple analysis of covariance (MANCOVA). For children with ADHD, differences in executive functioning among different subtypes were also examined. For working memory and planning, the performance of children and adolescents with ADHD did not differ from their non-ADHD peers at any age. For inhibition, children with ADHD performed more poorly than their typically developing peers at all ages except 13–15 years old. The group differences seemed to reflect a lag in executive function development because children with ADHD performed at the level of control children who were approximately 2 years younger. By ages 13–15 years, however, performance appeared to have stabilized and ADHD adolescents were performing at the same level as their typically developing peers. Differences in planning performance between ADHD and control children were seen at every age level, with children with ADHD performing at the level of typically developing children approximately 2 years younger. No differences in executive functioning as a function of ADHD subtype were observed. This study supports the idea that different executive functions develop at different rates. For children with ADHD, inhibition and planning development may lag behind that of their typically developing peers, rather than represent a complete deviation from normal development.

The role of development in the relations between ADHD trajectory and executive functions is of key interest and importance to the field, because further knowledge has the potential to lead to new and novel intervention strategies. Prospective longitudinal studies are sorely needed.

Several recent studies have investigated the degree to which various executive function deficits in children with ADHD can account for commonly seen functional impairments in these children.

Papaeliou, Maniadaki, and Kakouros (2012) investigated the effect of working memory, vocabulary, and grammar on narrative comprehension in 6- to 11-year-old children with ADHD. Participants were 25 children with ADHD and 25 typically developing comparison children matched for age and Performance IQ. Compared with the typically developing group, the ADHD group performed significantly lower on the Freedom from Distractibility index of the WISC (Digit Span and Arithmetic subtests used as a measure of working memory), the Grammar Comprehension Test, and the Sentence Recall test. Children with ADHD recalled less information from the stories than did typically developing children and were less sensitive to the importance of the information they recalled. Moreover, children with ADHD experienced problems in answering factual questions. Further analysis revealed that deficiencies in narrative comprehension in children with ADHD may be accounted for by problems in working memory.

Raiker, Rapport, Kofler, and Sarver (2012) examined the extent to which "objectively-measured" impulsivity in ADHD could be accounted for by deficits in working memory and/or inhibitory control. Children with ADHD (n = 21) and typically developing children (n = 20) were administered working memory tests assessing the domain-general central executive, as well as the more specific phonological loop and visuospatial sketchpad, and the Stop-Signal Task to measure behavioral inhibition. These indices served as potential mediators of ADHD-related impulsive responding as assessed by two laboratory tasks: commission errors on a rapid identical-pairs CPT and a visual matching to sample test. Bootstrapping analyses indicated that the working memory central executive mediated relations between ADHD and impulsivity, as measured by both tasks, even after accounting for inhibitory control. Inhibitory control, as measured by stop-signal reaction time, mediated the relation between ADHD and CPT measured impulsivity, but not after including the central executive score in the model. The authors concluded that working memory is the core deficit in ADHD. However, such a conclusion would be more firmly supported by a longitudinal design in which the purported neuropsychological mediators are acquired prior to the dependent measure.

Tseng and Gau (2013) investigated the extent to which executive functioning mediates the association between ADHD and social problems by examining ADHD symptoms, comorbidities, and executive functioning in 11- to 17-year-old ADHD youth with (n = 70) and without (n = 31) social problems, and a group of comparison children (n = 173). As compared to the comparison group, children with ADHD, irrespective of social problems, performed more poorly on tests of working memory, response inhibition, and planning, but not on a measure of set shifting. Furthermore, children with ADHD plus social problems performed more poorly on measures of inhibitory control compared to those with ADHD but no social problems. Finally, independent of age, gender, and IQ, measures of working memory and planning, but not set shifting or response inhibition, mediated the relations between ADHD and social problems. The authors concluded that some aspects of executive dysfunction may account for social problems often experienced by youth with ADHD. However, again, causal inferences are limited by the cross-sectional nature of the study.

Banaschewski et al. (2012) examined the extent to which cognitive and/or motivational factors play a role in the manifestation of emotional lability as is commonly seen in children with ADHD. In particular, they sought to determine whether emotional lability was predicted by specific patterns of performance on neuropsychological tasks and, if yes, whether relations between neuropsychological test performance and symptoms of emotional lability were mediated by ADHD symptoms. A multisite sample of 424 individuals with ADHD and 564 unaffected siblings and control participants, aged 6–18 years, was administered a neuropsychological test battery from which performance variables were aggregated as indices of processing speed, response variability, executive functions, choice impulsivity, and the influence of energetic and/or motivational factors. They found that with the exception of delay aversion (a motivational measure), all neuropsychological variables significantly predicted both ADHD and emotional lability symptoms with effect sizes generally in the low-to-moderate range. ADHD and emotional lability were most strongly predicted by measures of processing speed and response variability, followed by measures of executive functions (i.e., Go/No-go omission and commission errors). Notably, however, the association between neuropsychological indices and emotional lability was fully accounted for by variations in ADHD symptoms. In contrast, the relations between neuropsychological performance and ADHD symptoms remained significant after accounting for emotional lability symptoms. Thus, the authors concluded that the association between emotional lability and ADHD cannot be explained by deficits assessed using the cognitive or motivational measures administered in this study and that alternative mechanisms need to be considered.

Relatedly, Graziano, McNamara, Geffken, and Reid (2013) examined the degree to which "top-down" and "bottom-up" control processes can differentiate children with ADHD who have co-occurring aggression and/or internalizing symptoms in a sample of 74 children with ADHD aged 6–17 years. Top-down executive processes were assessed using two measures from the Delis–Kaplan Executive Function System (D-KEFS; Delis, Kaplan, & Kramer, 2001): the Number-Letter Switching condition on the Trail Making Test and the Inhibition/Switching condition of the Color-Word Interference Test. Bottom-up control processes were assessed via parent ratings on the Emotional Reactivity Checklist (Shields & Cicchetti, 1997). Results indicated that children with ADHD with more severe ADHD symptoms performed worse on executive function tasks and were reported by parents as being more emotionally labile, aggressive, and as having more internalizing symptoms. Emotional reactivity was also inversely associated with executive functioning, and positively associated with aggression and internalizing symptoms. Notably, executive functioning was found to be significantly associated with aggression but not internalizing symptoms, and emotional reactivity was associated with aggression irrespective of internalizing or ADHD symptom severity. Executive function deficits were less likely to occur in children with ADHD and co-occurring internalizing symptoms. The authors highlight the importance of integrating top-down and bottom-up regulatory measures when studying the multipathway models of ADHD and co-occurring problems.

Together these studies suggest that executive function deficits may account for some of the impairments characteristic of children with ADHD. In particular, working memory deficits were found to account for impulsivity, narrative comprehension difficulty, and social problems. However, neuropsychological measures do not appear to mediate the high rates of affective lability commonly seen in children with ADHD. All of these studies, however, used a cross-sectional design, which limits confidence in their conclusions.

SUBTYPES OF ADHD

DSM-IV defined three ADHD subtypes: (1) predominantly inattentive (at least six inattention and fewer than six hyperactive-impulsive symptoms), (2) predominantly hyperactive-impulsive (at least six hyperactive-impulsive and fewer than six inattention symptoms), and (3) combined type (at least six symptoms in both domains). However, their lack of temporal stability throughout childhood (Lahey, Pelham, Loney, Lee, & Willcutt, 2005) has raised questions regarding their validity and clinical utility. With the publication of DSM-V in 2013, the reliability and validity of ADHD subtypes has received considerable scrutiny in recent years. Focus has primarily been on the predominantly inattentive type and whether it differs from the combined type only in severity and/or whether a more restrictive definition, limiting the number of hyperactive-impulsive symptoms, would be more appropriate. Furthermore, it has been proposed that a variant of the predominantly inattentive type, characterized by "sluggish cognitive tempo (SCT)," might represent a distinct disorder.

Although proposals for revisions in the DSM-V to the subtype criteria for ADHD were put forth, in the final publication they remained largely the same. In recognition of their lack of temporal stability throughout the lifespan, the term "type" was changed to current "presentation." Nevertheless, the process of determining the structure of ADHD in the DSM-V generated considerable research.

One of several approaches used to assess the validity of ADHD subtypes has been to determine whether they differ on measures of neuropsychological functioning; perhaps surprisingly, this method was adopted by only a few researchers. Yang, Cheng, et al. (2013) examined the factor structure of the Chinese version of the WISC-IV as well as performance in a large sample (n = 334) of 6- to 12-year-old children with either ADHD Predominantly Inattentive (ADHD-PI) or ADHD Combined (ADHD-C) type; there was no non-ADHD comparison group. The WISC-IV four-factor model held-up in this Taiwanese sample. Overall, children with ADHD performed significantly worse relative to the normative means (i.e., approximately 0.5 SD below the mean), but there were no significant differences between those with ADHD-PI and ADHD-C. Nevertheless, using an ipsative analysis of strengths and weaknesses they found that relative to norms a disproportionate number of children with ADHD had weaknesses in Processing Speed, and this was even more so in those with ADHD-PI relative to those with ADHD-C.

Another area of executive function that has been examined is post-error slowing. Post-error slowing is the phenomenon in which individuals slow down or reduce their rate of responding on trials subsequent to committing an error. Post-error slowing on reaction time tasks is considered by many to represent consciously controlled self-regulation. Shiels, Tamm, and Epstein (2012) assessed post-error slowing in 7- to 11-year-old children with ADHD-C (n = 51), ADHD-PI (n = 53), and age/gender/ethnicity-matched comparison youth (n = 47). Children were administered a choice discrimination task and a variant of the Stop-Signal Task. Post-error slowing was found to be impaired in the ADHD-PI group on the choice discrimination task relative to both the ADHD-C and non-ADHD comparison groups. The researchers attribute the lack of post-error slowing in the ADHD-PI group as possibly being due to greater attentional difficulties and suggest that this deficiency may be present only in children with primary attentional difficulties.

An important dissociation that is emerging in the neuropsychological literature is the distinction between "hot" and "cold" executive functions (Zelazo & Müller, 2002). Hot executive functions are those associated with affective regulation and reward-related processes, which are mediated largely by circuits involving the ventromedial prefrontal cortex. Cold executive functions are more cognitive in nature and are associated more closely with neural systems involving the dorsolateral prefrontal cortex. Skogli, Egeland, Andersen, Hovik, and Øie (2013) compared "hot" and "cold" executive functions in 8- to 17-year-old youth with ADHD-PI (n = 44), ADHD-C (n = 36), and healthy control children (n = 50) using a battery of laboratory tests and the BRIEF (Gioia et al., 2000). Cold executive functions were assessed using the Letter-Number Sequencing subtest of the WISC-IV (working memory) as well as the Trail Making (cognitive flexibility), Color-Word Interference (controlled attention), Verbal Fluency, and Tower (planning) tests from the D-KEFS. Hot executive functions were assessed with the Hungry Donkey Task (Crone & van der Molen, 2004), which is a child version of the Iowa Gambling Task (Bechara, Damasio, Damasio, & Anderson, 1994). Children and adolescents with ADHD, irrespective of subtype, performed more poorly than comparison children on tests of working memory and verbal fluency. However, only the ADHD-PI group performed significantly worse than the comparison group on measures of controlled attention and cognitive flexibility. The ADHD-PI and ADHD-C groups did not differ significantly on any tests and there was no significant difference among the three groups in planning. Laboratory tests of hot executive functions yielded no significant group differences. The ADHD groups scored lower on all aspects of the BRIEF with Inhibit and Monitor scales worse in ADHD-C than ADHD-PI. Overall, few measures differentiated between ADHD subtypes. Furthermore, the hot executive function task was not significantly correlated with the other executive function measures, which the authors concluded indicates separate developmental trajectories.

In contrast to most other studies, Nikolas and Nigg (2013) posited that the use of single measures or narrowly focused batteries of neuropsychological tests to validate ADHD and/or ADHD subtypes is problematic because of the heterogeneity of the disorder and oftentimes poor reliability of single tests. Furthermore, they suggested that ADHD subtypes may not represent categorically distinct groups, but rather are indicative of differences in severity. To test these hypotheses, they used a large battery of neuropsychological tests to examine differences between 6- to 17-year-old youth with (n = 244) and without (n = 213) ADHD, between those with ADHD-C (n = 137) and ADHD-PI (n = 107), and between the DSM-V proposed restricted inattentive type of ADHD (n = 68). Confirmatory factor analysis of their test battery was used to generate latent measures of seven neuropsychological domains: (1) inhibition, (2) working memory, (3) memory span, (4) arousal, (5) processing speed, (6) response variability, and (7) temporal information processing. Youth with ADHD performed worse than control particpants on all domains, and those with ADHD-C performed worse than those with ADHD-PI on all domains. The authors interpreted these latter findings as being consistent with the hypothesis that subtype differences primarily reflect differences in severity. Those with the "restrictive inattentive" presentation of ADHD showed evidence of deficits in processing speed relative to the larger ADHD-PI group, but there were no other differences between them. Subtype × Sex and Subtype × Age interactions indicated greater differences between the ADHD-C and ADHD-PI subtypes in boys relative to girls, and in older relative to younger children. When all measures were included in the same model, inhibition, working memory, memory span, arousal, and response variability each provided unique incremental statistical prediction of ADHD symptom dimensions and of subtype. Temporal information processing and processing speed did not account for unique variance in distinguishing the groups. Based on these data, Nikolas and Nigg (2013) concluded that there are robust differences in neurocognitive performance between youth with and without ADHD, but these differences are cumulatively accounted for by only a subset of neuropsychological measures. Finally, they highlight the fact that composite and latent variables are superior to single neuropsychological measures for identifying weaknesses associated with ADHD.

Finally, two studies focused largely on the concept of SCT and its relation to the ADHD diagnosis. Children with SCT are characterized by behaviors that are linked to attentional difficulties, such as daydreaming, staring, lethargy, and hypoactivity, but distinct from those used to diagnose ADHD. Bauermeister, Barkley, Bauermeister, Martínez, and McBurnett (2012) examined a broad array of neuropsychological functions among children with ADHD (mixed subtypes), SCT, and control youth in a sample of 6- to 11-year-old children from Puerto Rico (n = 140). Confirmatory factor analysis of parent and teacher ratings of the 18 DSM-IV ADHD symptoms and four SCT symptoms yielded a three-factor solution (i.e., inattention, hyperactivity, and SCT) for both parent and teacher ratings. This supported the researchers' assumption that SCT can be constituted as its own separate domain. They then examined correlates of the three factors from each rater. Neuropsychological constructs assessed via tests were working memory, processing speed, memory retrieval, interference control, and planning/problem solving. Academic achievement was also evaluated. Inattention, as rated both by parent and teacher, was significantly correlated with virtually all neuropsychological domains, whereas SCT and hyperactivity, in general, were not correlated with neuropsychological measures. Unlike inattention symptoms, SCT was not correlated with executive dysfunction. With regard to psychiatric comorbidity, externalizing problems were most strongly associated with hyperactivity-impulsivity, whereas internalizing problems were most strongly associated with parent-rated SCT and teacher-rated Inattention. Based on these results, the authors concluded that inattention is likely the primary cause of impairment in ADHD and that further research is needed to study the validity and usefulness of SCT for distinguishing among several disorders of inattention.

Using a categorical approach to examine SCT, Capdevila-Brophy et al. (2012) recruited two groups of children between the ages of 7 and 12 years. One group consisted of children diagnosed with ADHD-PI who exhibited high levels of SCT (n = 19); the other comprised children diagnosed with ADHD-C or ADHD-PI who had low levels of SCT symptoms. The groups were compared on behavioral ratings (i.e., BRIEF and CBCL; Achenbach & Rescorla, 2001) and several neuropsychological tests (i.e., subtests from WISC-III, Conners' CPT, and NEPSY; Korkman, Kirk, & Kemp, 1998). There were no significant differences between the groups on neuropsychological tests measuring processing speed, visual attention, or perceptual reasoning. However, those without SCT performed more poorly on the CPT relative to those with SCT, suggesting poorer vigilance/sustained attention in that group. Additionally, those with SCT had significantly higher rates of anxiety and depression (internalizing problems). BRIEF ratings indicated that those with SCT had greater difficulties with self-monitoring, whereas those without SCT had more difficulties in inhibition and behavioral regulation. Overall, these data suggest that ADHD with high SCT symptoms can be somewhat distinguished from other ADHD groups on behavioral measures and vigilance tests, but not on other neuropsychological measures. Taken together, the two studies focusing on SCT indicate that this group is characterized by greater internalizing difficulties, but that the groups are not well differentiated by neuropsychological test performance.

Overall, the recent neuropsychological research provides only minimal data supporting a clear categorical distinction between children with ADHD-C and ADHD-PI, with the latter group perhaps having slower processing speed and greater attention dysfunction as measured by post-error slowing. The idea that they primarily represent differences in severity is also consistent with data showing small differences between the subtypes with the ADHD-C group performing somewhat worse. More research is necessary to determine whether those with SCT represent a distinct subgroup or diagnosis relative to those with ADHD-C and/or ADHD-PI.

HETEROGENEITY OF ADHD

It is well established that groups of children with ADHD perform more poorly than their typically developing peers in an array of neuropsychological domains—including, but not limited to executive functions (Halperin & Schulz, 2006). Furthermore, although these group differences are commonly observed, it is also clear that children with ADHD do not all experience deficits in the same areas, and some children show no deficits at all (Nigg et al., 2005). Given this striking heterogeneity in children's cognitive profiles, researchers have worked to better understand the nature of the variability in performance, and whether particular neuropsychological "subtypes" may correlate differentially with distinct behavioral symptoms and/or severity. Notably, seeming in support of the notion that neuropsychological impairment in children with ADHD is not limited to executive functions, most authors include several non-executive measures in their test batteries.

Sjöwall, Roth, Lindqvist and Thorell (2013) attempted to parse the heterogeneity of ADHD by examining three different neuropsychological domains in 102 children with ADHD aged 7–13 years and 102 matched comparison children: executive functions (i.e., working memory, inhibition, and shifting), delay aversion, and reaction time variability, as well as emotional regulation. Children with ADHD differed significantly from control participants on all measures, except delay aversion and recognition of disgust (part of emotion regulation). Closer examination of the specificity of these neuropsychological deficits indicated that 71% of the children with ADHD were shown to have at least one type of neuropsychological impairment as compared to 26% of controls. Among those with ADHD, 35% had poor executive functioning, 54% had high reaction time variability, and only 14% showed impaired delay aversion. Among the 68 children with impairment in either reaction time variability or executive functioning, there was substantial overlap (23 children having deficits in both), but there were also subgroups with impairment in either executive functioning (n = 13) or reaction time variability (n = 32). Overall, the authors concluded that executive functioning deficits and high reaction time variability are important characteristics of some, but not all, children with ADHD, and that when studying specific functions, reaction time variability and inhibition appeared to be of greatest importance.

Several studies have investigated the relation between patterns of neuropsychological performance and ADHD symptoms and/or severity. Yanez-Tellez et al. (2013) administered a large battery of neuropsychological tasks to 7- to 12-year-old boys with hyperactive/impulsive and combined types ADHD (n = 26) to better understand the cognitive profiles of these children, and to determine whether performance on these tasks was associated with behavioral symptoms. Compared to a control group of boys without learning or behavioral problems (n = 25), children with ADHD showed poorer performance on several of the tasks, including nonexecutive and executive functions. With respect to measures of executive function, boys with ADHD had poorer visual working memory performance, greater errors on the Wisconsin Card Sorting Task, and greater difficulty sustaining attention on a Continuous Task Execution. However, no differences as a function of diagnosis were observed on the Stroop or Tower of London tests. Thus, children with ADHD did not evidence deficits in all executive domains. Parents and teachers completed the Conners' ADHD Scale-Revised, and hyperactivity/impulsivity symptoms were regressed on tasks that showed significant group differences using backward multiple linear regression analysis. Errors and speed in naming colors and figures in rapid serial naming, understanding written instructions, arithmetic problems, and Wisconsin Card Sorting perseverative and total errors, and perseverative responses were the best combination of variables predicting hyperactive-impulsive symptoms.

Thaler, Bello, and Etcoff (2012) examined cognitive heterogeneity in children with ADHD using the WISC-IV. Specifically, they were interested in determining whether different WISC-IV profiles would predict diagnosis, symptom ratings, and adaptive functioning outcomes. Six- to 16-year-old children with ADHD-PI (n = 106) and ADHD-C (n = 83) were recruited from 564 children referred for neuropsychological evaluation. Children's cognitive functioning was assessed using the WISC-IV and their academic achievement was measured using the Woodcock-Johnson Test of Achievement, Third Edition (Woodcock, McGrew, & Mather, 2001). Parents completed behavioral rating scales. Cognitive heterogeneity among the four WISC-IV indices was examined using cluster analysis. A five-cluster solution was determined to be most optimal: Reduced Processing Speed Index (PSI; n = 79), High Average Perceptual Reasoning Index/PSI (n = 35), Below Average Working Memory Index/ PSI (n = 25), Superior Verbal Comprehension Index (n = 31), and Average PSI (n = 19). The Reduced PSI cluster contained the most children and was associated with more severe inattention ratings and higher rates of ADHD-PI diagnosis. Both the Reduced PSI and the Below Average Working Memory Index/PSI clusters were associated with poorer reading and math fluency achievement than the High Average Perceptual Reasoning Index/PSI and Superior Verbal Comprehension Index clusters. The authors suggested that findings support an association between deficits in processing speed and inattention, and that the WISC-IV may be a useful tool for predicting behavioral and adaptive outcomes in children with ADHD.

Based on the notion that poor working memory and slow processing speed are commonly found in children with a variety of neurodevelopmental disorders, Ek, Westerlund, and Fernell (2013) examined the extent to which indices of these cognitive functions were uniquely impaired relative to general cognitive ability in a heterogeneous sample of children and adolescents with an array of attentional and learning difficulties. In addition, they divided the group into those who met criteria for ADHD/subthreshold ADHD versus those with milder attentional difficulties. All children were administered the WISC-III. Verbal working memory was assessed via the Freedom from Distractibility Index (Digit Span and Arithmetic subtests), processing speed via the PSI (Coding and Symbol Search subtests), and general cognitive ability was measured by combining the Verbal Comprehension Index and Perceptual Organization indices. Across the entire group, verbal working memory and processing speed scores, which did not differ from each other, were significantly lower than general cognitive ability scores, and this difference was greater in boys than girls.

The pattern of scores was similar in both the ADHD/subthreshold ADHD and the milder attention problems group, but in addition, there was a trend such that those with milder attention problems performed better than those with ADHD/subthreshold ADHD in processing speed. The authors concluded that these types of cognitive differences need to be considered in children with different kinds of learning, behavior, and attention problems.

Rosch, Dirlikov, and Mostofsky (2013) examined speed and variability in responding during cognitive (Go/No-go) and motor (Finger Sequencing) tasks in 51 boys 8–12 years old, 28 with ADHD and 23 typically developing. Boys with ADHD were slower and more variable in both inter-tap interval on the Finger Sequencing task and reaction time on the Go/No-go task, with measures of speed and variability correlated across the two tasks. Variability in Finger Sequencing (motor) timing was found to be uniquely correlated with parent ratings of hyperactivity-impulsivity, whereas reaction time variability on the Go/No-go task uniquely predicted parent ratings of inattention. These findings implicate difficulties in motor control in the pathophysiology of ADHD, particularly as related to hyperactive-impulsive symptoms.

The above studies showed that particular neuropsychological domains were predictors of ADHD symptom profiles. In the following study, Fair, Bathula, Nikolas, and Nigg (2013) provide evidence that similar neuropsychological subtypes are observed in typically developing and ADHD populations, and that classifying children on the basis of neuropsychological data shows some promise only if done so within these subtypes (as opposed to across all children). The investigators administered a large battery of neuropsychological tests to 6- to 17-year-old youth with typical development (n = 213) and ADHD (n = 285). The neuropsychological tests were combined using confirmatory factor analysis to assess latent measures of working memory, inhibition, arousal/activation, response variability, temporal information processing, memory span, and processing speed. Not surprising, the ADHD and control groups differed significantly across all seven neuropsychological domains, but individual classification from the neuropsychological data was not good. However, they found several unique, but similar subtypes across both populations. Community detection yielded four neuropsychologically distinct subgroups of the typically developing children: (1) high response variability; (2) reduced working memory, memory span, inhibition, and output speed; (3) inaccurate temporal information processing; and (4) weak signal detection (interpreted as suboptimal arousal), and six distinct subgroups of children with ADHD that were highly similar to those detected in their non-ADHD counterparts. Notably, these subgroups, did not differ in symptom scores, IQ, age, or sex ratios, and as such did not represent more or less severe ADHD; rather they seemed to represent unique cognitive profiles within children who all have similar severity of ADHD. Further analyses examining individual classification indicated substantially better success at accurate classification of ADHD versus control status when examined within the context of the separate clusters. The authors concluded that typically developing children can be classified into distinct neuropsychological subgroups with high precision, and that some of the heterogeneity in individuals with ADHD might be "nested" in this normal variation.

More and more, researchers are attempting to delineate the cognitive heterogeneity in children with ADHD. It seems clear that when it comes to neuropsychological strengths and weaknesses, children with ADHD are not all cut from the same cloth. However, researchers have a lot of work in front of them to more precisely determine the nature of this heterogeneity, and its link to the behavioral expression of ADHD and associated impairment, as well as underlying neural and genetic heterogeneity, which is also likely to be characteristic of the disorder.

EXECUTIVE VERSUS NONEXECUTIVE

Several prominent theories propose that executive function deficits are central to the etiology of ADHD. For example, Barkley's (1997) theory argues that poor response inhibition is the core deficit in ADHD and that the difficulties in other neuropsychological domains (e.g., working memory) commonly observed in children with ADHD are downstream or secondary to deficits in inhibitory control. In contrast, Rapport, Chung, Shore, and Isaacs (2001) consider working memory to be the core deficit in ADHD. Others propose that given the heterogeneity observed in neuropsychological performance of children, working memory and response inhibition are candidate endophenotypes (Castellanos & Tannock, 2002). Thus, although each of these theories differs in which executive function is posited as most critical, all have in common the emphasis placed on higher-order cognitive dysfunction as central to ADHD etiology.

It is clear, however, that successful performance on putative executive function tasks does not solely depend on the higher-order cognitive ability of interest, but also on many nonexecutive processes (e.g., processing efficiency, motivation, alerting). For example, in the Stroop task, successful completion of the interference condition, during which an individual must inhibit the prepotent response of reading the word and instead name the ink color in which the word is printed, also requires color naming and single word reading. Thus, understanding the impact of these more basic processes on an individual's performance on purported higher-level tasks is critical if we are to know how and to what extent the higher-order deficit manifests in children with ADHD. This has been a common question in research published during the past 18 months—to what extent are executive function deficits mediated by nonexecutive processes? Evidence for mediation would be present if the relation between ADHD and executive dysfunction was no longer observed, or diminished in magnitude when more basic processes were included in the models.

To investigate this question, researchers have had children engage in tasks commonly used to assess executive functions, such as the Stop Signal Task and CPTs, but they have adopted novel analytic techniques to investigate findings. For example, ex-Gaussian distributional modeling, signal detection theory parameters, and diffusion modeling have all been used to better understand the processing of children with and without ADHD while completing executive function tasks.

Accuracy, errors, mean reaction time, and reaction time variability are generally the measures of interest when analyzing the performance of children on computerized and/or speeded neuropsychological tasks. Depending on task parameters (e.g., ratio of targets to nontargets), errors may be interpreted to reflect impulsive responding (failure of inhibitory control), attentional lapses, and so on. In conjunction with these classic measures of cognitive functioning, ex-Gaussian distribution models of reaction time and reaction time variability have been used to better understand processing speed in ADHD populations (e.g., Epstein et al., 2011; Leth-Steensen, Elbaz, & Douglas, 2000) and signal detection parameters have been used as a novel way to investigate the processing behind correct responses and errors (e.g., Epstein et al., 2003; Halperin, Trampush, Miller, Marks, & Newcorn, 2008; Losier, McGrath, & Klein, 1996).

Over the past 18 months, several studies have been published that have used ex-Gaussian distributional models. Briefly, ex-Gaussian analyses decompose the Gaussian (normally distributed) portion of the reaction time distribution from the tail to generate measures of mu (μ) and sigma (σ), which represent the mean and standard deviation of the Gaussian component of distribution, and tau (τ), which represents the exponential component, characterized by long reaction times in the tail of the distribution. Several studies of children with ADHD using ex-Gaussian analyses have suggested that the commonly reported elevated reaction time variability is due to increased tau or more very slow responses (i.e., outliers; e.g., Leth-Steensen et al., 2000; see Tamm et al., 2012 for a review). These very slow responses have been attributed to intermittent attentional lapses (Leth-Steensen et al., 2000) perhaps indicative of a failure to allocate sufficient effort (Douglas & Peters, 1979) or because of deficits in more basic regulatory (i.e., bottom-up) processes (Sergeant, 2005; Sonuga-Barke & Castellanos, 2007). The emphasis in recent studies has been to try to determine the extent to which this intra-individual variability in reaction time may account for children's performance on response inhibition and working memory tasks. For example, Borella, Ribaupierre, Cornoldi, and Chicherio (2013) had 9- to 12-year-old children with (n = 24) and without (n = 24) ADHD complete a computerized Stroop task and a simple reaction time task to examine the extent to which deficits were in interference control versus more basic processing deficits. When mean reaction time was assessed, no group differences in Stroop interference effects were found. However, across an array of measures children with ADHD had more variable reaction times, which the authors interpreted as indicating that children with ADHD have a more generalized deficit that then affects performance on measures of inhibitory and interference control. Specifically, they proposed that interference control may be a less fundamental characteristic of ADHD than previous empirical work led researchers to believe. Rather, findings suggest that children with ADHD exhibit self-regulatory deficits or a failure to allocate adequate effort to meet task demands.

Karalunas and Huang Pollock (2013) used an ex-Gaussian distribution approach to investigate whether reaction time parameters could predict inhibitory control and working memory performance. Children, 8–12 years old (mean age, 10 years), with and without ADHD completed four working memory tasks (Letter Span, Spatial Span, Digit Span Backwards, and Finger Windows Backwards) from which a single index was created, and the Stop Signal Task was used to measure inhibitory control.

Consistent with an abundance of literature in this area, working memory and inhibitory control was weaker for children with ADHD than their typically developing peers. Also consistent with the literature, children with ADHD showed greater tau values, indicating a greater number of very slow reaction times. Mediation analyses showed that tau mediated the relation between ADHD and inhibitory control. The relation between tau and working memory was in the expected direction, but model fit was poor. Therefore, these findings suggest that attentional lapses account for a substantial portion of the relation between ADHD and inhibitory control ability. However, the study was cross-sectional, and it is possible that ADHD is associated with attentional lapses through inhibitory control ability. Longitudinal studies are needed to test these predictions with greater precision.

Finally, the ex-Gaussian distribution model has been useful for better understanding the link between ADHD and behavioral performance during an academic exercise. In a sample of 147 children, 7–11 years old, with (combined and inattentive subtypes) and without ADHD, Antonini, Narad, Langberg, and Epstein (2013) monitored children's on-task and off-task behavior while they completed a math worksheet (approximately 20 minutes duration). Antonini et al. (2013) also had children complete several neuropsychological tasks, including a Choice Discrimination task, Rueda et al.'s (2004) child version of the Attention Network Test, a Go/No-go task, the Stop Signal Task, and an N-Back (n-1) task. Ex-Gaussian parameters were calculated along with the coefficient of variation (RTSD/mean RT). Children with ADHD were on task for a shorter duration during math than control children. Time on task was negatively associated with the coefficient of variation and tau, but not mu or sigma. The association between reaction time variability and on-task behavior was not moderated by ADHD status, suggesting that it is observed in children with ADHD as well as their typically developing peers. Although children who were more accurate on the computerized neuropsychological tests were on-task for longer periods of time during math, the negative association between tau and on-task behavior remained after controlling for neuropsychological task accuracy.

These studies, therefore, continue to demonstrate that intra-individual variability in reaction time is characteristic of children with ADHD, in line with the proposition that reaction time variability may be an endophenotype for ADHD (Castellanos, Sonuga-Barke, Milham, & Tannock, 2006). The field has been advanced, however, through the demonstration that there is a strong link between reaction time variability and executive functioning, and behavioral indicators of attention. Given this, it is critical to better understand the neural basis for this phenomenon (Kuntsi & Klein, 2011).

Another approach is to use signal detection parameters. Two primary measures, presumably reflecting nonexecutive processes, are derived from signal detection theory: discriminability (d') and response bias ($\ln\beta$). Discriminability is the ability to detect a target from a nontarget and provides an estimate of the sensitivity of information processing; total errors are inversely related to discriminability (Losier et al., 1996). Response bias provides a measure of how conservative an individual is in setting his or her response criteria for what is and is not a target.

More conservative individuals generate more errors of omission and fewer errors of commission, whereas the opposite pattern is observed for more liberal individuals (Losier et al., 1996).

Huang-Pollock, Karalunas, Tam, and Moore (2012) conducted a meta-analysis of 47 articles investigating children's CPT performance. Consistent with many studies in this area they found that children with ADHD made more errors of omission and commission, were slower to respond, and showed greater variability in their response times. Unlike other meta-analyses, however, they obtained large effect sizes, which they attributed to their correcting for both sampling and measurement error. They also found that when compared to typically developing peers, children with ADHD showed deficits in discriminability: that is, they were less able to detect targets from nontargets. No group differences in response bias were observed.

Signal detection parameters have been used for decades in psychological research, although originally they were used with unidimensional perceptual stimuli that differed along a gradient rather than with cognitive stimuli most often used in ADHD research today. Huang-Pollock et al. (2012) have argued that this is a significant limitation of the use of signal detection parameters to analyze performance on neuropsychological tasks, such as CPTs, because conceptually there is poor fit between the stimuli and the measures. Discriminability should be near ceiling for cognitive stimuli, perhaps limiting its value in aiding the understanding of differences in information processing between children who do and do not have ADHD (Huang-Pollock et al., 2012).

Recently, these types of measures have also been evaluated using Ratcliff's diffusion model (Ratcliff & McKoon, 2008). Where Ratcliff's model holds an advantage over other approaches is that it allows investigators to derive estimates of specific elements of information processing from two-choice decision tasks: drift rate (v), boundary separation (a) and nondecision time (T_{er}). Drift rate is the time it takes for an individual to acquire information from an encoded stimulus and to make a decision as to whether the stimulus is (or is not) a target. Drift rate is a property of the stimulus, such that more degraded stimuli result in slower accumulation of information (i.e., higher drift rate). Degree of boundary separation reflects how certain an individual needs to be to make a decision and is reflective of the degree of speed-accuracy trade-off. Nondecision time (T_{er}) reflects all other information processing not involved in stimulus discrimination, such as encoding, lexical access, response output, and so on.

Diffusion modeling has recently been used to better understand the cognitive processes involved in completing higher order tasks. For example, Karalunas, Huang-Pollack, and Nigg (2012) recruited two large, independent samples of children with and without ADHD, aged from 7 to 18 years of age. Participants completed a tracking version of the Stop Task; diffusion model parameters drift rate, boundary separation, and nondecision time were calculated from the choice reaction time "go" trials embedded within that task. When more classic measures of accuracy, mean reaction time, and reaction time standard deviation (i.e., variability) were analyzed, children with ADHD were less accurate and showed greater variability. Diffusion analyses indicated that these differences likely stemmed from significant group differences in drift rate (efficiency of information processing). No group differences in boundary separation or nondecision time were observed.

Similar findings were obtained by Huang-Pollock et al. (2012) in their meta-analysis of children's CPT performance, which used diffusion modeling to try to explain *why* children with ADHD performed more poorly than their typically developing peers. Drift rate was higher for children with ADHD, suggesting that they take longer to accumulate the information necessary from the encoded stimulus to decide if the stimulus is in fact a target.

Whereas Huang-Pollock et al. (2012) used diffusion modeling in the context of continuous performance tasks, Salum and colleagues (2013) used the approach to investigate inhibitory control deficits commonly observed in children with ADHD. They recruited a large sample (n = 704) of 6- to 12-year-old Brazilian children from the community and had them complete a 2-Choice Reaction Time task, a conflict control task and a go/no-go task. They aimed to investigate differences in basic information processing and inhibitory-based executive functions among children with ADHD only, other forms of psychopathology (nonoverlapping groups representing fear disorders, distress disorders, DBD, and ADHD plus DBD), and their typically developing peers, and to test whether deficits in inhibitory-based executive functions are observed above and beyond basic information processing deficits. Salum et al. found that children with ADHD had slower processing efficiency (i.e., longer drift rate) than their typically developing peers on both the 2-Choice Reaction Time task and the Conflict Control Task. In fact, poorer processing efficiency in the 2-Choice Reaction Time task differentiated the ADHD group from all other groups, indicating that this deficit was specific for ADHD. Furthermore, on both tasks, children with ADHD showed faster nondecision time (suggesting faster encoding, response output, and so on). On the 2-Choice Reaction Time task, children with ADHD also showed greater variability in processing efficiency and were more cautious in their response style. Thus, children with ADHD showed a number of deficits in basic information processing when compared to typically developing peers. When looking at classical parameters of inhibitory-based executive functions (i.e., percentage of correct responses in incongruent trials for the conflict control task and the percentage of correct inhibitions in No-Go trials of the Go/No-go tasks), children with ADHD also showed poorer performance than their typically developing peers. The key question, therefore, is whether the differences in these classical measures of inhibitory-based executive functions remained significant after controlling for deficits in basic information processes: the answer was no. Mediation analyses showed that 50% of classical inhibitory-based executive functions Go/No-go variables and 76% of the classical inhibitory-based executive functions conflict control task were mediated by processing efficiency. These findings led Salum et al. to conclude that children with ADHD are impaired in accumulating information required to perform a very simple decision.

Similarly, in conjunction with ex-Gaussian distribution modeling, Karalunas and Huang-Pollack (2013) used diffusion modeling to better understand children's performance on working memory and inhibitory control tasks. Recall that working memory and inhibitory control abilities were measured in ADHD and control children (mean age, 10 years), and that typically developing children performed better than ADHD children on these executive function measures. Once again, differences in basic information processing were observed between children with ADHD and their typically developing peers, such that drift rate was slower and nondecision time was faster for ADHD children. Furthermore, drift rate partially mediated the relation between ADHD and both inhibitory control and working memory.

Finally, Metin et al. (2013) also found that 6- to 17-year-old children with ADHD-C (n = 70) were no more likely to trade speed for accuracy (i.e., no group differences in boundary separation) than non-ADHD comparison youth (n = 50), which they interpreted to mean that the increased error rate of children with ADHD cannot be accounted for by an impulsive information processing style. Children with ADHD did, however, display slower drift rates and faster nondecision times than their non-ADHD counterparts. These findings occurred irrespective of task load. That is, findings were the same for the 2-Choice Reaction Time task, which required a simple perceptual decision, and the Conflict Control Task, during which suppression of a prepotent response was required on 25% trials. Why children with ADHD demonstrated faster nondecision times was unclear, but it could be related to encoding and/or motor preparation. The slower drift rate, however, was interpreted as evidence that children with ADHD exhibit an inefficient processing style. That this was observed independent of executive load was taken as further evidence that deficits are largely nonexecutive.

In summary, it seems that relative to their peers, children with ADHD perform significantly worse on a wide range of executive function measures. However, deficits in basic information processing are also seen, most consistently in the form of children with ADHD taking longer to accumulate information toward the decision point (i.e., longer drift rate). When these basic deficits are incorporated into models, the relation between ADHD and executive deficits is reduced.

Using more sensitive analyses to tease apart the role of executive and nonexecutive dysfunction has thus yielded exciting advances in the understanding of why children with ADHD perform more poorly on higher-order cognitive tasks. The next question, however, is what is driving the longer drift rates, and what exactly does faster nondecision time represent? Most commonly, longer drift rates are interpreted using the cognitive energetic model (Sergeant, 2000, 2005). That is, children's failure to allocate appropriate effort to these tasks results in their inefficient processing style (Huang-Pollock & Karalunas, 2012). Longer drift rate may also be reflective of deficiencies in the Default Mode Network (Gusnard & Raichle, 2001), whereby children fail to appropriately transition from the resting state to the task-positive network. Researchers appear to have more difficulty reconciling the group differences in nondecision time that are sometimes observed. Nondecision time may reflect encoding and/or motor preparation. To the extent that poor effort allocation affects the arousal and activation pools, Sergeant's cognitive energetic model may also be able to account for these findings; however, more work in this area is necessary.

Although focus thus far has been on processing efficiency, investigators have also assessed the degree to which motivational deficits may influence executive functioning performance. In a series of two studies, Strand et al. (2012) examined the extent to which working memory deficits in children with ADHD could be improved using incentives, which might imply a motivational component to the commonly observed neuropsychological deficit. In Study 1, a sample of 9- to 12-year-old boys with (n = 24) and without (n = 32) ADHD were administered a visuospatial N-Back task (0-back, 1-back, and 2-back conditions) and then re-administered the task 1 week later after being randomized to either an incentive or no-incentive condition. As expected, children with ADHD showed clear deficits in spatial working memory. However, incentives improved working memory performance, particularly among the children with ADHD, such that the provision of incentives reduced the ADHD-control group difference by about half, although it did not normalize working memory in the ADHD group. Study 2 examined the effect of incentives and stimulant medication (long-acting methylphenidate) on working memory performance in children with ADHD-combined type (n = 17). Both incentives and medication individually improved N-Back performance relative to the no-incentive, placebo condition. The combination of incentives and medication improved performance significantly more than either incentives or methylphenidate alone. Together, these studies indicate that, similar to stimulant medication, incentives can markedly improve working memory in children with ADHD, and highlights the role of motivation in studying cognitive deficits in ADHD.

Similar to Strand et al. (2012), a series of studies by Dovis, Van der Oord, Wiers, and Prins (2012, 2013) examined motivational factors relating to visuospatial working memory performance in youth with ADHD. Their initial study (Dovis et al., 2012) examined the effects of different reinforcers on working memory in 9- to 12-year-old children with (n = 30) and without (n = 31) ADHD. Children completed the Chessboard Task, a visuospatial working memory task based on Corsi blocks, and Letter-Number Sequencing, with four reinforcement conditions: Feedback-only, 1 euro, 10 euros, and a computer-game version of the task. Incentives significantly improved the working memory performance of children with ADHD, but even the largest reinforcers did not normalize these children's performance. In contrast, for control participants, only feedback was sufficient to yield optimal performance. The authors also investigated performance over time, and found that ADHD children, but not controls, showed poorer performance as the task progressed. Normalization of persistence was observed, but only when the strongest of incentives (10 Euro and videogame) were delivered. From this study, the authors concluded that both executive and motivational deficits give rise to visual-spatial working memory deficits in ADHD.

To further explore the nature of the visuospatial working memory deficit in children with ADHD and the impact of reward, Dovis et al. (2013) differentially assessed the short-term memory and central executive components of working memory. Eight- to 12 year-old children, 86 with ADHD-C and 62 control participants, were administered separate working memory tasks designed to differentially assess short-term memory and the central executive under reinforcement and non-reinforcement conditions. Not surprisingly, children with ADHD performed more poorly across tasks. Reinforcement improved short-term memory more in children with ADHD relative to control children, although it did not normalize their performance. Notably, reinforcement did not seem to improve the central executive-related performance in either group. Thus, the authors conclude that motivational deficits have a detrimental effect on visuospatial short-term memory performance of children with ADHD, but besides motivational deficits, both the visuospatial short-term memory and central executive of children with ADHD are impaired and give rise to their deficits in visuospatial working memory.

The role of attention was investigated by Casagrande et al. (2012), who attempted to look at the interaction among the different attention networks. They had children with (n = 18) and without (n = 18) ADHD complete the child version of the Attention Network Test on two occasions; during one session feedback was given following a response and during the second session no feedback was given. The order of the sessions was counterbalanced. During feedback trials, no differences in orienting or executive performance were seen between children with and without ADHD. A Group × Warning interaction was also seen during feedback trials, such that reaction time was slower in the no warning condition than when warning was present, but only for children with ADHD. For no feedback trials, the warning decreased reaction time of children with ADHD for incongruent trials only, suggesting that the conflict deficit was observed in the context of an alerting deficit. This finding adds further support to Sergeant's Cognitive-Energetic model (Sergeant, 2005).

Relatedly, and as discussed above, the increased reaction time variability characteristically seen in children with ADHD has typically been attributed to lapses in attention (e.g., Leth-Steensen et al., 2000). However, Klotz, Johnson, Wu, Isaacs, and Gilbert (2012) hypothesized that these slow and more variable responses may be at least in part accounted for by motor dysfunction. To test this, 19 children with ADHD and 16 healthy control participants, ages 8–14 years, were administered a simple reaction time task and a choice reaction time task. To decrease demands on sustained attention and fatigue, each of the tasks was limited to only two blocks of 10 trials each (i.e., 20 trials). Motor function was assessed with the Physical and Neurological Examination for Subtle Signs (PANESS; Denckla, 1985). Further, speed and variability of sequential finger movements in each hand were evaluated using a goniometer. Overall, children with ADHD had significantly poorer PANESS scores and slower and more variable simple and choice reaction times. Sequential finger-tapping rates, particularly in the nondominant (left) hand, were significantly slower in ADHD children. Longer reaction times on both tests were associated with worse PANESS scores and slower and more variable goniometer finger-sequencing values. More variable simple reaction times were also associated with poorer PANESS scores and more variable goniometer finger-sequencing values. Finally, stepwise regression analyses indicated that total motor development, as assessed using the PANESS, predicted both simple and choice reaction times, and that variability in timing in the left-hand finger tapping was the best predictor of reaction time variability. The authors suggest that the development of the motor system in childhood may provide an important window into the neurobiology of higher cognitive and behavioral functions.

Alderson, Rapport, Kasper, Sarver, and Kofler (2012) examined whether increased activity level associated with ADHD is secondary to inhibition deficits in 8- to 12-year-old boys with (n = 11) and without (n = 11) ADHD by assessing activity (using actigraphs) in five different conditions: (1) while using Paint program; (2) 2-Choice Reaction Time task; (3) 2-Choice Reaction Time task with periodic tone that is ignored; (4) Stop Signal Task; (5) Paint program again. Both groups increased activity level during the three active cognitive tasks, but the ADHD group did so to a greater extent. There was no greater increase in activity during the Stop Signal Task (inhibition task) relative to the other two active tasks. Thus, the authors concluded that increased activity is not secondary to a deficit in a limited resource inhibition system. Rather, it is associated with attentional processes. They further argued that taxing working memory in children with ADHD results in increased activity level.

The State Regulation Deficit model (Sergeant, 2000) proposes that children with ADHD have difficulty allocating appropriate effort to regulate arousal and activation. Based on this, it can be hypothesized that in tasks with slow event rate (ER), a pattern of underactivation and slow responding will be observed. Conversely, with fast ERs, a pattern of overactivation and fast responding will be observed. Metin, Roeyers, Wiersema, and van der Meere (2012) carried out a systematic review and meta-analyses of the effects of ER on performance on Go/No-go tasks to test predictions of State Regulation Deficit model on ADHD. When only using studies in which ER was manipulated as a within-subject variable, group × ER interactions were observed for both mean reaction time and errors of commission. That is, children with ADHD showed disproportionate slowing of responding on slow ER trials and a disproportionate increase in errors of commission on fast ER trials. Children with ADHD were more variable (greater reaction time SD) at both slow and fast ERs, but no group × ER interaction was observed. When studies using a between-subjects design were evaluated, it was again shown that children with ADHD responded more slowly than controls, particularly on slow trials. Children with ADHD made more errors of commission on both slow and fast ER trials than control children, and the trend for differentially more errors on fast ER trials was in the expected direction, but not significant. For reaction time, the between-study heterogeneity was partly, but not completely accounted for by age and ER. For both errors of commission and reaction time variability, ER was not a predictor of heterogeneity. Thus, the authors concluded that the findings were best explained with the state regulation deficit model, but the fact that differences in responding between children with and without ADHD persist after accounting for ER, lends further support to the heterogeneity observed in ADHD.

Finally, Takacs et al. (2014) assessed verbal (Syllable Span) and nonverbal (Corsi Blocks) working memory, inhibitory control (Stroop), and verbal fluency (semantic and phonemic), as well as strategic thinking used in the completion of verbal fluency tasks in 8- to 12-year-old typically developing children (n = 22) and 22 children with ADHD. As expected, children with ADHD performed significantly more poorly across the neuropsychological measures and domains. Further analyses indicated that children with ADHD had a different temporal pattern of responding relative to their typically developing peers; specifically, they made fewer responses in the first 15 seconds of verbal fluency, but after that there were no significant differences in the number of words generated. Finally, qualitative analyses of lexical and executive strategies (word clustering and switching) suggested that the reduced efficiency of children with ADHD in semantic fluency was due to suboptimal shifting between word clusters and a deficient ability to produce new clusters of items. The authors concluded that the group difference is at the level of accessing and/or activating common words, whereas the executive process of searching the lexicon is largely intact.

Overall, recent findings suggest that when more basic nonexecutive processes are taken into account, differences in executive performance between children with and without ADHD are either no longer observed or their magnitude is substantially diminished. These findings lend support to theories that implicate nonexecutive processes as central to ADHD etiology (Halperin & Schulz, 2006; Sergeant, 2000; Sonuga-Barke & Castellanos, 2007).

COMORBIDITY AND DISSOCIATION OF ADHD FROM OTHER DISORDERS

A substantial number of papers published in the recent past have focused on the extent to which executive deficits are uniquely associated with ADHD relative to other psychiatric disorders and whether the presence of psychiatric comorbidity, which is the rule rather than the exception in ADHD, impacts neuropsychological functioning. Results from studies such as these are not only valuable for characterizing the nature of the specific deficits linked to ADHD (and other disorders), but have important implications for the validity of the syndrome and parsing its heterogeneity. Most of these studies have focused on comorbidity with other disruptive behavior disorders (DBD; ODD and CD), anxiety disorders, autism spectrum disorders (ASDs), and language and learning disorders. However, other less common comorbidities are also considered.

Disruptive Behavior Disorders

The DBDs, ODD, and CD, commonly co-occur with ADHD and as such are an important source of clinical heterogeneity. Due to their considerable overlap, the field has struggled to determine the unique neuropsychological deficits associated with each disorder.

In one of the few studies to look at neuropsychological functioning in preschool children, Schoemaker et al. (2012) examined a sample of 3.5- to 5.5-year-old children classified as either having ADHD (n = 61), a DBD without ADHD (n = 33), ADHD plus DBD (n = 52), or being typically developing (n = 56). These preschoolers were administered a battery of five tests, which factor analysis indicated tapped into two domains: inhibitory control (Go/No-go, Modified Snack Delay, Shape

School—Inhibit) and working memory (Delayed Alternation, Nine Boxes task). Robust group differences in inhibitory control emerged that were associated with the presence of ADHD rather than DBD, with effect sizes being similar for the ADHD and comorbid groups. In contrast, few group differences in working memory were found. The authors suggest that working memory differences may emerge later in development.

Martel, Roberts, and Gremillion (2013) also examined a preschool sample of 98 children aged 3–6 years divided into those with ADHD (n = 17), ODD (n = 18), both disorders (n = 39), and neither disorder (n = 24). Their aim was to evaluate associations among differing types of control processes and ODD and ADHD during early childhood. Affect control was assessed via clinician report following a 3-hour session with the child as well as with a laboratory-based task in which the child had to withhold touching a wrapped "gift." Temperamental effortful control was measured using the Child Behavior Questionnaire (Rothbart, Ahadi, Hershey, & Fisher, 2001), and cognitive control was assessed using a variety of tasks administered to the child designed to measure response inhibition, working memory, and set-shifting. Correlational analyses revealed that affective but not effortful control was associated with cognitive control, and that together they correlated with ADHD but not ODD symptom severity. The authors suggest that early affective control deficits may lead to later cognitive control deficits in ADHD.

Rhodes, Park, Seth, and Coghill (2012) examined working memory in older, 7- to 13-year-old boys, divided into those with ADHD (n = 21), ODD (n = 21), ADHD plus ODD (n = 27), and typically developing peers (n = 26). The children were all administered a battery of verbal and spatial memory tests from the CANTAB. Confirmatory factor analysis indicted presence of five factors: (1) verbal functioning, (2) spatial functioning, (3) working memory storage, (4) working memory central executive, and (5) long-term memory. Boys with ODD and ADHD plus ODD, but not ADHD only, performed poorly on verbal memory tasks; the performance of the ADHD group on verbal memory tasks was similar to the comparison group. In contrast, all three clinical groups had lower scores on spatial memory tasks, as well as on the storage and central executive working memory factors, and the long-term memory factor. These findings are in line with Schoemaker et al.'s hypothesis that working memory deficits emerge later than the preschool years. These results are unique in that previous studies have not reported working memory deficits uniquely associated with ODD and the suggestion that verbal working memory deficits are associated with ODD but not ADHD.

Munkvold, Manger, and Lundervold (2014) compared performance on the Conners' CPT-II across 7- to 9-year-old children with ADHD (n = 59), ODD (n = 10), ADHD plus ODD (n = 15), and normal control children (n = 160) and examined the degree to which group differences could be explained by IQ. The majority of the seven measures from the Conners' CPT-II were moderately intercorrelated and none of them distinguished between any of the clinical groups. The group with ADHD, but not ODD, differed significantly from the control group on omission errors and reaction time variability (two of seven measures), although these group differences disappeared when controlling for IQ. The authors conclude that although diagnostic criteria for ADHD involve behavioral descriptions of inattention and impulsivity, such behavior is not manifested as poorer performance on the Conners CPT-II. They suggested that, consistent with Willcutt et al.'s (2005) meta-analysis, their results indicate that neurocognitive deficits are neither necessary nor sufficient to identify ADHD in children and that scores from the Conners' CPT-II should be interpreted cautiously when part of a diagnostic evaluation. Furthermore, although using different measures and assessing different constructs, unlike Rhodes et al. (2012), they report no evidence for neurocognitive dysfunction in ODD, as this group did not differ from the control group on any measure.

Dolan and Lennox (2013) examined "hot" and "cool" executive functions using a computerized battery in 72 adolescents with CD and 35 with CD plus ADHD who were recruited from "secure care" or prisons, as well as in 20 healthy control participants. They found no significant differences between the CD groups with and without ADHD on measures of hot (i.e., delay of gratification, risk taking, motivational control) or cool (i.e., planning, set-shifting, behavioral inhibition) executive functions. Relative to the control group, the comorbid group, but not the CD-only group, tended to perform more poorly on some cool executive function measures. However, on hot executive function measures both CD groups performed poorly relative to controls, particularly on the delay of gratification test. Despite limited significant group differences, several measures of hot and cool executive functions were significantly correlated with externalizing problems as measured by the Child Behavior Checklist (Achenbach, 1991). These data suggest that ADHD may not affect executive functioning in children with CD, and the authors suggest that a dimensional approach may be more sensitive to neuropsychological dysfunction in children with CD.

Recent evidence, therefore, appears to suggest that when executive dysfunction is observed, it is related to ADHD but not the DBDs (but see Rhodes et al., 2012). However, the age of children who are studied is likely critical, given developmental differences in executive abilities. Children with DBDs do tend to perform more poorly than their non-afflicted peers on tasks assessing temporal discounting, but no differences in the capacity of children with DBDs to delay gratification are seen between those with and without comorbid ADHD.

Anxiety Disorders

Although not as common as comorbid DBDs, a very substantial portion of children with ADHD present with co-occurring anxiety disorders and to date, the extent to which this comorbidity affects neurocognitive function remains unclear. Thus, this is a ripe area for investigation in which we have identified four recent studies.

Jarrett, Wolff, Davis, Cowart, and Ollendick (2012) examined neurocognitive differences in a clinically referred sample of 6- to 17-year-old youth with ADHD (n = 41), anxiety disorders (i.e. generalized anxiety disorder, separation anxiety, specific phobia; n = 62), and those with comorbid ADHD plus anxiety (n = 31). Children with ODD and CD were excluded from the study. All children were administered the

Conners' CPT to assess vigilance; the Wechsler Digit Span Backwards test served as an index of working memory. Regardless of comorbid anxiety, children with ADHD had more variable reaction time on a CPT task than the anxiety-only group, while mean reaction time and hit rate did not differ among the three groups. This is consistent with considerable literature that suggests that reaction time variability is greater in children with ADHD (Epstein et al., 2003). Notably, the ADHD plus anxiety group performed significantly worse than the ADHD-only group, but not the anxiety-only group on Digit Span Backwards. The authors note that few studies have examined neurocognitive characteristics of children with anxiety and that working memory may be an important area to examine further in future studies of child anxiety.

Whereas Jarrett et al. (2012) assessed verbal working memory, Vance, Ferrin, Winther, and Gomez (2013) comprehensively evaluated spatial working memory in 6- to 16-year-old youth with ADHD alone (n = 163), ADHD plus anxiety (n = 243), anxiety disorders alone (n = 69), and an age- and gender-matched healthy control group (n = 116). Along with a variety of rating scales, participants were administered the Spatial Working Memory and Spatial Span tests from the CANTAB. The two groups with ADHD performed more poorly than the anxiety-only group, who in turn performed more poorly than control participants on both measures of spatial working memory. It is notable that despite the fact that anxiety disorders alone were associated with impaired spatial working memory and spatial span compared to control participants, there was no evidence of an additive effect of ADHD and anxiety on spatial working memory measures.

To examine the differential nature of attentional problems in children and adolescents Weissman, Chu, Reddy, and Mohlman (2012) compared children with ADHD but not anxiety disorders (n = 23) and anxiety disorders but not ADHD (n = 24) on tests of general and emotion-based attention processes. General attention processes were assessed using the Conners CPT-II and the Stroop Color-Word test. Emotion-based attention was measured using a Faces Dot Probe Task, which requires an individual to press a button in response to a stimulus in the context of two faces: one neutral and one happy, sad, or angry. As expected, children with ADHD performed more poorly on measures of general attention (i.e., the CPT and Stroop), but youth with anxiety disorders had greater attentional bias toward angry faces on the visual probe task, but not toward happy or sad faces. The authors conclude that children with ADHD have general attention problems, whereas attentional difficulties in anxious children may be specific to threatening stimuli. They suggest a possible role for neuropsychological assessment in differential diagnosis.

Finally, Bloemsma et al. (2013) assessed the impact of comorbid anxiety on several domains of neurocognitive functioning in children and adolescents with ADHD. Five- to 19-year-old children and adolescents with ADHD-C (n = 238; mean age, 11.5 years) and their typically developing peers (n = 271; mean age, 11.2) were recruited as part of the International Multicenter ADHD Genetics project (IMAGE). Anxiety was assessed using parent and teacher ratings and child self-report. After at least a 48-hour medication-free period, children completed a large battery of neurocognitive tests measuring several constructs, including behavioral inhibition, cognitive flexibility, interference control, time production and reproduction, visuospatial and verbal working memory, motor control, motor speed, and response speed. Linear structural equation modeling was used to estimate the effect of comorbid anxiety on children's and adolescents' neurocognitive functioning. Parent- and teacher-rated anxiety yielded few significant relations; parent-reported anxiety was not associated with any of the neurocognitive functions and teacher-rated anxiety was only associated with poorer time production. Child and adolescent self-reported anxiety, however, was associated with slower motor speed, slower response speed, and better behavioral inhibition. The authors concluded that when it comes to assessing anxiety, the child and adolescent himself or herself is a critical source of information. Furthermore, given that results suggest that anxiety offsets some of the negative neurocognitive effects associated with ADHD, Bloemsma et al. (2013) also emphasize the need to take into account comorbid disorders when assessing the neurocognitive functioning of children and adolescents with ADHD.

It seems, therefore, that the neurocognitive profile of children with ADHD may be moderated by comorbid anxiety. Exactly which executive functions are affected by the presence of anxiety in children with ADHD seems to vary across studies, although there is evidence for differences in working memory, behavioral inhibition, and also for the nonexecutive process of response speed. Differences in findings may, in part, reflect the way in which anxiety is assessed (i.e., adult vs. child report) and how anxiety is included in analyses (i.e., categorical vs. dimensional approaches).

Autism Spectrum Disorders

The considerable overlap between ADHD and ASD has become apparent in recent years and formally recognized with the recent publication of the DSM-V. Unlike in previous editions, ADHD can now be concurrently diagnosed with ASD. Reflecting this change, a handful of studies have recently been published focusing on executive functioning in relation to ASD and ADHD comorbidity.

To improve accuracy in differential diagnosis, Mayes, Calhoun, Mayes, and Molitoris (2012) determined the degree to which the symptoms of ADHD and autism overlap and whether the groups could be differentiated using neuropsychological measures. The sample for this study consisted of 1,005 children ages 2–16 years. Among these, 23 had high-functioning autism (IQ > 80), 324 had low-functioning autism (IQ < 80), 112 had ADHD-C, and 46 had ADHD-PI. The four groups were compared on an array of clinical symptoms as well as on measures of working memory and processing speed as measured by the WISC-IV indices, vigilance as measured by a CPT, and visuomotor integration as measured by the Developmental Test of Visual-Motor Integration (Beery, 1997). Those with ADHD and autism were easily distinguished by checklists of ASD symptoms, with very few of these symptoms being reported in children with ADHD. In contrast, ADHD symptoms were very common in the children with autism; those with high- and low-functioning autism did not differ significantly on maternal ratings of inattention, impulsivity, and hyperactivity from youth with ADHD-C. Also notable is the fact that there were no significant group differences on any of the neuropsychological measures. Collectively, these data suggest that children with ASD display symptoms of ADHD, which the authors suggest are part of the disorder, but children with ADHD do not typically display symptoms of autism, which makes these two disorders relatively distinguishable. Notably, this study was conducted using DSM-IV criteria for ASD and ADHD; it would be of interest to know what portion of the children with autism would meet criteria for ASD plus ADHD as now included in DSM-V.

Salcedo-Marin, Moreno-Granados, Ruiz-Veguilla, and Ferrin (2013) also compared ADHD-only (n = 80) and ASD-only (n = 23) groups using tasks measuring planning (Zoo Map), inhibitory control (Stroop), attention (Digit Span Forwards), processing speed (Coding), working memory (Digit Span), and motor coordination (Grooved Pegboard). There were no significant differences between the two groups on any of the executive function skills tested. However, a particular focus of this manuscript was on the evaluation of planning ability. Following detailed analyses, it is suggested that children with ADHD and ASD present with different patterns of planning function. Overall, this study showed that although there were no differences on the majority of executive functions between ASD and ADHD, the ASD group did have poorer planning skills.

Lundervold et al. (2012) sought to characterize aspects of executive function and attention, as assessed by the Conners CPT-II, in children with combined ASD plus ADHD (n = 11), and to determine whether performance could be differentiated from that of children with either diagnosis alone (ADHD, n = 38; ASD, n = 9) and children with neither diagnosis (n = 134). In general, the ADHD plus ASD group was more similar to the ADHD-only group than to the ASD-only group. Relative to the ASD-only group, both the ASD plus ADHD group and the ADHD-only group had a more impulsive response style (greater speed-accuracy tradeoff), greater variability, and lower consistency. Post hoc paired group comparisons were difficult to evaluate due to the small number of participants in several groups. There were no group differences on measures of sustained attention or vigilance. Importantly, however, the relations between IQ and CPT-II performance varied as a function of group. Among those with ASD, most CPT-II measures were highly correlated with IQ. In contrast, only reaction time was correlated with IQ in the ADHD group. Because children with ASD represent a wide range in intellectual functioning, the authors suggest that CPT results should be interpreted very cautiously in children with ASD.

Taken together, the previously reviewed papers suggest that children with ADHD and ASD do not differ substantially with regard to executive functions, except perhaps for subtle differences in planning ability and reaction time variability. It will be of interest to see whether findings change as a function of the recent publication of the DSM-V, which now permits the comorbid condition to be formally diagnosed. This will likely allow for more studies that include both the comorbid group and groups of youth with ASD but low levels of ADHD symptoms. For now, however, the recent literature suggests that differences between the two disorders do not stem from differences in executive function.

Learning and Language Disorders

The overlap between diagnoses of ADHD and learning disabilities is considerable (e.g., Mayes & Calhoun, 2013); this is of tremendous concern given the heightened risk these children face of adverse educational outcomes (e.g., Faraone, Biederman, Monuteaux, Doyle, & Seidman, 2001). Researchers have devoted considerable energy to better understanding the nature of these comorbidities and mechanisms contributing to their occurrence.

Although decoding difficulties are common in children who have ADHD, the literature is inconsistent as to whether children with ADHD have particular deficits in reading comprehension. Miller et al. (2013) noted that in part, these inconsistencies are due to several key methodological differences across studies. To address these limitations, the authors investigated whether the "centrality deficit" (i.e., fewer ideas central to text are retained because individuals have difficulty forming connections among ideas within text; Miller & Kennan, 2009) is observed in children with ADHD. If present, they sought to determine whether neuropsychological variables might be able to explain the phenomenon. Nine- and 10-year-old children with a primary subtype of ADHD (n = 27) and 8- to 11-year-old typically developing children (n = 76) read aloud a passage from the Qualitative Reading Inventory-III (Leslie & Caldwell, 2001) and then had to immediately recall it. They also answered six open-ended questions about the passage. In addition to this reading comprehension task, children completed measures of general intellectual functioning, working memory, processing speed, and inhibition. To assess whether children with ADHD showed deficits in comprehension due to decoding difficulties, their performance on the reading comprehension task was compared to 27 children selected from the control group whose word-reading level matched that of ADHD children. All children, irrespective of ADHD status, recalled more central ideas than peripheral ideas, but a significant Group × Centrality interaction emerged, showing that control children recalled significantly more central ideas than ADHD children. A series of regressions were carried out using the whole sample to assess whether any of the neuropsychological variables assessed were able to predict the proportion of central ideas recalled, after controlling for word reading skill and gender. Only working memory emerged as a significant predictor; furthermore, working memory significantly mediated the relation between ADHD severity and the recall of central ideas. The authors concluded that children with ADHD have difficulties forming a coherent mental representation of the text that they read, and that this appears to be related to working memory difficulties.

Differential diagnosis of ADHD and reading disability (RD) is complicated by the fact that both groups have been shown to present with deficits in attention. Miranda et al. (2013) used the Conners CPT to determine whether it could differentiate between children with ADHD (n = 52) and dyslexia (n = 32) in relation to a Brazilian standardization sample (n = 475). Importantly, the groups differed significantly in age and sex distribution. Relative to the standardization sample, children with ADHD performed poorly on 10 out of the 15 CPT measures. Children with

ADHD made more omission and commission errors, had more variable reaction times and more perseveration responses, and were less able to discriminate target from nontarget stimuli (d'). They did not differ from the standardization sample in reaction time and response bias. Relative to the standardization sample, the dyslexia group had increased commission errors, variability, perseveration responses, and inconsistency in the reaction time over the six time blocks (Hit SE block). In general, the ADHD group performed more poorly than the dyslexia group. Relative to those with dyslexia, children with ADHD displayed greater attention deficits (higher omission errors), more variable reaction times, a higher rate of anticipatory responses (perseverations), and less consistent reaction times with longer stimulus intervals. The authors conclude that their results "confirm that Conners' CPT has considerable potential for measuring attention problems, can distinguish ADHD from dyslexia, can distinguish both of these from clinical controls, and can be used as a diagnostic instrument for ADHD and LD" (p. 96). However, these conclusions seem premature given that sensitivity and specificity were not evaluated.

Gooch, Snowling, and Hulme (2012), using more sophisticated ex-Gaussian analyses, sought to determine the mechanisms underpinning the more variable responses on the Stop Signal Task in children with ADHD relative to their typically developing peers, and to examine the impact of comorbid dyslexia on Stop Signal Task responding. An ex-Gaussian approach had not previously been used to examine children with dyslexia. Using the Stop Signal Task as their primary outcome measure, Gooch et al. (2012) compared four groups of children aged between 6 and 14.75 years of age: (1) 17 with ADHD symptoms-only, (2) 17 with dyslexia-only, (3) 25 with ADHD symptoms plus dyslexia, and (4) 38 typically developing comparison children. Using 2×2 [ADHD (yes/no) $\times$ Dyslexia (yes/no)] analyses of variance to analyze the data they found surprisingly few significant results. There were no significant main effects or interactions for mu or tau, although they detected a weak, nonsignificant trend for children with ADHD symptoms to have larger values for tau than those without ADHD symptoms. They did find a significant main effect for ADHD for sigma such that those with ADHD had more variable responses. None of the planned comparisons for the comorbid group (ADHD symptoms plus dyslexia) to each of the separate clinical groups were significant. These findings suggest that children with ADHD do not show generalized slowing of all responses but are more variable in their responding. However, in contrast to findings of most studies (e.g., Leth-Steensen et al., 2000; Epstein et al., 2011) these data suggest that the increased variability is not due to more outliers or abnormally slow responding (attentional lapses) as would be indicated by increased tau. They suggest that the increased variability in response times may be due to impairments in response preparation or motor timing. Notably, on all measures, children with dyslexia responded similarly to their typically developing peers.

To further explore similarities and differences between ADHD, RD, and the comorbid condition (ADHD plus RD), de Jong, Licht, Sergeant, and Oosterlaan (2013) examined the extent to which these conditions are etiologically distinct by comparing them on measures of lexical route processing, sublexical route processing, and rapid naming. The sample consisted of 10- to 13-year-old children with RD (n = 27),

ADHD (n = 18), RD plus ADHD (n = 20), and 29 typically developing comparison children. Lexical route processing was assessed using an orthographic processing task in which letter strings were presented on a computer screen; the child had to determine whether or not each string represented a correctly spelled word. Sublexical route processing was assessed using a phonological decision task; the child had to determine whether letter strings, if pronounced, sounded like read words. Rapid naming was assessed using the Rapid Automatized Naming task (Denckla, 1973). Children with ADHD and children with RD demonstrated orthographic and phonological impairments as measured by number of errors, although deficits seemed to be greater in those with RD as evidenced by slower processing on both tasks. There were no significant ADHD × RD interactions, suggesting that effects were additive in the comorbid group. Furthermore, as expected, rapid naming differed as a function of both ADHD and RD, indicating slower rapid naming in both groups. Again, the RD by ADHD interaction was not significant. The authors concluded that ADHD and RD appear to be overlapping disorders with shared deficits in lexical route processing, sublexical route processing, and rapid naming, but RD can be dissociated from ADHD by lexical and sublexical speed. Their data did not support the notion that ADHD plus RD is a separable clinical entity distinct from both ADHD and RD.

Noting the high comorbidity between ADHD and academic underachievement, Gremillion and Martel (2013) were interested in identifying possible mechanisms accounting for this phenomenon. A large sample of 6- to 12-year-old children with ADHD (n = 266) and their typically developing peers (n = 207), as well as a group of children with subthreshold ADHD symptoms (n = 73) were recruited from the community. Children completed a battery of tests designed to measure semantic language (WISC-IV Vocabulary), verbal working memory (WISC-IV Digit Span Backwards), and math and reading achievement (WIAT-II Math Reasoning and Reading Comprehension, respectively). Group comparisons between children with a primary ADHD diagnosis and their typically developing peers showed that children with ADHD performed more poorly on measures of semantic language, verbal working memory, and math achievement, but surprisingly no group differences in reading achievement were observed. Mediation analyses using the whole sample assessed whether semantic language and verbal working memory (dimensional raw scores) accounted for the negative relation between ADHD (continuous symptom counts) and academic achievement (dimensional raw scores), after covarying for gender. Together, semantic language and verbal working memory fully mediated the relation between ADHD symptoms and reading achievement, and partially mediated the relation between ADHD symptoms and math achievement. For both of these analyses, the effect of semantic language was stronger than for verbal working memory. The authors suggested that given the role that semantic language and verbal working memory play in conferring risk for academic underachievement in children with more severe ADHD symptoms, these areas are potential targets for intervention.

Using a large battery of tests that were closely linked to distinct aspects of Baddeley's model of working memory (Baddeley, 2006; Baddeley & Hitch, 1974), Hutchinson, Bavin, Efron, and Sciberras (2012) examined differences between children with

ADHD and those with specific language impairment (SLI). The sample consisted of 18 children with SLI, 16 with ADHD, 11 with ADHD plus SLI, and 24 typically developing children. The children ranged in age from 6 to 9 years old. Multiple tests in their battery assessed the phonological loop, visual-spatial sketchpad, central executive, and the episodic buffer, as defined by Baddeley. Both SLI groups performed significantly lower than the typically developing group on tasks assessing the phonological loop, but no impairments on these measures were detected in children with ADHD only. There were no significant group differences for any of the measures assessing the visual-spatial sketchpad. On the single task assessing Baddeley's episodic buffer, the SLI and comorbid groups, but not the ADHD group, performed significantly below the typically developing comparison group. The poor performance of the children with SLI on the episodic buffer task was inferred to be due to difficulties in chunking verbal information into syntactic units. Finally, the typically developing group performed significantly better than all three clinical groups on two of the three central executive tasks. Together, the results indicate that children with SLI have deficits in phonological processing, the episodic buffer, and the central executive, as defined in Baddeley's model, whereas ADHD is characterized by selective deficits in the executive component of working memory. The authors concluded that ADHD and SLI likely develop independently because the comorbid condition did not appear to have a unique profile or an additive affect. Relative to ADHD, the presence of SLI resulted in poorer working memory, as indicated by the number of components impaired. Furthermore, the authors posit that children with SLI and children with ADHD have poor academic outcomes, perhaps due to working memory deficits.

Finally, although much research is devoted to better understanding cognitive correlates of comorbidity between ADHD and learning disabilities (LD), other research has investigated the link between ADHD, LD, and other psychopathology. It is well established that children with ADHD are at greater risk for other psychiatric comorbidities as compared to their non-ADHD peers; however, the risk for other psychopathology (outside of ADHD) in children with LD is less clear. Mattison and Mayes (2013) investigated whether differences in parent- and teacher-rated psychopathology are seen between ADHD children with and without comorbid LD. In this retrospective cross-sectional study, the authors reviewed the charts of a large sample of 6- to 16-year-old children with ADHD (n = 595) who presented at an outpatient clinic for a psychoeducational evaluation. The presence of psychopathology in children was measured using the Pediatric Behavior Scale (Lindgren & Koeppl, 1987), which was completed by both mothers and teachers. Children completed a battery of general cognitive, neuropsychological, and academic achievement tests, including the WISC-III/WISC-IV; WIAT/WIAT-II; the Gordon Diagnostic System (Gordon, 1983), which is a CPT; and the Developmental Test of Visual-motor Integration (Beery, 1997). In this sample of children with ADHD, 75% had a comorbid LD (math, 30.3%; reading, 39.9%; or written expression disability, 62.4%), based on predicted achievement by IQ. Compared to children with ADHD alone, those who had ADHD plus LD performed more poorly in several domains including visual-motor integration, working memory, and processing speed, and they achieved a lower executive function composite score. No group differences were observed in verbal comprehension, perceptual reasoning, or on the CPT. Furthermore, no group differences in psychopathology were observed for either parent or teacher report. Next, the authors looked at the relations among cognitive/neuropsychological measures, and parent- and teacher-rated psychopathology across the whole sample. Few significant relations were obtained, but lower executive function composite scores and lower academic achievement were significantly (yet weakly) associated with the teacher-rated general domains, ADHD, Depression-Anxiety, Inappropriate Social, and for the executive function composite only, Conduct. The achievement composite score was regressed on FSIQ, the executive function composite, visual-motor integration, and parent and teacher ADHD composite ratings. Full ScaleIQ, executive functioning, and teacher-rated ADHD emerged as significant, independent predictors of academic achievement. Thus, it seems that children with ADHD plus LD show poorer executive functioning than children with ADHD alone. However, comorbidity does not appear to confer greater risk for additional psychopathology than ADHD alone, at least as measured using parent and teacher ratings on the Pediatric Behavior Scale (Lindgren & Koeppl, 1987).

Other Less Common Comorbid Conditions

Throughout the past decade there has been a substantial increase in the rate at which bipolar disorder has been diagnosed in children (Blader & Carlson, 2007), with a sizable portion of these youth also meeting criteria for ADHD. Furthermore, differential diagnosis is complicated by the fact that bipolar disorder and ADHD have several overlapping features, including high energy, hyperactivity, excessive talking, emotional lability, and impulsivity. Two recent studies by Udal et al. (2012a, 2012b) have examined differences in executive functioning in youth with ADHD, bipolar disorder, and co-occurring ADHD plus bipolar disorder. In one study, Udal et al. (2012a) predicted that the nature of executive function deficits would differ between children with bipolar disorder and ADHD, and that such deficits would be most evident in those with bipolar disorder and a history of psychotic symptoms. Furthermore, they posited that all three clinical groups would have slow processing speed, which might account for the apparent executive function deficits. To assess this, they compared groups of 6- to 19-year-old children with bipolar disorder (n = 24), ADHD (n = 26), ADHD plus bipolar disorder (n = 13), and control participants (n = 68) on measures of working memory (i.e., Digit Span and Knox Cube Test), cognitive flexibility (i.e., Wisconsin Card Sort Test), inhibition (i.e., Conners CPT-II, Stroop interference condition and Children's Checking Task), and processing speed (i.e., Stroop color naming and word naming conditions). Relative to controls, all three clinical groups showed evidence of executive deficits with the combined group being most impaired. There were no significant differences between any of the clinical groups, although executive impairment in the bipolar group varied as a function of history of psychotic symptoms. The nonpsychotic bipolar group only evidenced deficits in processing speed. After controlling for processing speed, working memory scores improved and interference control scores normalized in both bipolar and ADHD patients. The authors concluded that executive deficits in bipolar disorder are more closely associated with a history of psychotic symptoms than comorbid ADHD. Furthermore, they suggested that apparent executive function deficits in both ADHD and bipolar disorder may be at least partially accounted for by slow processing speed.

In another study (Udal et al., 2012b) this same group sought to differentiate memory deficits (working memory and declarative memory) between children with early onset bipolar disorder and ADHD-C. For this study, the final sample consisted of 23 children with bipolar disorder, 26 with ADHD, 15 with bipolar plus ADHD, and 68 healthy controls. Memory was assessed in all participants using Digit Span, the Rey Auditory Verbal Learning Test, and the California Verbal Learning Test-II (CVLT-II). Children with ADHD performed significantly worse than control participants on measures of working memory and free recall trials 1-5 of the CVLT-II. Recognition did not differ between ADHD and control groups. In contrast, children with bipolar disorder did not differ from controls on measures of working memory, but did differ from them on multiple memory measures suggesting impaired learning and recognition. The comorbid group performed worse on all free recall trials, working memory, and recognition. Notably, none of the clinical groups differed on short and long delay recall of the CVLT-II. Children with ADHD and bipolar disorder did not differ from each other on any measures. As in the previous study, they compared children with bipolar disorder and a history of psychotic episodes/features versus all of the other groups, and in general, found the most severe deficits in this group. These data suggest that youth with bipolar disorder and a history of psychotic symptoms have inefficient encoding of verbal material, whereas memory problems in ADHD are characterized by impaired free recall and working memory.

Deficits in response inhibition are characteristic of children with ADHD and traumatic brain injury (TBI). Furthermore, adolescents with ADHD are at increased risk for automobile crashes and other accidents (Barkley, Murphy, & Kwasnik, 1996), which in turn places them at increased risk for TBI, and children with TBI often present with ADHD-like symptoms following their brain injury (Max et al., 2004). To more carefully examine inhibitory control in these two groups of children, Ornstein et al. (2013) administered the Stop-Signal task to a sample of 6- to 14-year-old children consisting of 92 with ADHD, 103 TBI, and 79 of their typically developing peers. Among those with TBI, injury severity ranged from mild to severe. Children with both ADHD and TBI showed deficient inhibitory control as measured by the stop-signal reaction time, and those with ADHD had somewhat greater deficits than those with TBI, irrespective of whether the latter group met criteria for secondary ADHD (diagnosed as a consequence of the head injury). It is notable that the development of secondary ADHD symptoms in the TBI group was not related to poorer inhibitory control. Although ADHD and TBI appear to share a common cognitive deficit, the underlying neural mechanisms leading to this impairment remain to be determined, as well as whether or not it is the same or different in the two groups.

ADHD frequently co-occurs with tic disorders, yet little is known about the impact of this comorbidity on executive functioning in children with ADHD. Lin, Lai, and Gau (2012) compared ADHD children with (n = 40) and without (n = 40) a co-occurring tic disorder, to a non-tic/non-ADHD comparison group (n = 40) on a large battery of executive function measures (i.e., reaction time, sustained attention, spatial working memory, planning, set-shifting) from the CANTAB. Children ranged in age from 8 to 16 years. Although there were several differences between the clinical groups and control participants, there were no significant differences between the ADHD-only group and the comorbid group. This suggests that the presence of a tic disorder does not further impair executive functioning in children with ADHD.

Neurofibromatosis type 1 (NF1) is a genetic disorder that, among other things, affects neurocognitive development (Payne, Hyman, Shores, & North, 2011). Children with NF1 display frequent difficulty with planning, impulsivity, and organization, and oftentimes present with comorbid ADHD. Payne, Arnold, Pride, and North (2012) examined whether spatial working memory and inhibitory control are impaired in children with NF1 who do not have ADHD and whether the presence of ADHD exacerbates these executive difficulties in children with NF1. A sample of 7- to 15-year-old children with NF1 only (n = 49), NF1 plus ADHD (n = 35), and 30 unaffected comparison children were administered the Spatial Working Memory and Stop-Signal tasks from the CANTAB. Relative to the comparison group, both NF1 groups showed significant impairments in spatial working memory and inhibition as measured by the stop-signal reaction time. The NF1-only and NF1 plus ADHD groups did not differ on either measure, indicating that having a comorbid ADHD diagnosis does not contribute to deficits in working memory or inhibitory control in children with NF1. Furthermore, these data suggest that executive impairments are not unique contributors to ADHD symptomatology in NF1. The study did not include an ADHD-only group, so further research needs to be carried out to determine what role a co-occurring NF1 diagnosis has on ADHD-related executive deficits.

Focusing on another group with significant developmental difficulties, Ware et al. (2012) examined the impact of prenatal exposure to alcohol on executive and adaptive functioning in children with ADHD, and the degree to which executive deficits can account for poor adaptive functioning in these children. As part of a multisite study, three groups of 8- to 18-year-old children were tested: (1) 142 with a history of heavy prenatal alcohol exposure (60% had ADHD), (2) 82 children with ADHD who were not exposed to alcohol prenatally, and (3) 133 typically developing comparison children without ADHD or a history of prenatal alcohol exposure. Children completed the Verbal Fluency-Switching, Design Fluency-Switching, Trail Making Test-Switching, and Color-Word Interference-Inhibition/Switching tasks from the D-KEFS. Only conditions involving switching conditions were used for this study, because the authors indicate that they are the most sensitive to impairments in higher-order cognitive flexibility and set shifting abilities. In addition, parents were administered the Vineland Adaptive Behavior Scales-II (Sparrow, Cicchetti, & Balla,

2005) to assess the children's adaptive functioning. Results indicated a significant main effect of group on all four D-KEFS measures such that those with ADHD irrespective of prenatal alcohol exposure performed more poorly than the comparison children. There were no significant differences on any of the executive function measures between the ADHD groups with and without prenatal exposure to alcohol. In contrast, those with alcohol exposure had poorer adaptive functioning relative to those with ADHD but not exposure, who in turn had poorer adaptive functioning than controls. Furthermore, regression analyses indicated that executive function measures were predictive of adaptive functioning, and notably, significant interactions suggested that these relations differed as a function of group. For the ADHD without prenatal alcohol exposure group, the relation between adaptive abilities and executive function was broad-based, with three of the four D-KEFS measures predicting the Vineland composite adaptive score. For the group with ADHD plus alcohol exposure the relation was specific to nonverbal executive function measures (i.e., Trail Making and Spatial Fluency). In the unaffected control group, test performance did not predict adaptive functioning scores after controlling for age. These results support the notion that executive function deficits are predictive of poorer adaptive functioning irrespective of prenatal alcohol exposure.

White, Mous, and Karatekin (2013) attempted to tease out specific aspects of spatial working memory in children and adolescents with ADHD (n = 33) and nonaffective psychoses (n = 25). A typically developing control group (n = 58) was also recruited. Participants, aged 8–20 years, performed an oculomotor delayed-response task and memory-guided saccades were measured following delays of 2, 8, and 20 seconds. During the delay periods, participants were presented with words from different semantic categories and they had to respond when a word appeared that did not belong to the category "food." Performance was compared to a control condition in which the target location was always the same. Participants with ADHD had larger distance errors than control participants at 20-seconds delay. Children and adolescents with psychosis had larger distance errors than control participants at all delay periods, and larger distance errors than children with ADHD at 8-seconds delay. For the distractor task, both clinical groups made more errors than the control group. The authors suggested that their findings support encoding impairments in children and adolescents with psychosis and a delay-dependent deficit in those with ADHD.

Children with ADHD are at elevated risk of urinary problems, including nocturnal enuresis (Duel, Steinberg-Epstein, Hill, & Lerner, 2003). Yang, Huang, et al. (2013) investigated the neuropsychological performance of 6- to 10-year-old ADHD children with (n = 15) and without (n = 38) nocturnal enuresis. The relation between nocturnal enuresis and neuropsychological performance in children with ADHD was also assessed. No differences in alertness as a function of group were observed. However, children with ADHD and nocturnal enuresis had faster reaction time on measures of working memory, inhibitory control, and auditory sustained attention than children with ADHD alone. The authors conclude that there is evidence for a different neuropsychological profile of ADHD children with nocturnal enuresis compared to those who do not have nocturnal enuresis. However, the pattern of findings was not in the expected direction and the mechanism for why children with ADHD and nocturnal enuresis would have faster reaction times on neuropsychological tasks is not clear.

Overall, it is evident that despite the fact that children with ADHD can be differentiated from their typically developing peers on a wide array of neuropsychological measures, including those of nonexecutive and executive functions, differentiation from youth with other psychiatric and neurodevelopmental disorders is far more difficult. Some data suggest that increased reaction time variability and slow processing speed may be more specifically associated with ADHD, but executive function deficits seem to be characteristic of children with a wide array of behavioral, psychiatric, and/or developmental disorders.

STRENGTHS AND WEAKNESSES OF THE RECENTLY PUBLISHED LITERATURE

Within the past 2 years, a plethora of research has been conducted to elucidate the role of executive functions and their neural substrates in the pathophysiology of ADHD. Importantly, a major strength of recent research is the shift away from simple comparisons of children with and without ADHD on various tests of executive function. Rather, compelling questions related to the mechanisms accounting for disparate performance on tests, the degree to which poor performance is specific to children with ADHD, and how performance relates to functioning in the real world have become the focus of recent publications. Also, recent research reflects the growing appreciation for the heterogeneity of ADHD and the fact that children with ADHD are far from a homogeneous group. As a result of these lines of research, a notable shift in the conceptualization of ADHD as an "executive function disorder" is beginning to emerge.

A compelling body of research continues to demonstrate poor performance by children and adolescents with ADHD on an array of executive function measures, most prominently in the areas of inhibitory control and working memory. Notably, differences in the domains of inhibitory control and working memory are typically observed despite the myriad tasks that researchers have used to assess the constructs. Furthermore, these executive deficits are evident across the different subtypes (DSM-IV) and presentations (DSM-V) of ADHD suggesting that, at least from a neurocognitive perspective, they are more similar than different. To the extent that executive abilities represent a relatively stable trait, this finding is not surprising given the fact that, as now recognized in DSM-V, children who are repeatedly evaluated often change subtype across evaluations (Lahey et al., 2005). The extent to which such switches is due to developmental factors, environmental factors, or measurement error is unknown, but recent findings suggest that it is not due to changing patterns of executive dysfunction.

Of importance is the recent application of analytic techniques designed to elucidate the neuropsychological heterogeneity of ADHD and the fact that many, but not all children with ADHD have executive function deficits, and that those with such deficits often differ in the nature of their difficulties (e.g., working memory vs. inhibitory control). There is no doubt that a number of disparate neural mechanisms can lead to the phenotypic presentation of ADHD (i.e., inattention, impulsiveness, and overactivity). Such research has the potential to lead to tailored treatments based upon the nature of the individual's dysfunction.

Serious questions have also been raised in the past 2 years regarding the degree to which executive dysfunction represents a core etiological factor in the emergence of ADHD. More sophisticated research strategies that integrate lower-level processing measures with higher-order executive tests are beginning to suggest that poor performance on these latter tests might be due to lower-level deficiencies in arousal, processing efficiency, or other nonexecutive abilities. Although this is not necessarily a new idea (e.g., Halperin & Schulz, 2006; Marks et al., 2005; Sergeant, 2000; Sonuga-Barke & Castellanos, 2007), the quality of recent research addressing this essential question is quite exceptional.

Finally, notable in recent research is the relative lack of specificity of executive function deficits to ADHD. Although a limited number of papers reported greater executive function impairments in youth with ADHD relative to other disorders (Jarrett et al., 2012; Schoemaker et al., 2012), most studies that included multiple clinical groups tended to find few, if any, significant differences between them. Thus, similar to children with ADHD, executive deficits were reported in children with ODD (Rhodes et al., 2012), autism (Mayes et al., 2012), bipolar disorder (Udal, 2012a), dyslexia (Miranda et al., 2013), SLI (Hutchinson et al., 2012), and NF1 (Payne et al., 2012). This lack of specificity suggests the need for extreme caution when using neuropsychological tests for differential diagnostic purposes and underscores the necessity of comprehensive clinical evaluation.

Considerable progress related to the understanding of the neuropsychological bases of ADHD has been made in the past 1–2 years. However, a major weakness that runs through much of this research is the lack of prospective longitudinal designs. Although several studies demonstrate an appreciation for the importance of developmental factors, all are cross-sectional in nature. ADHD is a neurodevelopmental disorder and it is quite likely that the relationship between cognitive and behavioral functions changes as children age. Furthermore, several very important studies have used mediation to elucidate the underlying determinants of functional impairments as well as executive function deficits. Longitudinal data would substantially strengthen the ability to make causal inferences. It should be noted that this review focused on categorical studies focusing on children diagnosed with ADHD, and within that framework we did not identify any recent neuropsychological longitudinal studies focusing on childhood. However, recent dimensional studies have used longitudinal designs (Rajendran et al., 2013a; 2013b). Longitudinal data such as these are necessary to elucidate the evolving role of executive functions in ADHD over the lifespan.

FUTURE DIRECTIONS

As the field moves forward, it is critical to use developmentally sensitive longitudinal designs focusing on the degree to which neuropsychological heterogeneity represents stable individual differences over time as well as the extent to which such heterogeneity predicts or is associated with variations in course and outcome. Mediation studies that attempt to infer causality must also be strengthened by the use of longitudinal designs, which will allow for the evaluation of the temporal order of strengths and deficits as they emerge over development. What we have learned about the neuropsychology of ADHD needs to be applied to the development of novel interventions that improve and enhance treatment.

REFERENCES

Achenbach, T. M. (1991). *Manual for the Child Behavior Checklist/4-18 and 1991 Profile.* Burlington, VT: Department of Psychiatry, University of Vermont.

Achenbach, T. M., & Rescorla, L. A. (2001). *Manual for the ASEBA school-age forms & profiles.* Burlington, VT: University of Vermont, Research Center for Children, Youth, and Families.

Alderson, R. M., Rapport, M. D., Kasper, L. J., Sarver, D. E., & Kofler, M. J. (2012). Hyperactivity in boys with attention deficit/hyperactivity disorder (ADHD): The association between deficient behavioral inhibition, attentional processes, and objectively measured activity. *Child Neuropsychology, 18,* 487–505.

Antonini, T. N., Narad, M. E., Langberg, J., & Epstein, J. N. (2013). Behavioral correlates of reaction time variability in children with and without ADHD. *Neuropsychology, 27,* 201–209.

Baddeley, A. D. (2006). The episodic buffer: A new component of working memory. *Trends in Cognitive Sciences, 4,* 417–423.

Baddeley, A. D., & Hitch, G. (1974). Working memory. In G. A. Bower (Ed.), *Recent advances in learning and motivation* (8 ed., pp. 47–89). New York: Academic Press.

Banaschewski, T., Jennen-Steinmetz, C., Brandeis, D., Buitelaar, J. K., Kuntsi, J., Poustka, L., et al. (2012). Neuropsychological correlates of emotional lability in children with ADHD. *The Journal of Child Psychology and Psychiatry, 53,* 1139–1148.

Barkley, R. A. (1997). Behavioral inhibition, sustained attention, and executive function: Constructing a unified theory of ADHD. *Psychological Bulletin, 121,* 65–94.

Barkley, R. A., Grodzinsky, G., & DuPaul, G. J. (1992). Frontal lobe functions in attention deficit disorder with and without hyperactivity: A review and research report. *Journal of Abnormal Child Psychology, 20,* 168–188.

Barkley, R. A., Koplowitz, S., Anderson, T., & McMurray, M. B. (1997). Sense of time in children with ADHD: Effects of duration, distraction, and stimulant medication. *Journal of the International Neuropsychological Society, 3,* 359–369.

Barkley, R. A., Murphy, K. R., & Kwansik, D. (1996). Motor vehicle driving competencies and risks in teens and young adults with attention deficit hyperactivity disorder. *Pediatrics, 98,* 1089–1095.

Bauermeister, J. J., Barkley, R. A., Bauermeister, J. A., Martínez, J. V., & McBurnett, K. (2012). Validity of the sluggish cognitive tempo, inattention and hyperactivity symptom dimensions: Neuropsychological and psychosocial correlates. *Journal of Abnormal Child Psychology, 40,* 683–697.

Bechara, A., Damasio, A. R., Damasio, H., & Anderson, S. W. (1994). Insensitivity to future consequences following damage to human prefrontal cortex. *Cognition, 1-3,* 7–15.

Beery, K. E. (1997). *The Beery-Buktenica Developmental Test of Visual-motor Integration (VMI).* (4th, rev. ed.) Parsippany, NJ: Modern Curriculum Press.

Benson, D. F. (1991). The role of frontal dysfunction in attention deficit hyperactivity disorder. *Journal of Child Neurology, 6*, S9–S12.

Bioulac, S., Lallemand, S., Rizzo, A., Philip, P., Fabrigoule, C., & Bouvard, M. P. (2012). Impact of time on task on ADHD patient's performances in a virtual classroom. *European Journal of Paediatric Neuropsychology, 16*, 514–521.

Blader, J. C., & Carlson, G. A. (2007). Increased rates of bipolar disorder diagnoses among US child, adolescent, and adult inpatients, 1996-2004. *Biological Psychiatry, 62*, 107–114.

Bloemsma, J. M., Boer, F., Arnold, R., Banaschewski, T., Faraone, S. V., Buitelaar, J. K., et al. (2013). Comorbid anxiety and neurocognitive dysfunctions in children with ADHD. *European Child and Adolescent Psychiatry, 22*, 225–234.

Bolden, J., Rapport, M. D., Raiker, J. S., Sarver, D. E., & Kofler, M. J. (2012). Understanding phonological memory deficits in boys with attention-deficit/hyperactivity disorder (ADHD): Dissociation of short-term storage and articulatory rehearsal processes. *Journal of Abnormal Child Psychology, 40*, 999–1011.

Borella, E., de Ribaupierre, A., Cornoldi, C., & Chicherio, C. (2013). Beyond interference control impairment in ADHD: Evidence from increased intraindividual variability in the color-Stroop test. *Child Neuropsychology, 19*, 495–515.

Capdevila-Brophy, C., Artigas-Pallarés, J., Navarro-Pastor, J. B., García-Nonell, K., Rigau-Ratera, E., & Obiols, J. E. (2012). ADHD predominantly inattentive subtype with high sluggish cognitive tempo: A new clinical entity? *Journal of Attention Disorders, 20*, 1–10.

Casagrande, M., Martella, D., Ruggiero, M. C., Maccari, L., Paloscia, C., Rosa, C., et al. (2012). Assessing attentional systems in children with attention deficit hyperactivity disorder. *Archives of Clinical Neuropsychology 27*(1), 30–44.

Casey, B. J., Castellanos, F. X., Giedd, J. N., Marsh, W. L., Hamburger, S. D., Schubert, A. B., et al. (1997). Implication of right frontostriatal circuitry in response inhibition and attention-deficit/hyperactivity disorder. *Journal of the American Academy of Child & Adolescent Psychiatry, 36*, 374–383.

Castellanos, F. X., Sonuga-Barke, E. J., Milham, M. P., & Tannock, R. (2006). Characterizing cognition in ADHD: Beyond executive dysfunction. *Trends in Cognitive Sciences, 10*, 117–123.

Castellanos, F. X., & Tannock, R. (2002). Neuroscience of attention-deficit/hyperactivity disorder: The search for endophenotypes. *Nature Reviews Neuroscience, 3*, 617–628.

Chelune, G. J., Ferguson, W., Koon, R., & Disckey, R. O. (1986). Frontal lobe dysinhibition in attention-deficit disorder. *Child Psychiatry and Human Development, 16*, 221–234.

Conners, C. K., & Staff, M. (2000). Conners' Continuous Performance Test II: Computer program for windows technical guide and software manual. North Tonawanda, NY: Multi-Health Systems.

Crone, E. A., & van der Molen, M. W. (2004). Developmental changes in real life decision making: Performance on a gambling task previously shown to depend on the ventromedial prefrontal cortex. *Developmental Neuropsychology, 25*, 251–279.

de Jong, C. G. W., Licht, R., Sergeant, J. A., & Oosterlaan, J. (2013). RD, ADHD, and their comorbidity from a dual route perspective. *Child Neuropsychology, 18*, 467–486.

Delis, D. C., Kalpan, E., & Kramer, J. H. (2001). D-KEFS executive function system: Examiners manual. San Antonio, TX: Pearson.

Denckla, M. B. (1973). Colour-naming in dyslexic boys. *Cortex, 8*, 164–176.

Denckla, M. B. (1985). Revised neurological examination for subtle signs. *Psychopharmacology Bulletin, 21*, 773–800.

Dolan, M., & Lennox, C. (2013). Cool and hot executive function in conduct-disordered adolescents with and without co-morbid attention deficit hyperactivity disorder: Relationships with externalizing behaviours. *Psychological Medicine*. doi:10.1017/S0033291712003078, Published online: 30 January 2013.

Douglas, V. I., & Peters, T. J. (1979). Toward a clearer definition of attentional deficit of hyperactive children. In G. A. L. M. Hale (Ed.), *Attention and cognitive development* (pp. 173–243). New York: Plenum Press.

Dovis, S., Van der Oord, S., Wiers, R. W., & Prins, P. J. M. (2012). Can motivation normalize working memory and task persistence in children with attention-deficit/hyperactivity disorder? The effects of money and computer-gaming. *Journal of Abnormal Child Psychology, 40*, 669–681.

Dovis, S., Van der Oord, S., Wiers, R. W., & Prins, P. J. M. (2013). What part of working memory is not working in ADHD? Short-term memory, the central executive and effects of reinforcement. *Journal of Abnormal Child Psychology, 41*, 901–917.

Duel, B. P., Steinberg-Epstein, R., Hill, M., & Lerner, M. (2003). A survey of voiding dysfunction in children with attention deficit-hyperactivity disorder. *The Journal of Urology, 170*, 1521–1523.

Ek, U., Westerlund, J., & Fernell, E. (2013). General versus executive cognitive ability in pupils with ADHD and with milder attention problems. *Neuropsychiatric Disease and Treatment, 9*, 163–168.

Emslie, H., Wilson, C. F., Burden, V., Nimmo-Smith, I., & Wilson, A. B. (2003). Behavioral Assessment of the Dysexecutive Syndrome in Children (BADS-C). San Antonio, TX: Pearson.

Epstein, J. N., Erkanli, A., Conners, C. K., Klaric, J., Costello, J. E., & Angold, A. (2003). Relations between Continuous Performance Test performance measures and ADHD behaviors. *Journal of Abnormal Child Psychology, 31*, 543–554.

Epstein, J. N., Langberg, J., Rosen, P. J., Graham, A., Narad, M. E., Antonini, T. N., et al. (2011). Evidence for higher reaction time variability for children with ADHD on a range of cognitive tasks including reward and event rate manipulations. *Neuropsychology, 25*, 427–441.

Eysenck, S. B. G., Easting, G., & Pearson, P. R. (1984). Age norms for impulsiveness, venturesomeness, and empathy in children. *Personality and Individual Differences, 5*, 315–321.

Fair, D. A., Bathula, D., Nikolas, M. A., & Nigg, J. T. (2013). Distinct neuropsychological subgroups in typically-developing youth inform heterogeneity in children with ADHD. *Proceedings of the National Academy of Sciences, 109*, 6769–6774.

Faraone, S. V., Biederman, J., Monuteaux, M. C., Doyle, A. E., & Seidman, L. J. (2001). A psychometric measure of learning disability predicts educational failure four years later in boys with attention-deficit/hyperactivity disorder. *Journal of Attention Disorders, 4*, 220–230.

Ferrin, M., & Vance, A. (2012). Examination of neurological subtle signs in ADHD as a clinical tool for the diagnosis and their relationship to spatial working memory. *Journal of Child Psychology and Psychiatry, 53*, 290–400.

Frazier, T. W., Demaree, H. A., & Youngstrom, E. A. (2004). Meta-analysis of intellectual and neuropsychological test performance in attention-deficit/hyperactivity disorder. *Neuropsychology, 18*, 543–555.

Fried, R., Hirshfield-Becker, D., Petty, C., Batchelder, H., & Biederman, J. (2012). How informative is the CANTAB to assess executive functioning in children with ADHD?

A controlled study. *Journal of Attention Disorders*. doi:10.1177/1087054712457038. Published online 24 August 2012.

Fuster, J. M. (1997). Network memory. *Trends in Neuroscience, 20*, 451–459.

Gau, S. S., & Chiang, H. (2013). Association between early attention-deficit/hyperactivity symptoms and current verbal and visuo-spatial short-term memory. *Research in Developmental Disabilities, 34*, 710–720.

Gioia, G. A., Isquick, P. K., Guy, S., & Kenworthy, L. (2000). BRIEF: Behavior Rating Inventory of Executive Function. Lutz, FL: PAR

Gooch, D., Snowling, M., & Hulme, C. (2012). Reaction time variability in children with ADHD symptoms and/or dyslexia. *Developmental Neuropsychology, 37*, 453–472.

Gordon, M. (1983). *The Gordon Diagnostic System*. DeWitt, NY: Gordon Systems.

Graziano, P. A., McNamara, J. P., Geffken, G. R., & Reid, A. M. (2013). Differentiating co-occurring behavior problems in children with ADHD: Patterns of emotional reactivity and executive functioning. *Journal of Attention Disorders, 17*, 249–260.

Gremillion, M. L., & Martel, M. M. (2013). Semantic language as a mechanism explaining the association between ADHD symptoms and reading and mathematics underachievement. *Journal of Abnormal Child Psychology, 40*, 1339–1349.

Gusnard, D. A., & Raichle, M. E. (2001). Searching for a baseline: Functional imaging and the resting human brain. *Nature Reviews Neuroscience, 2*, 685–694.

Halperin, J. M., & Schultz, K. P. (2006). Revisiting the role of the prefrontal cortex in the pathophysiology of attention-deficit/hyperactivity disorder (ADHD). *Psychological Bulletin, 132*, 560–581.

Halperin, J. M., Trampush, J. W., Miller, C. J., Marks, D. J., & Newcorn, J. H. (2008). Neuropsychological outcome in adolescents/young adults with childhood ADHD: Profiles of persisters, remitters and controls. *Journal of Child Psychology and Psychiatry, 49*, 958–966.

Hasson, R., & Fine, J. D. (2012). Gender differences among children with ADHD on continuous performance tests: A meta-analytic review. *Journal of Attention Disorders, 16*, 190–198.

Huang-Pollock, C. L., Karalunas, S. L., Tam, H., & Moore, A. N. (2012). Evaluating vigilance deficits in ADHD: A meta-analysis of CPT performance. *Journal of Abnormal Psychology, 121*, 360–371.

Hutchinson, E., Bavin, E., Efron, D., & Sciberras, E. (2012). A comparison of working memory profiles in school-aged children with specific language impairment, attention deficit/hyperactivity disorder, comorbid SLI and ADHD and their typically developing peers. *Child Neuropsychology, 18*, 190–207.

Jarrett, M. A., Wolff, J. C., Davis, T. E., III, Cowart, M. J., & Ollendick, T. H. (2012). Characteristics of children with ADHD and comorbid anxiety. *Journal of Attention Disorders*. doi:10.1177/1087054712452914. Published online 3 August 2012.

Karalunas, S. L., Huang-Pollock, C. L., & Nigg, J. T. (2012). Decomposing attention-deficit/hyperactivity disorder (ADHD)-related effects in response speed and variability. *Neuropsychology, 26*, 684–694.

Karalunas, S. L., & Huang-Pollock, C. L. (2013). Integrating impairments in reaction time and executive function using a diffusion model framework. *Journal of Abnormal Child Psychology, 41*, 837–850.

Kasper, L. J., Alderson, R. M., & Hudec, K. L. (2012). Moderators of working memory deficits in children with attention-deficit/hyperactivity disorder (ADHD): A meta-analytic review. *Clinical Psychology Review, 32*, 605–617.

Klotz, J. M., Johnson, M. D., Wu, S. W., Isaacs, K. M., & Gilbert, D. L. (2012). Relationship between reaction time variability and motor skill development in ADHD. *Child Neuropsychology, 18*, 576–585.

Korkman, M., Kirk, U., & Kemp, S. (1998). *NEPSY: A developmental neuropsychological assessment.* San Antonio, TX: Psychological Corporation.

Kuntsi, J., & Klein, C. (2011). Intraindividual variability in ADHD and its implications for research of causal links. In C. Stanford, & R. Tannock (Eds.), *Behavioral neuroscience of attention deficit hyperactivity disorder and its treatment, current topics in behavioral neurosciences* (9 ed.) (pp. 67–91). Berlin/Heidelberg: Springer-Verlag.

Lahey, B. B., Pelham, W. E., Jr., Loney, J., Lee, S. S., & Willcutt, E. G. (2005). Instability of the DSM-IV subtypes of ADHD from preschool through elementary school. *Archives of General Psychiatry, 62*, 896–902.

Leslie, L., & Caldwell, J. (2001). *Qualitative Reading Inventory—3.* New York: Addison Wesley Longman, Inc.

Leth-Steensen, C., Elbaz, Z. K., & Douglas, V. I. (2000). Mean response times, variability, and skew in the responding of ADHD children: A response time distributional approach. *Acta psychologica, 104*, 167–190.

Lin, Y., Lai, M., & Gau, S. S. (2012). Youths with ADHD with and without tic disorders: Comorbid psychopathology, executive function and social adjustment. *Research in Developmental Disabilities, 33*, 951–963.

Lindgren, S. D., & Koeppl, G. K. (1987). Assessing child behavior problems in a medical setting: Development of the Pediatric Behavior Scale. In R. J. Prinz (Ed.), *Advances in behavioral assessment of children and families* (pp. 57–90). Greenwich, CT: JAI.

Losier, B. J., McGrath, P. J., & Klein, R. M. (1996). Error patterns on the continuous performance test in non-medicated and medicated samples of children with and without ADHD: A meta-analytic review. *Journal of Child Psychology and Psychiatry, 37*, 971–978.

Lundervold, A. J., Stickert, M., Hysing, M., Sørensen, L., Gillberk, C., & Posserud, M. (2012). Attention deficits in children with combined autism and ADHD: A CPT study. *Journal of Attention Disorders.* doi:10.1177/1087054712453168. Published online 31 August 2012.

Marks, D. J., Berwid, O. G., Santra, A., Kera, E. A., Cyrulnik, S. E., & Halperin, J. M. (2005). Neuropsychological correlates of AD/HD symptoms in preschoolers. *Neuropsychology, 19*, 446–455.

Martel, M. M., Roberts, B., & Gremillion, M. L. (2013). Emerging control and disruptive behavior disorders during early childhood. *Developmental Neuropsychology, 38*, 153–166.

Martinussen, R., Hayden, J., Hogg-Johnson, S., Tannock, R. (2005). A meta-analysis of working memory impairments in children with attention-deficit/hyperactivity disorder. *Journal of the American Academy of Child & Adolescent Psychiatry, 44*, 377–384.

Mattes, J. A. (1980). The role of frontal lobe dysfunction in childhood hyperkinesis. *Comparative Psychology, 21*, 358–369.

Mattison, R. E., & Mayes, S. D. (2013). Relationships between learning disability, executive function, and psychopathology in children with ADHD. *Journal of Attention Disorders, 16*, 138–146.

Max, J. E., Lansing, A. E., Castillo, C. S., Bokura, H., Schachar, R., Collings, N., et al. (2004). Attention deficit hyperactivity disorder in children and adolescents following traumatic brain injury. *Developmental Neuropsychology, 25*, 159–177.

Mayes, S. D., & Calhoun, S. L. (2013). Frequency of reading, math, and writing disabilities in children with clinical disorders. *Learning and Individual Differences, 16*, 145–157.

Mayes, S. D., Calhoun, S. L., Mayes, R. D., & Molitoris, S. (2012). Autism and ADHD: Overlapping and discriminating symptoms. *Research in Autism Spectrum Disorders, 6*, 277–285.

Metin, B., Roeyers, H., Wiersema, J. R., & van der Meere, J. J. (2012). A meta-analytic study of event rare effects on go/no-go performance in attention-deficit/hyperactivity disorder. *Biological Psychiatry, 72*, 990–996.

Metin, B., Roeyers, H., Wiersema, J. R., van der Meere, J. J., Thompson, M., & Sonuga-Barke, E. J. (2013). ADHD performance reflects inefficient but not impulsive information processing: A diffusion model analysis. *Neuro, 27*, 193–200.

Miller, A. C., & Keenan, J. M. (2009). How word reading skill impacts text memory: The centrality deficit and how domain knowledge can compensate. *Annals of Dyslexia, 59*, 99–113.

Miller, A. C., Keenan, J. M., Betjemann, R. S., Willcutt, E. G., Pennington, B. F., & Olson, R. K. (2013). Reading comprehension in children with ADHD: Cognitive underpinnings of the centrality deficit. *Journal of Abnormal Child Psychology, 41*, 473–483.

Miller, C. J., Newcorn, J. H., & Halperin, J. M. (2010). Fading memories: Retrospective recall inaccuracies in ADHD. *Journal of Attention Disorders, 14*, 7–14.

Miranda, M. C., Barbosa, R., Muszkat, M., Rodrigues, C. C., Sinnes, E. G., Coelho, L. F. S., et al. (2013). Performance patterns in Conners' CPT among children with attention deficit hyperactivity disorder and dyslexia. *Arquivos de Neuro-Psiquiatria, 70*, 91–96.

Munkvold, L. H., Manger, T., & Lundervold, A. J. (2014). Conners' continuous performance test (CCPT-II) in children with ADHD, ODD, or a combined ADHD/ODD diagnosis. *Child Neuropsychology, 20*(1), 106–126. doi:10.1080/09297049.20 12.753997.

Nigg, J. T., Willcutt, E. G., Doyle, A. E., & Sonuga-Barke, E. J. (2005). Causal heterogeneity in attention-deficit/hyperactivity disorder: Do we need neuropsychologically impaired subtypes? *Biological Psychiatry, 57*, 1224–1230.

Nikolas, M. A., & Nigg, J. T. (2013). Neuropsychological performance and attention-deficit hyperactivity disorder subtypes and symptom dimensions. *Neuropsychology, 27*, 107–120.

Ornstein, T. J., Max, J. E., Schachar, R., Dennise, M., Barnes, M., Ewing-Cobbs, L., et al. (2013). Response inhibition in children with and without ADHD after traumatic brain injury. *Journal of Neuropsychology, 7*, 1–11.

Papaeliou, C. F., Maniadaki, K., & Kakouros, E. (2012). Association between story recall and other language abilities in schoolchildren with ADHD. *Journal of Attention Disorders*. 2012 Jul 26. [Epub ahead of print]. PMID: 22837548

Payne, J. M., Arnold, S. S., Pride, N. A., & North, K. N. (2012). Does attention-deficit-hyperactivity disorder exacerbate executive dysfunction in children with neurofibromatosis type 1? *Developmental Medicine & Child Neurology, 54*, 898–904.

Payne, J. M., Hyman, S. L., Shores, E. A., & North, K. N. (2011). Assessment of executive function and attention in children with neurofibromatosis type 1: Relationships between cognitive measures and real-world behavior. *Child Neuropsychology, 17*, 313–329.

Pontius, A. A. (1973). Dysfunction patterns analogous to frontal lobe system and caudate nucleus syndromes in some groups of minimal brain dysfunction. *Journal of the American Medical Women's Association, 28*, 285–292.

Qian, Y., Shuai, L., Chan, R. C. K., Qian, Q., & Wang, Y. (2013). The developmental trajectories of executive function of children and adolescents with attention deficit hyperactivity disorder. *Research in Developmental Disabilities, 34*, 1434–1445.

Raiker, J. S., Rapport, M. D., Kofler, M. J., & Sarver, D. E. (2012). Objectively-measured impulsivity and attention-deficit/hyperactivity disorder (ADHD): Testing competing predictions from the working memory and behavioral inhibition models of ADHD. *Journal of Abnormal Child Psychology, 40*, 699–713.

Rajendran, K., Rindskopf, D., O'Neill, S., Marks, D. J., Nomura, Y., & Halperin, J. M. (2013a). Neuropsychological functioning and severity of ADHD in early childhood: A four-year cross-lagged study. *Journal of Abnormal Psychology*. 122 (4), 1179–1188.

Rajendran, K., Trampush, J. W., Rindskopf, D., Marks, D. J., O'Neill, S., & Halperin, J. M. (2013b). Association between variation in neuropsychological development and trajectory of ADHD severity in early childhood. *American Journal of Psychiatry, 170*(10), 1205–1211.

Rapport, M. D., Chung, K., Shore, G., & Isaacs, P. (2001). A conceptual model of child psychopathology: Implications for understanding attention deficit hyperactivity disorder and treatment efficacy. *Journal of Clinical Child Psychology, 30*, 48–58.

Ratcliff, R., & McKoon, G. (2008). The diffusion decision model: Theory and data for two-choice decision tasks. *Neural Computation, 20*, 813–922.

Rauch, W. A., Gold, A., & Schmitt, K. (2012). Combining cognitive and personality measures of impulse control in the assessment of childhood ADHD. *European Journal of Psychological Assessment, 28*, 208–215.

Rhodes, S. M., Park, J., Seth, S., & Coghill, D. R. (2012). A comprehensive investigation of memory impairment in attention deficit hyperactivity disorder and oppositional defiant disorder. *Journal of Child Psychology and Psychiatry, 53*, 128–137.

Robbins, T. W., James, M., Owen, A. M., Sahakian, B. J. L., & Rabbitt, P. (1994). Cambridge Neuropsychological Test Automated Battery (CANTAB): A factor analytic study of a large sample of normal elderly volunteers. *Dementia, 5*, 266–281.

Rommelse, N., Altink, M. E., De Sonneville, L. M., Buschgens, C. J., Buitelaar, J. K., Oosterlaan, J., et al. (2007). Are motor inhibition and cognitive flexibility dead ends in ADHD? *Journal of Abnormal Child Psychology, 35*, 957–967.

Rosch, K. S., Dirlikov, B., & Mostofsky, S. H. (2013). Increased intrasubject variability in boys with ADHD across tests of motor and cognitive control. *Journal of Abnormal Child Psychology, 41*, 485–495.

Rothbart, M. K., Ahadi, S. A., Hershey, K. L., & Fisher, P. (2001). Investigations of temperament at three to seven years: The Children's Behavior Questionnaire. *Child Development, 72*, 1394–1408.

Rueda, M. R., Fan, J., McCandliss, B. D., Halparin, J. D., Gruber, D. B., Lercari, L. P., et al. (2004). Development of attentional networks in childhood. *Neuropsychologia, 42*, 1029–1040.

Salcedo-Marin, M. D., Moreno-Granados, J. M., Ruiz-Veguilla, M., & Ferrin, M. (2013). Evaluation of planning dysfunction in attention deficits hyperactivity disorder and autistic spectrum disorders using the Zoo Map Task. *Child Psychiatry and Human Development, 44*, 166–185.

Salum, G. A., Sergeant, J. A., Sonuga-Barke, E. J., Vandekerckhove, J., Gadelha, A., Pan, P. M., et al. (2013). Specificity of basic information processing and inhibitory control in attention deficit hyperactivity disorder. *Psychological Medicine*. 2013 Apr 8:1–15. [Epub ahead of print].

Schoemaker, K., Bunte, T., Wiebe, S. A., Espy, K. A., Dekovic, M., & Matthys, W. (2012). Executive function deficits in preschool children with ADHD and DBD. *Journal of Child Psychology and Psychiatry, 53,* 111–119.

Sergeant, J. A. (2000). The cognitive-energetic approach to attention deficit hyperactivity disorder. *Neuroscience & Biobehavioral Reviews, 24,* 7–12.

Sergeant, J. A. (2005). Modeling attention-deficit/hyperactivity disorder: A critical appraisal of the cognitive-energetic model. *Biological Psychiatry 57,* 1248–1255.

Shields, A., & Cicchetti, D. (1997). Emotion regulation among school-age children: The development and validation of a new criterion Q-sort scale. *Developmental Psychology, 33,* 906–916.

Shiels, K., Tamm, L., & Epstein, J. N. (2012). Deficient post-error slowing in children with ADHD is limited to the inattentive subtype. *Journal of the International Neuropsychological Society, 18,* 612–617.

Shimoni, M., Engel-Yeger, B., & Tirosh, E. (2012). Executive dysfunctions among boys with attention deficit hyperactivity disorder (ADHD): Performance-based test and parents report. *Research in Developmental Disabilities, 33,* 858–865.

Shue, K. L., & Douglas, V. I. (1992). Attention deficit hyperactivity disorder and the frontal lobe syndrome. *Brain and Cognition, 20,* 104–124.

Sjöwall, D., Roth, L., Lindqvist, S., & Thorell, L. B. (2013). Multiple deficits in ADHD: Executive dysfunction, delay aversion, reaction time variability, and emotional deficits. *Journal of Child Psychology and Psychiatry,* 54(6):619–27.

Skogli, E. W., Egeland, J., Andersen, P. N., Hovik, K. T., & Øie, M. (2013). Few differences in hot and cold executive functions in children and adolescents with combined and inattentive subtypes of ADHD. *Child Neuropsychology.* 2013 Jan 2. [Epub ahead of print]. PMID: 23281923

Sonuga-Barke, E. J. (2003). The dual pathway model of AD/HD: An elaboration of neuro-developmental characteristics. *Neuroscience & Biobehavioral Reviews, 27,* 593–604.

Sonuga-Barke, E. J., & Castellanos, F. X. (2007). Spontaneous attentional fluctuations in impaired states and pathological conditions: A neurobiological hypothesis. *Neuroscience & Biobehavioral Reviews, 31,* 977–986.

Sparrow, S. S., Cicchetti, D., & Balla, D. A. (2005). *Vineland Adaptive Behavior Scales.* (2 ed.) Circle Pines, MN: AGS Publishing.

Strand, M. T., Hawk, L. W., Jr., Bubnik, M., Shiels, K., Pelham, W. E., Jr., & Waxmonsky, J. G. (2012). Improving working memory in children with attention-deficit/hyperactivity disorder: The separate and combined effects of incentives and stimulant medication. *Journal of Abnormal Child Psychology, 40,* 1193–1207.

Takács, Á., Kóbor, A., Tárnok, Z., & Csépe, V. (2014). Verbal fluency in children with ADHD: Strategy using and temporal properties. *Child Neuropsychology, 20*(4), 415–429.

Tamm, L., Narad, M. E., Antonini, T. N., O'Brien, K. M., Hawk, L. W., Jr., & Epstein, J. N. (2012). Reaction time variability in ADHD: A review. *Neurotherapeutics, 9,* 500–508.

Taylor, E., Schachar, R., Thorley, G., & Wieselberg, M. (1986). Conduct disorder and hyperactivity: I. Separation of hyperactivity and antisocial conduct in British child psychiatric patients. *British Journal of Psychiatry, 149,* 760–767.

Thaler, N. S., Bello, D. T., & Etcoff, L. M. (2012). WISC-IV profiles are associated with differences in symptomatology and outcome in children with ADHD. *Journal of Attention Disorders, 17*, 291–301.

Toplak M. E., Rucklidge, J. J., Hetherington, R., John, S. C., & Tannock, R. (2003). Time perception deficits in attention-deficit/hyperactivity disorder and comorbid reading difficulties in child and adolescent samples. *Journal of Child Psychology and Psychiatry, 44*, 888–903.

Tseng, W., & Gau, S. S. (2013). Executive function as a mediator in the link between attention-deficit/hyperactivity disorder and social problems. *Journal of Child Psychology and Psychiatry, 54*(9), 996–1004.

Udal, A. H., Øygarden, B., Egeland, J., Malt, E. F., Løvdahl, H., Pripp, A. H., et al. (2012a). Executive deficits in early onset bipolar disorder versus ADHD: Impact of processing speed and lifetime psychosis. *Clinical Child Psychology and Psychiatry, 18*, 284–299.

Udal, A. H., Øygarden, B., Egeland, J., Malt, E. F., & Grøholt, B. (2012b). Memory in early onset bipolar disorder and attention-deficit/hyperactivity disorder: Similarities and differences. *Journal of Abnormal Child Psychology, 40*, 1179–1192.

Vance, A., Ferrin, M., Winther, J., & Gomez, R. (2013). Examination of spatial working memory performance in children and adolescents with attention deficit hyperactivity disorder, combined type (ADHD-CT) and anxiety. *Journal of Abnormal Child Psychology, 41*, 891–900.

Walg, M., Oepen, J., & Prior, H. (2012). Adjustment of time perception in the range of seconds and milliseconds: The nature of time-processing alterations in children with ADHD. *Journal of Attention Disorders*. 2012 Jul 30. [Epub ahead of print]. PMID: 22851208

Ware, A. L., Crocker, N., O'Brien, J. W., Deweese, B. N., Roesch, S. C., Coles, C. D., et al. (2012). Executive function predicts adaptive behavior in children with histories of heavy prenatal alcohol exposure and attention-deficit/hyperactivity disorder. *Alcoholism: Clinical and Experimental Research, 36*, 1431–1441.

Weissman, A. S., Chu, B. C., Reddy, L. A., & Mohlman, J. (2012). Attention mechanisms in children with anxiety disorders and in children with attention deficit hyperactivity disorder: Implications for research and practice. *Journal of Clinical Child and Adolescent Psychology, 41*(2), 117–126.

White, T., Mous, S., & Karatekin, C. (2013). Memory-guided saccades in youth-onset psychosis and attention deficit hyperactivity disorder (ADHD). *Early Intervention in Psychiatry*. 2013 Feb 28. doi:10.1111/eip.12038. [Epub ahead of print]

Willcutt, E. G., Doyle, A. E., Nigg, J. T., Faraone, S. V., & Pennington, B. F. (2005). Validity of the executive function theory of attention-deficit/hyperactivity disorder: A meta-analytic review. *Biological Psychiatry, 57*, 1336–1346.

Woodcock, R. W., McGrew, K. S., & Mather, N. (2001). Examiner's manual. In *Woodcock-Johnson III Tests of Achievement*. Itasca, IL: Riverside.

Yang, P., Cheng, C., Chang, C., Liu, T., Hsu, H., & Yen, C. (2013). Wechsler Intelligence Scale for Children 4th edition-Chinese version index scores in Taiwanese children with attention-deficit/hyperactivity disorder. *Psychiatry and Clinical Neurosciences, 67*, 83–91.

Yang, T., Huang, K., Chen, S., Chang, H., Yang, H., & Guo, Y. (2013). Correlation between clinical manifestations of nocturnal enuresis and attentional performance in children with attention deficit hyperactivity disorder (ADHD). *Journal of the Formosan Medical Association, 112,* 41–47.

Yañez-Téllez, G., Romero-Romero, H., Rivera-García, L., Prieto-Corona, B., Bernal-Hernández, J., Marosi-Holczberger, E., et al. (2013). Cognitive and executive functions in ADHD. *Actas Españolas de Psiquiatría, 40,* 293–298.

Zelazo, P. D., & Müller, U. (2002). Executive function in typical and atypical development. In U. Goswami (Ed.), *Handbook of childhood cognitive development* (pp. 445–469). Oxford: Blackwell.

7

NEUROPSYCHOLOGY OF ATTENTION

An Update

Diane B. Howieson

INTRODUCTION

Not just one, but multiple cognitive processes are activated during any behavior. As examples, speed of information processing, working memory capacity, and executive functions influence attention and the associations are bidirectional. Attention, in turn, affects memory and other downstream cognitive processes. This chapter discusses the particular relationships of attention with other aspects of cognition. It is beyond the scope of this chapter to review these cognitive functions in other contexts. Although attention is divided into a number of types, multiple types of attention are deployed to perform the cognitive tests described in this chapter. As much as possible, the tests are discussed in relation to the dominant type of attention necessary for test success.

HISTORICAL BACKGROUND

The concept of attention exists throughout the ages. The systematic study of attention started in the 19th and early 20th centuries with the emerging discipline of experimental psychology. The Stroop task, frequently used to this day to measure the effects of interference on attention, was developed in 1935 (Stroop, 1935). By the 1950s researchers were interested in learning how the brain regulates attention in real time. Hubel, Henson, Rupert, and Galambos (1959), using single-cell recordings from a cat's cortex, identified cells that responded only when the cat paid attention to a sound source. Soon after evoked responses in humans were being used to record cortical areas responsive to attention (Haider et al., 1964). Patients with focal brain injuries resulting from stroke, tumors, or penetrating brain injuries have offered opportunities to explore the role of specific brain areas for attention (Robertson & Rafal, 2000). Studies exploring various aspects of attention have escalated since the 1980s along with the growth of interest in experimental and clinical neuropsychology.

Since the 1990s major advances have occurred with the advent of functional neuro-imaging and other new technologies that allow for a study of brain networks involved in attention. The influential work of Petersen and Posner (2012) and Posner's book *Cognitive Neuroscience of Attention* (Posner, 2012) present a comprehensive review of current models of attention. The basic model proposes that three networks control attention: (1) an alerting network that supports sustained vigilance; (2) an orient-ing network; and (3) an executive network that regulates attention processes, such as selective attention, set shifting, conflict resolution, and inhibitory control. The ever-increasing research on attention is understandable given the central importance of attention for behavior.

ATTENTION COMPONENTS

Many tests of attention are computer based because of the ability to measure small differences accurately in response speed and consistency in a standardized fashion.

Alertness

Alertness is often described as watchfulness of the environment in expectation of an event. This anticipation is also termed readiness, responsivity, or vigilance. Typically, alertness is measured by how fast a person responds to a stimulus. The presence of the warning signal facilitates reactions, often measured as reaction time. Alerting cues are particularly beneficial when examining individuals at their off-peak time of day (Knight & Mather, 2013). Excessively high states of alertness can result in increased errors when responses are based on information not com-pletely processed (Posner, 1978).

Orienting

Orienting is a form of attention that prioritizes sensory input by selecting a modality or location (Peterson & Posner, 2012). The role of orienting is well illustrated by the observation that patients with damage to certain brain areas, particularly in the right hemisphere, may fail to orient or respond to a stimulus in the opposite side of space despite intact sensory and motor abilities (Heilman, Watson, & Valenstein, 2012). Testing for orienting often compare the speed of responding when a person is given a spatial cue where the impending stimulus will appear (e.g., the left or the right side of the screen). With spatial cues, response times are faster in the cued direction, than when no cue is given. When the cue opposes the correct direction, response times are slowed. The type of stimulus also affects orienting as demonstrated by the find-ing that socially relevant stimuli (e.g., faces) enhance orienting (Federico et al., 2013). Once attention is directed to a location, normal subjects have a reduced probability of returning attention to the already examined locations (Posner, Rafal, Choate, & Vaughan, 1988), although the size of this phenomenon depends on such variables as target duration and the presence of an intervening event (Martin-Arévalo, Chica, & Lupianez, 2013).

Although counterintuitive, there is evidence to suggest that alerting and orienting can occur without awareness. In one study, a high-frequency flicker that did not produce conscious awareness nevertheless produced alerting and orienting effects (Lu et al., 2012). In another paradigm, attention was directed to the naturally anticipated location of a subliminally moving target showing that an object can still attract attention in the absence of awareness (Hsieh & Colas, 2012). In this experiment subjects were presented with a subliminal moving cue and asked to indicate the orientation of a stimulus at the naturally anticipated location of the cue's trajectory and at off-trajectory locations. The subliminal moving cue enhanced subjects' performance on this orientation-discrimination task. Discriminability at locations in the vicinity of the final position of the cue was significantly better than at distal locations, showing that a moving object can still attract attention when presented subliminally (Hsieh & Colas, 2012). Subjects' ability to guess whether or not the cue was present did not differ from chance.

Sustained Attention

Sustained attention requires maintaining alertness and focus over time, which is important for many everyday tasks. Some occupations are defined by sustained attention, such as air traffic control. Tests designed to measure sustained attention often require response to every occurrence of an irregular appearing stimulus. Success requires freedom from distractions. Adding a nontarget distractor makes the task more difficult. Response accuracy, speed, and consistency serve as measures of sustained attention. Because maintaining focus during monotonous and repetitive tasks is more difficult than cognitively challenging ones, most continuous performance tests are lengthy and intentionally boring (Robertson & O'Connell, 2010). The Continuous Performance Test II (Conners, 2000) is a repetitive, monotonous task taking 14 minutes to complete. Using the Sustained Attention to Response Task, which requires withholding key presses to one of nine target stimuli, researchers showed that excessive daytime sleepiness can hinder performance (Van Schie et al., 2012). Sustaining attention over short intervals can be a problem as, for example, when attentional shifts lead to mind wandering (Smallwood, 2013). Many elders complain that they go into a room to do something, but forget why they are there because their thoughts have moved on.

Divided Attention

The attention system has limited capacity so that attention to one stimulus or task can interfere with attending to another (Lavie, 2001). Studies have shown that performing a cognitive task while walking (Camicioli, Howieson, Lehman, & Kaye, 1997) or stepping (Zheng et al., 2012) slows motor performance and may contribute to falls in the elderly. In this era of media multitasking, researchers studied whether frequent use of multiple forms of media simultaneously, such as television, telephone or text messaging, and video games, has a beneficial or detrimental affect on attention. Researchers studied the effect of media multitasking experience on one's ability to perform two tasks simultaneously and to switch between two tasks using a reaction time task (Alzahabi & Becker, 2013). Subjects viewed a number and a letter on a screen and indicated whether the number was odd or even and whether the letter was a consonant or a vowel. In the dual-task condition the participants were asked to classify both the number and letter on each trial. In the task-switch condition, a cue for each trial indicated whether the number or letter was to be classified. In this study, heavy media multitaskers were not better at the dual task but they were better able to switch between tasks in the task-switching condition. Not all results coming from this relatively young area of research are consistent. In a previous study using similar procedures heavy media multitaskers were worse at task switching (Ophir, Nass, & Wagner, 2009).

Executive Control of Attention

More challenging demands on attention require using executive control of attention. Control may involve selecting where attention is guided while avoiding distractions, shifting attention as appropriate, directing attention away from an engaging but nontarget stimulus, or all of these according to personal goals. Executive dysfunction can influence many aspects of behavior and impairments observed on attention tests may be representative of broader cognitive problems.

Selective Attention

Selective attention is the active directing of attention to a stimulus and often involves ignoring irrelevant stimuli. Under conditions of simultaneous presentation of similar and dissimilar visual and auditory stimuli with instructions to attend to one and not the other, researchers found slower response times when the stimuli were dissimilar (Donohue, Todisco, & Woldorff, 2013). This finding was interpreted as showing that attention was captured by the incongruent irrelevant modality rather than the relevant modality. The authors concluded that selective attention is often unable to filter out distracting stimuli from another modality.

So-called "flanker" tests measure spatial selective attention. A target stimulus is accompanied on a screen by nontarget stimuli. A common setup presents a fixation point on a screen followed by a row of five arrows, and respondents are instructed to indicate the direction of the central arrow (Figure 7.1). The reaction times for responding to the target when the accompanying stimuli are congruent versus incongruent are compared. The task assesses the ability to selectively focus while ignoring irrelevant stimuli.

The Attention Network Test (ANT; Fan et al., 2002) is a flanker task using five arrows as shown in Figure 7.1; the task is to indicate whether the central arrow points

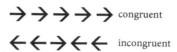

FIG 7.1 Flanker test. The top row shows that the target and nontarget items point in the same direction (congruent stimuli), whereas the bottom row shows that the directions for the target and nontarget are conflicting (incongruent stimuli).

left or right. For this test trials are either cued or uncued and stimuli are either congruent, incongruent, or neutral in which a center arrow is flanked by horizontal lines. Reaction times are compared for the various combinations of conditions. Alerting is measured by comparing conditions in which a cue appears on the screen indicating that a target will soon follow to trials with no cues. The orienting condition compares trials with spatial cues indicating whether the arrows will appear above or below a fixation point to trials with no spatial cues. Executive control compares trials with congruent and incongruent flankers. Responses are fastest when trials are cued and the distractors are either neutral or congruent with the target (Fan et al., 2002; Weinbach & Henik, 2012). Looking at data from intact adults, a high split-half reliability was reported for all conditions (Mahoney et al., 2010), although another report found the reliability of executive control was moderately high while alerting and orienting measures had low reliability (MacLeod et al., 2010). Using more trials increases the reliability of network scores (Ishigami & Klein, 2011). The reliabilities of both orienting and executive control were good in a study of patients with multiple sclerosis (MS) with repeated administrations over 6 months (Ishigami, Fisk, Wojtowicz, & Klein, 2013). An ANT-Revised (Fan et al., 2009) was designed to examine the additional effect of manipulating whether or not the spatial cue provides information about the direction of the target. The researchers found that a valid spatial cue enhanced response speed and an invalid cue slowed response speed, thereby having the expected negative effect on executive control.

The NIH-TB Flanker Inhibition Control and Attention Test (Weintraub et al., 2013) is a flanker test similar to the ANT. It was selected because this brief test (takes about 4 minutes) measures ability to focus, select, sustain, and shift attention. These operations important for daily functioning are impaired in neuropsychological disorders, such as attention-deficit/hyperactivity disorder (ADHD), and are mediated by well-studied, distributed large-scale neuroanatomic networks, described later. The task presents a fixation point on a screen followed by a row of five arrows. The patient is instructed to indicate the direction of the central arrow (Figure 7.1). The scoring integrates accuracy and reaction time differences between trials with congruent and incongruent flankers. Clinical data from this newly released test have not been reported but age effects have been demonstrated (Figure 7.2).

Set Shifting

Often daily situations require that attention shift among stimuli, such as monitoring traffic while driving. Studies of attention shifting often ask participants to switch

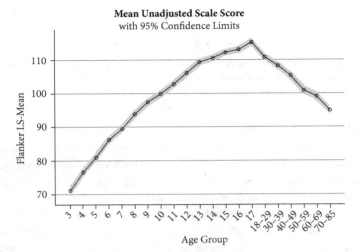

Mean Unadjusted Scale Score
with 95% Confidence Limits

FIG 7.2 The NIH-TB Flanker Inhibition Control and Attention Test least square means by age group.

From the National Institutes of Health and Northwestern University, with permission.

attention between two or more types of stimuli. In a study described previously, subjects viewed a number and a letter on a screen and indicated whether the number was odd or even and whether the letter was a consonant or a vowel (Alzahabi & Becker, 2013). In the task-switch condition, a cue for each trial indicated whether the number or letter was to be classified. In this study, heavy media multitaskers were better at switching between tasks than light media multitaskers.

Conflict and Inhibitory Control

Some situations require attending to stimuli that are not the most prominent or most frequent. Paradigms for testing inhibitory control include classic "go/no-go" tasks. The no-go items are infrequent or they require inhibiting a prepotent response. Flanker tests measure inhibitory control by assessing the ability to ignore distracting stimuli.

Several continuous performance tests have a condition that requires withholding responses to infrequent nontarget items. The Sustained Attention to Response test described previously has such a condition. About 20% of the numbers that appear on a screen are items that should not elicit a response. Evidence suggests that this test places higher demands on response inhibition than sustained attention (Carter, Russell, & Helton, 2013). The soon to be released Continuous Performance Test III has a new ratio of nontargets to targets to improve the test's sensitivity to impulsivity problems and has a new impulsivity score. The use of target and nontarget stimuli allows for measures of commission as well as omission with these tests. As expected, speed-accuracy trade-offs affect performance on these tasks (Seli et al., 2013).

ATTENTION NETWORKS

Advances in functional imaging techniques have begun to uncover the complex set of interactions within networks of brain regions that direct attention and thereby mental processes. Much of the work has involved studying attention to visual stimuli. Visual tasks are easier to manipulate for research purposes compared to other modalities, although similarities exist across stimulus modalities (Sturm & Willmes, 2001). Three major attention systems have been proposed: (1) alerting, (2) orienting, and (3) executive control (Fan et al., 2009). According to current models, alerting is been associated with activity of thalamic, frontal, and parietal regions. Orienting is associated with superior and inferior parietal lobes; frontal eye fields; and subcortical areas including the superior colliculi, the pulvinar, and reticular nuclei of the thalamus.

Selective attention has been shown to involve two sets of regions in the dorsal and ventral frontoparietal cortex that are recruited under varying conditions (Corbetta, Patel, & Shulman, 2008). When selective attention based on internal goals or expectations is engaged, a bilateral dorsal network is activated involving the frontoparietal regions, frontal eye fields, and the middle temporal complex. This system is often described as top-down control of attention.

To be adaptive, attention must disengage and change focus so that new relevant stimuli can be monitored. Under these conditions, a second, largely right-hemisphere ventral network involving the frontoparietal regions, the temporoparietal junction, the ventral frontal cortex, and insula is coactivated so that attention is reoriented to a behaviorally relevant environmental stimulus, such as an unexpected loud noise (Corbetta et al., 2008). This bottom-up attention system interacts with the top-down system to allow for adaptive control of attention (Figure 7.3). Dysfunction of these networks appears important for the phenomenon of spatial neglect or inattention (Corbetta & Shulman, 2011; Rengachary, He, Shulman, & Corbetta, 2011).

A similar network has been described for sustained attention on monotonous tasks that use mainly right-sided regions including dorsomedial, mid- and ventrolateral prefrontal cortex, anterior insula, parietal areas including the temporoparietal junction, and subcortical structures (Langner & Eickhoff, 2013). Based on a review of functional neuroimaging data, these authors conclude that sustained attention involves mixtures of top-down control processes related to task maintenance and transient stimulus-driven, bottom-up processes related to target-driven reorienting of attention as needed. As such, sustained attention for boring tasks is a multicomponent process.

When adaptive attention requires detecting and resolving conflict, the anterior cingulate cortex (Bush, Luu, & Posner, 2000; Petersen & Posner, 2012), anterior insula (Sridharan, Levitin, & Menon, 2008), and lateral prefrontal cortex are involved (Fan et al., 2003; Matsumoto & Tanaka, 2004). For instance, functional imaging studies have shown that the anterior cingulate cortex plays a role in Stroop performance (Mead et al., 2002; Ravnkilde et al., 2002).

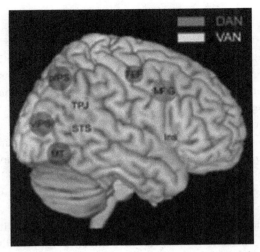

FIG 7.3 Regions of interest are colored according to whether they belong to the dorsal attention network (DAN) or ventral attention network (VAN). Doral areas include frontal eye fields (FEF), posterior intraparietal sulcus (pIPS), ventral intraparietal sulcus (vIPS), and middle temporal region (MT). Ventral areas are temporal parietal junction (TPJ), superior temporal sulcus (STS), and insula (Ins). The hatched pattern of the middle frontal gyrus (MFG) indicates that activation of this region is correlated with both attention networks.

Adapted from Ptak and Schnider (2011), The attention network of the human brain: Relating structural damage associated with spatial neglect to functional imaging correlates of spatial attention, *Neuropsychologia, 49,* 3063–3070, with permission from Elsevier, Copyright (2011) and the author.

ATTENTION DISORDERS IN CLINICAL SYNDROMES

Aging

Psychomotor slowing and slowed cognitive processing can account for much of the measured changes in performance that decline with age (Lezak, Howieson, Bigler, & Trahan, 2012). Any attention test requiring speed will put older adults at a disadvantage. Alerting and orienting are relatively intact in older adults (Mahoney et al., 2010) but age-related changes have been observed on alerting tasks in some cases (Jennings, Dagenbach, Engle, & Funke, 2007; Zhou et al., 2011). The greatest age-related changes are on tasks requiring executive control. Selective attention abilities of older adults were tested by examining their ability to ignore words superimposed on a picture, or visa versa, in a 1-back task. Older adults were more distracted than younger adults by the overlapping words during the 1-back task, and they subsequently showed more priming for these words on an implicit memory task (Campbell, Grady, Ng, & Hasher, 2012). Older adults' performance on a selective attention task also was adversely affected compared to younger adults by increasing stimulus (visual) load, although older adults benefited from cueing more in the high than low visual load condition (Muller-Oehring et al., 2013). Age effects on the ANT have been greatest on the selective attention condition in which flanker arrows point in the opposite direction of the target arrow (Mahoney et al.,

2010; Zhou et al., 2011; Figure 7.2). These researchers have speculated that executive control is weaker in older adults because of the deteriorating prefrontal cortex function with increasing age. Reduced executive control of attention in older adults also has been linked with white matter pathology (Hedden et al., 2012).

Attention Deficit Disorder

ADHD is a developmental disorder characterized by excessive levels of inattention, hyperactivity, impulsiveness, or a combination of these problems. Although expressed in childhood, it endures into adulthood in about 65% of adults diagnosed as children, although often in a lesser form (Faraone, Biederman, & Mick, 2006). In a meta-analytic review of adults with ADHD, moderate effect sizes were found for measures of sustained attention, selective attention, and response inhibition (Hervey, Epstein, & Curry, 2004). Attention deficits appear to stem from problems with executive functioning (Mapou, 2009). A comparison of adults with ADHD and other psychiatric disorders found that ADHD adults performed more poorly on set-shifting tasks: D-KEFS color-word switching, category switching, and the Navon Task (Holst & Thorell, 2013). Other group differences were observed for inhibition and fluency. Recent work has attempted to further refine the nature of the attention impairments in ADHD. Adults with ADHD were asked to identify two visual targets under conditions of distractors with visual crowding or no crowding (Stevens et al., 2012). Although the ADHD group was impaired relative to control subjects by the presence of nearby distractors, this interference appeared to result from failure to suppress distractors under conditions of perceptual interference rather than a problem with selective attention.

Another factor influencing attention performance is the ability to maintain multiple items in working memory, which constrains attention selection (Finke et al., 2011). In this study of the effect of working memory, the number of letters displayed on a screen constituted working memory load and adults with ADHD were unable to report more than three letters from working memory, whereas most subjects in the control group could report four. Memory acquisition also is affected. A meta-analytic review of adult ADHD concluded that memory deficits reflect deficient memory encoding but not retrieval or retention (Skodzik, Holling, & Pedersen, 2013). The authors conclude that the core encoding problem may result from impaired attention, executive functioning, working memory, or self-regulation.

Of the brain regions studied, the most consistent data identify the dorsal anterior cingulate cortex as dysfunctional in ADHD (Bush, 2010). Many other areas have been studied with particular emphasis on dysfunction of the lateral prefrontal cortex and the striatum. A meta-analytic review of functional magnetic resonance imaging studies of ADHD concluded that characteristic findings are hypoactivation in the frontoparietal executive control network, putamen, and ventral attention network as well as hyperactivation of the default network and visual circuits (Cortese et al., 2012).

Schizophrenia

Schizophrenia is a generally catastrophic mental disorder. Delusions and hallucinations are core features that cause inward directed attention. Abnormal attention, though not a defining sign, is a major feature. Yet attention disturbance is not confined to psychotic episodes (Wohlberg & Kornetsky, 1973), and deficits occur in most domains of attention. Disturbances in sustained and selective attention are well documented (Harvey & Keefe, 2009). Impairments are seen when the person with schizophrenia is confronted with excessive task demands or becomes overloaded with information (Cohen, Salloway, & Sweet, 2008). In studies using the ANT persons with schizophrenia performed as well as control subjects on the alerting and orienting conditions but were impaired on the conflict condition where flanker arrows pointed in the opposite direction of the target (Breton et al., 2011; Orellana, Slachevsky, & Pena, 2012). The findings were interpreted as showing that schizophrenia impairs executive control of attention, an interpretation supported by the additional finding of impairment on the Stroop conflict task (Breton et al., 2011). However, a different finding was obtained with a modified version of the ANT with an auditory alerting signal (Amado et al., 2011). Persons with schizophrenia were slower overall than control subjects but they benefited from the alerting effect in the incongruent flanker condition when their attention was validly oriented. Cognitive Neuroscience Treatment Research to Improve Cognition in Schizophrenia has divided selective attention into two components: input selection and rule selection (Luck, Ford, Sarter, & Lustig, 2012). The latter refers to creating a link between the selected input and the processing systems in which the implementation of attention will occur, for example storing stimulus input in memory or other response selection. One theory proposes that persons with schizophrenia are impaired with input selection but not rule selection. As a test of this theory, a schizophrenia group was compared to control subjects on a sustained attention task under conditions of either distraction or no distraction (Demeter et al., 2013). As predicted the schizophrenia group was disproportionally vulnerable to distraction. By contrast, patients' sustained attention without distraction was relatively unimpaired supporting the theory that input selection control is impaired in schizophrenia. Impaired speed of processing also is a major obstacle to control of attention for persons with schizophrenia (Dickinson, Ramsey, & Gold, 2007).

Traumatic Brain Injury

Problems with attention are common after traumatic brain injury (TBI), particularly with sustained and controlled attention. Impaired sustained attention may show up as inconsistency in performance over time. TBI patients performed worse than control subjects on the Psychomotor Vigilance Test with slower response times, increased response variability, and attention lapses (Sinclair, Ponsford, Rajaratnam, & Anderson, 2013). Abnormalities in sustained attention were seen in patients with moderate to severe TBI using a go/no-go sustained attention task (Kim et al., 2012).

In addition to impaired performance, cerebral blood flow was different between patients and control subjects at rest and on task. TBI patients also show deficits when executive control of attention is required. These researchers found, as others have, that slowed information processing appeared to contribute to poor attention performance. Impairment in Stroop performance was reported in severely head-injured patients an average of 9 months postinjury, supporting previous suggestions of executive control deficits (Merkley et al., 2013). Using the ANT, researchers found as expected that TBI patients compared to control subjects were impaired on the conflict resolution condition (Rodriguez-Bailon, Trivino, & Lupianez, 2012).

Several reasons may account for the attention deficits observed in people with TBI. Data from a sustained attention study suggested that in addition to generalized cognitive slowing, fatigue, sleep disturbance, and depression can influence performance (Sinclair et al., 2013). Injury to the frontal lobes that is common following at least moderate TBI has been proposed as an obvious possibility because of the important role of frontal areas in executive control (Rodriguez-Bailon et al., 2012). Bonnelle and colleagues (2011) provided evidence from diffusion tensor imaging that white matter injury likely causes disconnection within attention networks.

Although more common and lasting following moderate to severe TBI, attention problems may be present acutely and subacutely after milder injury. Changes in brain function have even been observed in asymptomatic patients following mild TBI. In a functional magnetic resonance imaging study, mild TBI patients differed from control subjects in modulation of bilateral dorsolateral prefrontal and bilateral visual streams despite near normal performance on a modified Stroop task requiring selective attention and inhibitory control (Mayer et al., 2012). Patients also lacked the expected task-induced deactivation within the default node network under conditions of higher attentional load. A similar alteration in network connectivity was observed in acute TBI patients with severity ranging from mild to moderate/severe during a sustained attention task (Bonnelle et al., 2011).

MS

Attention is one of the cognitive domains most commonly impaired in MS (Guimaraes & Sa, 2012). The slowing of information processing probably compounds this problem (Genova, Deluca, Chiaravalloti, & Wylie, 2013). The Paced Serial Attention Test (PASAT) is frequently included in the examination of MS patients and its demands on selective attention, working memory, and speed make it sensitive to cognitive dysfunction. A comparison of MS patients' performance on the PASAT and Stroop test found that patients were slow on both, but speed on the Stroop conflict task more closely related to patients' disability status (Lynch, Dickerson, & Denney, 2010). The ANT has been used with MS patients to examine types of attention with mixed results. Two studies of MS patients found that they were less efficient on the alerting task but performed as well as control subjects for orienting and executive control except when interference produced by flankers was enhanced by nonspatial cueing (Crivelli et al., 2012; Urbanek et al., 2010). Using a modified version of the ANT

(ANT-I) in which an auditory cue was used for alerting, researchers found that MS patients were particularly impaired on the executive control condition but not the other two conditions (Wojtowicz, Omisade, & Fisk, 2013). PASAT scores were more predictive of group membership (MS vs. control subjects) than the executive control ANT-I score; however, intraindividual variability across all trials of the ANT-I was the best predictor of group membership. MS patients frequently are also impaired on attention shifting tasks, such as slow performance on the Trail Making Test (Genova et al., 2013).

Dementia

Alzheimer disease produces broad cognitive deficits. The most prominent loss is memory of new information and evidence suggests that after the usual amnestic stage in Alzheimer disease, attention is the first nonmemory domain to be affected (Grady et al., 1988; Perry & Hodges, 1999). Support for the early impairment in divided attention as a result of Alzheimer disease was obtained during a study of people with a rare form of autosomal-dominant disease (MacPherson et al., 2012). These participants had verbal learning impairments but no other cognitive deficits on a wide range of clinical tests. They were impaired on the divided attention task used by Baddeley involving reciting digits while performing a visuographic tracking task. In this case, the dual-task performance was better than memory tests at detecting cognitive symptoms. The findings suggest that Alzheimer patients have limited attention load capacity. Alzheimer patients with moderate dementia perform below control subjects on a variety of attention tests with divided attention and set-shifting particularly affected (Baddeley, Baddeley, Bucks, & Wilcock, 2001; Perry & Hodges, 1999).

Mild cognitive impairment is a description of cognitive impairment greater than expected for age but not qualifying for a diagnosis of dementia. It is often a precursor to Alzheimer disease, particularly when the prominent impairment involves memory. A study of participants classified as having mild cognitive impairment showed they had slower latencies than intact adults on the CANTAB (Sahakian & Owen, 1992) sustained and selective attention measures (Saunders & Summers, 2011).

Alzheimer disease produces a major decrement in the neurotransmitter acetylcholine. Hence, mild Alzheimer disease treatment often relies on drugs that increase acetylcholine levels. The beneficial effects of these cholinergic agonists may be based on the vital role acetylcholine plays in the top-down control of attention orienting and stimulus discrimination (Klinkenberg, Sambeth, & Blokland, 2011).

Fluctuating attention is considered characteristic of dementia with Lewy bodies. Attention deficits are seen early in the disease process (Molano et al., 2010). Compared to Alzheimer patients, people with Lewy body dementia show greater impairment in attention, particularly the sustained, selective, and divided types (Calderon et al., 2001). Behavioral variant of frontotemporal dementia is a syndrome that includes disinhibition, cognitive rigidity, and inappropriate behavior (Salmon & Stuss, 2013), features that affect attention (Stopford et al., 2012). On a slightly abbreviated version of the National Institutes of Health Cognitive-TB flanker test, both Alzheimer and frontotemporal dementia patients performed worse than control subjects, showing that selective attention was affected by conflicting stimuli for both groups (Possin et al., 2013).

IMPLICATIONS FOR TREATMENT
OF ATTENTION DISORDERS

Evidence for the benefits of rehabilitation of attention problems has been disappointing. A meta-analysis of the effects of rehabilitation of attention impairment of stroke patients found immediate benefits for measures of divided and selective attention but insufficient evidence of benefits on measures of global attention or functional outcomes in the long term (Loetscher & Lincoln, 2013). Few studies report long-term evaluations of treatment effectiveness. Most research designs use a pretraining and posttraining evaluation, sometimes with an additional short-term evaluation a few months later (e.g., Cerasa et al., 2013; Flavia et al., 2010). Research in this area also is hampered by small sample sizes and methodological differences between studies, preventing conclusions based on a reasonable number of studies (Penner & Kappos, 2006). The disappointing results have led to the suggestion that rather than attempting to train specific types of attention, it may be more beneficial to train people on specific functional skills, such as vocational duties (Michel & Mateer, 2006).

FUTURE DIRECTIONS

Traditional neuropsychological tests do not adequately identify the component operations underlying attention control processes. Most clinical tests require a complex of cognitive operations working in concert or sequentially. The use of tests designed to focus on a particular attention process, such as the reaction time test described in this chapter, often lead to a better identification of specific attention deficits than traditional tests. Understanding an individual's specific strengths and weaknesses could lead to more effective individualized treatment programs. For example, people who have mild cognitive impairment benefit, at least in the short term, by training strategies designed to boost this system (Carretti, Borella, Fostinelli, & Zavagnin, 2013).

New technological advances allow for an examination of how neural networks are activated by task demands and how training affects neural processing (Chen et al., 2011). These advances raise the possibility that it may be possible to train specific neural networks to improve attention. This area of study still has many unknowns. Opportunities exist for studying tasks that activate brain regions other than those currently studied and that activate cognitive processes not yet well studied (Bush, 2010).

The study of neurotransmitters associated with specific attention tasks could lead to better treatment options for persons with attention problems. It has been shown that the alerting system is largely regulated by norepinephrine (Posner & Petersen,

1990), orienting by acetylcholine (Klinkenberg et al., 2011), and executive control of attention by dopamine (Fan et al., 2005).

Genetic associations with attention disorders are being uncovered that may lead to treatment strategies. For example, a nucleotide polymorphism within the ANK3 gene has been associated with impaired performance on the Continuous Performance Test (Hatzimanolis et al., 2012). Healthy young adults with this polymorphism had reduced sensitivity for target detection, increased errors of commission, and atypical response latency variability. Another study found an association between a nucleotide polymorphism associated with a dopamine gene and alerting performance on the ANT (Zhu et al., 2013). An association between genes and attention deficits has been found for ADHD (Franke et al., 2012), schizophrenia (Ohi et al., 2013), and bipolar disorder (Franke et al., 2012).

SUMMARY

Impaired attention is one of the most common and debilitating consequences of many neuropsychological disorders. Researchers are integrating data from multiple sources, including attention task performance, neuroimaging, genetics, and neurochemistry to better understand attention processes in healthy and diseased brains. The hope is that advances in understanding the nature of attention disorders will lead to better treatments.

REFERENCES

Alzahabi, R., & Becker, M. W. (2013). The association between media multitasking, task-switching, and dual-task performance. *Journal of Experimental Psychology: Human Perception and Performance, 39*, 1485–1495.

Amado, I., Lupianez, J., Chirio, M., Landgraf, S., Willard, D., Olié, J. P., & Krebs, M. O. (2011). Alertness can be improved by an interaction between orienting attention and alerting attention in schizophrenia. *Behavoiral and Brain Functions, 7*, 24.

Baddeley, A. D., Baddeley, H. A., Bucks, R. S., & Wilcock, G. K. (2001). Attentional control in Alzheimer's disease. *Brain, 124*, 1492–1508.

Bonnelle, V., Leech, R., Kinnunen, K. M., Ham, T. E., Beckmann, C. F., De Boissezon, X., . . . Sharp, D. J. (2011). Default mode network connectivity predicts sustained attention deficits after traumatic brain injury. *Journal of Neuroscience, 31*, 13442–13451.

Breton, F., Plante, A., Legauffre, C., Morel, N., Adès, J., Gorwood, P., . . . Dubertret, C. (2011). The executive control of attention differentiates patients with schizophrenia, their first-degree relatives and healthy controls. *Neuropsychologia, 49*, 203–208.

Bush, G. (2010). Attention-deficit/hyperactivity disorder and attention networks. *Neuropsychopharmacology, 35*, 278–300.

Bush, G., Luu, P., & Posner, M. I. (2000). Cognitive and emotional influences in anterior cingulate cortex. *Trends in Cognitive Sciences, 4*, 215–222.

Calderon, J., Perry, R. J., Erzinclioglu, S. W., Berrios, G. E., Dening, T. R., & Hodges, J. R. (2001). Perception, attention, and working memory are disproportionately impaired in dementia with Lewy bodies compared with Alzheimer's disease. *Journal of Neurology, Neurosurgery and Psychiatry, 70,* 157–164.

Camicioli, R., Howieson, D., Lehman, S., & Kaye, J. (1997). Talking while walking: the effect of a dual task in aging and Alzheimer's disease. *Neurology, 48,* 955–958.

Campbell, K. L., Grady, C. L., Ng, C., & Hasher, L. (2012). Age differences in the frontoparietal cognitive control network: implications for distractibility. *Neuropsychologia, 50,* 2212–2223.

Carretti, B., Borella, E., Fostinelli, S., & Zavagnin, M. (2013). Benefits of training working memory in amnestic mild cognitive impairment: specific and transfer effects. *International Psychogeriatrics, 25,* 617–626.

Carter, L., Russell, P. N., & Helton, W. S. (2013). Target predictability, sustained attention, and response inhibition. *Brain and Cognition, 82,* 35–42.

Cerasa, A., Gioia, M. C., Valentino, P., Nisticò, R., Chiriaco, C., Pirritano, D. . . . Quattrone, A. (2013). Computer-assisted cognitive rehabilitation of attention deficits for multiple sclerosis: a randomized trial with FMRI correlates. *Neurorehabilitation and Neural Repair, 27,* 284–295.

Chen, A. J., Novakovic-Agopian, T., Nycum, T. J., Song, S., Turner, G. R., Hills, N. K., . . . D'Esposito, M. (2011). Training of goal-directed attention regulation enhances control over neural processing for individuals with brain injury. *Brain, 134,* 1541–1554.

Cohen, R. A., Salloway, S., & Sweet, L. H. (2008). Neuropsychaitric aspects of disorders of attention. In S. C. Yudofsky & R. E. Hales (Eds.), *Textbook of neuropsychiatry and behavioral neurosciences* (5th ed.) (pp. 405–444). Washington, DC: American Psychiatric Publishing.

Conners, C. K. (2000). *Conner's Continuous Performance Test (CPT-II) Version 5.* San Antonio, TX, PsychCorp.

Corbetta, M., Patel, G., & Shulman, G. L. (2008). The reorienting system of the human brain: from environment to theory of mind. *Neuron, 58,* 306–324.

Corbetta, M., & Shulman, G. L. (2011). Spatial neglect and attention networks. *Annual Review of Neuroscience, 34,* 569–599.

Cortese, S., Kelly, C., Chabernaud, C., Proal, E., Di Martino, A., Milham, M. P., & Castellanos, F. X. (2012). Toward systems neuroscience of ADHD: a meta-analysis of 55 fMRI studies. *American Journal of Psychiatry, 169,* 1038–1055.

Crivelli, L., Farez, M. F., Gonzalez, C.D., Fiol, M., Amengual, A., Leiguarda, R., & Correale, J. (2012). Alerting network dysfunction in early multiple sclerosis. *Journal of the International Neuropsychological Society, 18,* 757–763.

Demeter, E., Guthrie, S. K., Taylor, S. F., Sarter, M., & Lustig, C. (2013). Increased distractor vulnerability but preserved vigilance in patients with schizophrenia: evidence from a translational Sustained Attention Task. *Schizophrenia Research, 144,* 136–141.

Dickinson, D., Ramsey, M. E., & Gold, J. M. (2007). Overlooking the obvious: a meta-analytic comparison of digit symbol coding tasks and other cognitive measures in schizophrenia. *Archives of General Psychiatry, 64,* 532–542.

Donohue, S. E., Todisco, A. E., & Woldorff, M. G. (2013). The rapid distraction of attentional resources toward the source of incongruent stimulus input during multisensory conflict. *Journal of Cognitive Neuroscience, 25,* 623–635.

Fan, J., Flombaum, J. I., McCandliss, B. D., Thomas, K.M., & Posner, M.I. (2003). Cognitive and brain consequences of conflict. *Neuroimage, 18,* 42–57.

Fan, J., Gu, X., Guise, K. G., Liu, X., Fossella, J., Wang, H., & Posner, M. I. (2009). Testing the behavioral interaction and integration of attentional networks. *Brain and Cognition, 70*, 209–220.

Fan, J., McCandliss, B. D., Fossella, J., Flombaum, J. I., & Posner, M. I. (2005). The activation of attentional networks. *Neuroimage, 26*, 471–479.

Fan, J., McCandliss, B. D., Sommer, T., Raz, A., & Posner, M. I. (2002). Testing the efficiency and independence of attentional networks. *Journal of Cognitive Neuroscience, 14*, 340–347.

Faraone, S. V., Biederman, J., & Mick, E. (2006). The age-dependent decline of attention deficit hyperactivity disorder: a meta-analysis of follow-up studies. *Psychological Medicine, 36*, 159–165.

Federico, F., Marotta, A., Adriani, T., Maccari, L., & Casagrande, M. (2013). Attention network test--the impact of social information on executive control, alerting and orienting. *Acta Psychologica, 143*, 65–70.

Finke, K., Schwarzkopf, W., Muller, U., Frodl, T., Müller, H. J., Schneider, W. X., . . . Hennig-Fast, K. (2011). Disentangling the adult attention-deficit hyperactivity disorder endophenotype: parametric measurement of attention. *Journal of Abnormal Psychology, 120*, 890–901.

Flavia, M., Stampatori, C., Zanotti, D., Parrinello, G., & Capra, R. (2010). Efficacy and specificity of intensive cognitive rehabilitation of attention and executive functions in multiple sclerosis. *Journal of the Neurological Sciences, 288*, 101–105.

Franke, B., Faraone, S. V., Asherson, P., Buitelaar, J., Bau, C. H., Ramos-Quiroga, J. A., . . . International Multicentre persistent ADHD Collaboration. (2012). The genetics of attention deficit/hyperactivity disorder in adults, a review. *Molecular Psychiatry, 17*, 960–987.

Genova, H. M., Deluca, J., Chiaravalloti, N., & Wylie, G. (2013). The relationship between executive functioning, processing speed, and white matter integrity in multiple sclerosis. *Journal of Clinical and Experimental Neuropsychology, 35*, 631–641.

Grady, C. L., Haxby, J. V., Horwitz, B., Sundaram, M., Berg, G., Schapiro, M., . . . Rapoport, S. I. (1988). Longitudinal study of the early neuropsychological and cerebral metabolic changes in dementia of the Alzheimer type. *Journal of Clinical and Experimental Neuropsychology, 10*, 576–596.

Guimaraes, J., & Sa, M. J. (2012). Cognitive dysfunction in multiple sclerosis. *Frontiers in Neurology, 3*, 74.

Haider, M., Spong, P., & Lindsley, D. B. (1964). Attention, Vigilance, and Cortical Evoked-Potentials in Humans. *Science, 145*, 180–182.

Harvey, P. D., & Keefe, R. S. E. (2009). Clinical neuropsychology of schizophrenia. In E. Grant & K. M. Adams (Eds.), *Neuropsychological assessment of neuropsychiatric and neuromedical disorders* (3rd ed.) (pp. 507–522). New York, NY: Oxford University Press.

Hatzimanolis, A., Smyrnis, N., Avramopoulos, D., Stefanis, C. N, Evdokimidis, I., & Stefanis, N. C. (2012). Bipolar disorder ANK3 risk variant effect on sustained attention is replicated in a large healthy population. *Psychiatric Genetics, 22*, 210–213.

Hedden, T., Van Dijk, K. R., Shire, E. H., Sperling, R. A, Johnson, K. A, & Buckner, R. L. (2012). Failure to modulate attentional control in advanced aging linked to white matter pathology. *Cerebral Cortex, 22*, 1038–1051.

Heilman, K. M., Watson, R. T., & Valenstein, E. (2012). Neglect and related disorders. In K. M. Heilman & E. Valenstein (Eds.), *Clinical neuropsychology* (5th ed.) (pp. 296–348). New York, NY: Oxford University Press.

Hervey, A. S., Epstein, J. N., & Curry, J. F. (2004). Neuropsychology of adults with attention-deficit/hyperactivity disorder: a meta-analytic review. *Neuropsychology, 18*, 485–503.

Holst, Y., & Thorell, L. B. (2013). Neuropsychological Functioning in Adults With ADHD and Adults With Other Psychiatric Disorders: The Issue of Specificity. *Journal of Attention Disorders*, Oct 17 {Epub ahead of print}, PMID 24134875.

Hsieh, P. J., & Colas, J. T. (2012). Awareness is necessary for extracting patterns in working memory but not for directing spatial attention. *Journal of Experimental Psychology: Human Perception and Performance, 38*, 1085–1090.

Hubel, D. H., Henson, C. O., Rupert, A., & Galambos, R. (1959). Attention units in the auditory cortex. *Science, 129*, 1279–1280.

Ishigami, Y., Fisk, J. D., Wojtowicz, M., & Klein, R. M. (2013). Repeated measurement of the attention components of patients with multiple sclerosis using the Attention Network Test-Interaction (ANT-I): stability, isolability, robustness, and reliability. *Journal of Neuroscience Methods, 216*, 1–9.

Ishigami, Y., & Klein, R. M. (2011). Repeated Measurement of the Components of Attention of Older Adults using the Two Versions of the Attention Network Test: Stability, Isolability, Robustness, and Reliability. *Frontiers in Aging Neuroscience, 3*, 17.

Jennings, J. M., Dagenbach, D., Engle, C. M., & Funke, L. J. (2007). Age-related changes and the attention network task: an examination of alerting, orienting, and executive function. *Neuropsychology, Development, and Cognition. Section B, Aging, Neuropsychology and Cognition, 14*, 353–369.

Kim, J., Whyte, J., Patel, S., Europa, E., Slattery, J., Coslett, H. B., & Detre, J. A. (2012). A perfusion fMRI study of the neural correlates of sustained-attention and working-memory deficits in chronic traumatic brain injury. *Neurorehabilitation and Neural Repair, 26*, 870–880.

Klinkenberg, I., Sambeth, A., & Blokland, A. (2011). Acetylcholine and attention. *Behavioural Brain Research, 221*, 430–442.

Knight, M., & Mather, M. (2013). Look out-it's your off-peak time of day! Time of day matters more for alerting than for orienting or executive attention. *Experimental Aging Research, 39*, 305–321.

Langner, R., & Eickhoff, S. B. (2013). Sustaining attention to simple tasks: A meta-analytic review of the neural mechanisms of vigilant attention. *Psychological Bulletin, 139*, 870–900.

Lavie, N. (2001). Capacity limits to selective attention: Behavioral evidence and implications for neural activity. In J. Braun & C. Koch (Eds.), *Visual attention and cortical circuits* (pp. 49–68). Cambridge, MA: MIT Press.

Lezak, M. D., Howieson, D., Bigler, E. D., & Trahan, D. E. (2012). *Neuropsychological assessment* (5th ed.). New York, NY: Oxford University Press.

Loetscher, T., & Lincoln, N. B. (2013). Cognitive rehabilitation for attention deficits following stroke. Cochrane Database of Systematic Reviews, Issue 5. Art.No.: CD002842.

Lu, S., Cai, Y., Shen, M., Zhou, Y., & Han, S. (2012). Alerting and orienting of attention without visual awareness. *Consciousness and Cognition, 21*, 928–938.

Luck, S. J., Ford, J. M., Sarter, M., & Lustig, C. (2012). CNTRICS final biomarker selection: Control of attention. *Schizophrenia Bulletin, 38*, 53–61.

Lynch, S. G., Dickerson, K. J., & Denney, D. R. (2010). Evaluating processing speed in multiple sclerosis: a comparison of two rapid serial processing measures. *The Clinical Neuropsychologist, 24*, 963–976.

MacLeod, J. W., Lawrence, M. A., McConnell, M. M., Eskes, G.A., Klein, R.M., & Shore, D. I. (2010). Appraising the ANT: Psychometric and theoretical considerations of the Attention Network Test. *Neuropsychology, 24*, 637–651.

MacPherson, S. E., Parra, M. A., Moreno, S., Lopera, F., & Della Sala, S. (2012). Dual task abilities as a possible preclinical marker of Alzheimer's disease in carriers of the E280A presenilin-1 mutation. *Journal of the International Neuropsychological Society, 18*, 234–241.

Mahoney, J. R., Verghese, J., Goldin, Y., Liptdon, R., & Holtzer, R. (2010). Alerting, orienting, and executive attention in older adults. *Journal of the International Neuropsychological Society, 16*, 877–889.

Mapou, R. L. (2008). *Adult learning disabilities and ADHD: Research-informed assessment.* New York, NY: Oxford University Press.

Martin-Arevalo, E., Chica, A. B., & Lupianez, J. (2013). Task dependent modulation of exogenous attention: effects of target duration and intervening events. *Attention, Perception, & Psychophysics, 75*, 1148–1160.

Matsumoto, K., & Tanaka, K. (2004). Neuroscience. Conflict and cognitive control. *Science, 303*, 969–970.

Mayer, A. R., Yang, Z., Yeo, R. A., Pena, A, Ling, J. M, Mannell, M. V., . . . Mojtahed, K. (2012). A functional MRI study of multimodal selective attention following mild traumatic brain injury. *Brain Imaging Behav, 6*, 343–354.

Mead, L. A., Mayer, A. R., Bobholz, J. A., Woodley, S. J., Cunningham, J. M., Hammeke, T. A., & Rao, S. M. (2002). Neural basis of the Stroop interference task: response competition or selective attention? *Journal of the International Neuropsychological Society, 8*, 735–742.

Merkley, T. L., Larson, M. J., Bigler, E. D., Good, D. A., & Peristein, W. M. (2013). Structural and functional changes of the cingulate gyrus following traumatic brain injury: relation to attention and executive skills. *Journal of the International Neuropsychological Society, 19*, 899–910.

Michel, J. A., & Mateer, C. A. (2006). Attention rehabilitation following stroke and traumatic brain injury. A review. *Europa Medicophysica, 42*, 59–67.

Molano, J., Boeve, B., Ferman, T., Smith, G., Parisi, J., Dickson, D., . . . Petersen, R. (2010). Mild cognitive impairment associated with limbic and neocortical Lewy body disease: a clinicopathological study. *Brain, 133*, 540–556.

Müller-Oehring, E. M., Schulte, T., Rohlfing, T., Pfefferbaum, A., & Sullivan, E. V. (2013). Visual search and the aging brain: discerning the effects of age-related brain volume shrinkage on alertness, feature binding, and attentional control. *Neuropsychology, 27*, 48–59.

Ohi, K., Hashimoto, R., Yasuda, Y., Fukumoto, M., Nemoto, K., Ohnishi, T., . . . Takeda, M. (2013). The AKT1 gene is associated with attention and brain morphology in schizophrenia. *The World Journal of Biological Psychiatry, 14*, 100–113.

Ophir, E., Nass, C., & Wagner, A. D. (2009). Cognitive control in media multitaskers. *Proceedings of the National Academy of Sciences of the United States of America, 106*, 15583–15587.

Orellana, G., Slachevsky, A., & Pena, M. (2012). Executive attention impairment in first-episode schizophrenia. *BMC Psychiatry, 12*, 154.

Penner, I. K., & Kappos, L. (2006). Retraining attention in MS. *Journal of the Neurological Sciences, 245*, 147–151.

Perry, R. J., & Hodges, J. R. (1999). Attention and executive deficits in Alzheimer's disease. A critical review. *Brain, 122*(Pt 3), 383–404.

Petersen, S. E., & Posner, M. I. (2012). The attention system of the human brain: 20 years after. *Annual Review of Neuroscience, 35*, 73–89.

Posner, M. I. (1978). *Chronometric explorations of mind*. Englewood Heights, NJ: Erlbaum.

Posner, M. I. (2012). Progress in attention research. In M. I. Posner (Ed.), *Cognitive neuroscience of attention* (2nd ed) (pp. 1–8). New York, NY: Guilford Press.

Posner, M. I., & Petersen, S. E. (1990). The attention system of the human brain. *Annual Review of Neuroscience, 13*, 25–42.

Posner, M. I., Rafal, R. D., Choate, L. S., & Vaughan, J. (1988). Inhibition of return: Neural basis and function. *Cognitive Neuropsychology, 2*, 211–228.

Possin, K. L., Feigenbaum, D., Rankin, K. P., Smith, G. E., Boxer, A. L., Wood, K., ... Kramer, J. H. (2013). Dissociable executive functions in behavioral variant frontotemporal and Alzheimer dementias. *Neurology, 80*, 2180–2185.

Ravnkilde, B., Videbech, P., Rosenberg, R., Gjedde, A., & Gade, A. (2002). Putative tests of frontal lobe function: a PET-study of brain activation during Stroop's Test and verbal fluency. *Journal of Clinical and Experimental Neuropsychology, 24*, 534–547.

Rengachary, J., He, B. J., Shulman, G. L., & Corbetta, M. (2011). A behavioral analysis of spatial neglect and its recovery after stroke. *Frontiers in Human Neuroscience, 5*, 29.

Robertson, I. H., & O'Connell, R. G. (2010). Vigilant attention. In A. C. Nobre & J. T. Coull (Eds.), *Attention and time* (pp.79–88). Oxford, UK: Osfored University Press.

Robertson, L. C., & Rafal, R. (2000). Disorders of visual attention. In M. S. Gazzaniga (Ed.), *The new cognitive neurosciences* (2nd ed.) (pp. 633–650). Cambridge, MA: MIT Press.

Rodriguez-Bailon, M., Trivino, M., & Lupianez, J. (2012). Executive attention and personality variables in patients with frontal lobe damage. *The Spanish Journal of Psychology, 15*, 967–977.

Sahakian, B. J., & Owen, A. M. (1992). Computerized assessment in neuropsychiatry using CANTAB: discussion paper. *Journal of the Royal Society of Medicine, 85*, 399–402.

Salmon, D. P., & Stuss, D. T. (2013). Executive functions can help when deciding on the frontotemporal dementia diagnosis. *Neurology, 80*, 2174–2175.

Saunders, N. L., & Summers, M. J. (2011). Longitudinal deficits to attention, executive, and working memory in subtypes of mild cognitive impairment. *Neuropsychology, 25*, 237–248.

Seli, P., Jonker, T. R., Solman, G. J., Cheyne, J. A., & Smilek, D. (2013). A methodological note on evaluating performance in a sustained-attention-to-response task. *Behavior Research Methods, 45*, 355–363.

Sinclair, K. L., Ponsford, J. L., Rajaratnam, S. M., & Anderson, C. (2013). Sustained attention following traumatic brain injury: use of the Psychomotor Vigilance Task. *Journal of Clinical and Experimental Neuropsychology, 35*, 210–224.

Skodzik, T., Holling, H., & Pedersen, A. (2013). Long-Term Memory Performance in Adult ADHD: A Meta-Analysis. *Journal of Attention Disorders*, Nov 14 [Epub ahead of print], PMID 24232170.

Smallwood, J. (2013). Distinguishing how from why the mind wanders: a process-occurrence framework for self-generated mental activity. *Psychological Bulletin, 139*, 519–535.

Sridharan, D., Levitin, D. J., & Menon, V. (2008). A critical role for the right fronto-insular cortex in switching between central-executive and default-mode networks. *Proceedings of the National Academy of Sciences of the United States of America, 105*, 12569–12574.

Stevens, A. A., Maron, L., Nigg, J. T., Cheung, D., Ester, E. F., & Awh, E. (2012). Increased sensitivity to perceptual interference in adults with attention deficit hyperactivity disorder. *Journal of the International Neuropsychological Society, 18*, 511–520.

Stopford, C. L., Thompson, J. C., Neary, D., Richardson, A. M., & Snowden, J. S. (2012). Working memory, attention, and executive function in Alzheimer's disease and fronto-temporal dementia. *Cortex, 48*, 429–446.

Stroop, J. R. (1935). Studies of interference in serial verbal reactions. *Journal of Experimental Psychology, 18*, 643–662.

Sturm, W., & Willmes, K. (2001). On the functional neuroanatomy of intrinsic and phasic alertness. *Neuroimage, 14*, S76–84.

Urbanek, C., Weinges-Evers, N., Bellmann-Strobl, J., Bock, M., Dörr, J., Hahn, E., . . . Paul, F. (2010). Attention Network Test reveals alerting network dysfunction in multiple sclerosis. *Multiple Sclerosis, 16*, 93–99.

Van Schie, M. K., Thijs, R. D., Fronczek, R., Van Schie, M. K, Thijs, R. D, Fronczek, R., . . . Van Dijk, J. G. (2012). Sustained attention to response task (SART) shows impaired vigilance in a spectrum of disorders of excessive daytime sleepiness. *Journal of Sleep Research, 21*, 390–395.

Weinbach, N., & Henik, A. (2012). The relationship between alertness and executive control. *Journal of Experimental Psychology: Human Perception and Performance, 38*, 1530–1540.

Weintraub, S., Dikmen, S. S., Heaton, R. K., Tulsky, D. S, Zelazo, P. D, Bauer, P. J., . . . Gershon, R. C. (2013). Cognition assessment using the NIH Toolbox. *Neurology, 80*, S54–64.

Wohlberg, G. W., & Kornetsky, C. (1973). Sustained attention in remitted schizophrenics. *Archives of General Psychiatry, 28*, 533–537.

Wojtowicz, M., Omisade, A., & Fisk, J. D. (2013). Indices of cognitive dysfunction in relapsing-remitting multiple sclerosis: intra-individual variability, processing speed, and attention network efficiency. *Journal of the International Neuropsychological Society, 19*, 551–558.

Zheng, J. J., Delbaere, K., Close, J. C., Sachdev, P., Wen, W., Brodaty, H., & Lord, S. R. (2012). White matter hyperintensities and impaired choice stepping reaction time in older people. *Neurobiology of Aging, 33*, 1177–1185.

Zhou, S. S., Fan, J., Lee, T. M., Wang, C. Q., & Wang, K. (2011). Age-related differences in attentional networks of alerting and executive control in young, middle-aged, and older Chinese adults. *Brain and Cognition, 75*, 205–210.

Zhu, B., Chen, C., Moyzis, R. K., Dong, Q., Chen, C., He, Q., . . . Lin, C. (2013). The DOPA decarboxylase (DDC) gene is associated with alerting attention. *Progress in Neuro-Psychopharmacology and Biological Psychiatry, 43*, 140–145.

INDEX

Page numbers followed by *f* or *t* indicate figures or tables, respectively.